From the Big Bang to Your Cells: The Remarkable Story of Minerals

An Exciting Journey through Space, Time, and the Dawn of Life

First Edition

Published in the United States of America.
Fathom Publishing, Salt Lake City, Utah.

ISBN: 978-0578166117

Cover design by Kathleen F. Goodrun
Index by Clive Pyne Book Indexing

Table of Contents

Introduction

It was a hot summer afternoon in 2004 when I held in my hand a large, reddish-brown apple from a local grocery store. Sitting there next to the others in the basket, there was something peculiar about this apple. It was larger, firmer, and had different patterns of color, and seemed to have its own unique shape. I paused for a moment to examine the apples closer and I noticed some similarities and irregularities between all of them. Even though this bunch of apples was of the same species and from the same orchard, this one seemed to stand out from the rest.

After purchasing the apple I began to wonder what makes an apple grow differently than another, even if they are from the same orchard. In fact, what makes a plant grow in the first place? And what makes it produce fruit? Is there something besides water and sunlight that controls the health of a plant? These thoughts had never dawned on me before and I was determined to find out what was contained inside this apple.

If I handed you a piece of food and told you that it contained aluminum, arsenic, lithium, lead, mercury, nickel, and tin, would you eat it? Most people would refuse without question. However, people don't realize that these elements are found in fruits and vegetables every day. The piece of food I am referring to is that apple.

I decided to find out what was contained in this apple, so I submitted it to a local university laboratory for a mineral analysis. Days later I received their report that listed all the minerals that it contained. As expected, minerals considered essential such as magnesium, calcium, and potassium were found, but I was astonished to learn that aluminum, nickel, tin, barium, strontium, lead, arsenic, and lithium were also found.

There had to be some kind of explanation. All my life I had heard that these minerals were harmful and should be avoided. What were they doing in a healthy looking apple? Were these minerals absorbed from the soil inadvertently? And what benefit, if any, could they possibly have in a plant?

THE BREAKTHROUGH

Just as Isaac Newton's curiosity was inspired by an apple, I also began to ask questions, but I wanted to know what was responsible for the growth of an apple tree and the color, shape, aroma, and flavor of its fruit. My determination to find answers was so intense that I acquired and studied every book about minerals that I could find, as well as various university and laboratory research on how minerals affect living organisms. Through my independent study and research I realized that every book had its own emphasis about minerals. Astronomy books discussed how the universe and Earth were created. Geology books talked about rocks, crystals, mountains, and volcanoes. Soil science books explained how rocks break down in the soil. And plant physiology books showed how plant roots seek out and absorb minerals from the soil and carry them into their tissues.

I eventually realized that there were not any books out there that explained the entire panoramic history of minerals, beginning from the creation of the universe until today, and comprising all the amazing things they perform in both plants and humans. So I challenged myself to write it.

When I sat down that summer to begin writing this book I was finally coming closer to the answers that had sparked my curiosity in the first place. The task was great, but the rewards were certain. Not only did I learn the individual characteristics of each element but I also learned that a plant cannot grow, produce a harvest, or even survive extreme weather conditions unless certain minerals are present in its tissues. But there was more to learn so I continued studying biology, chemistry, and nutrition books to see what role minerals also have in people. This is when I began to see a very interesting pattern. The same minerals that strengthen plant cells, defend them from infections, and help the plants grow and produce a healthy crop are the same minerals that perform similar functions in our bodies.

The big picture started coming together. It became clear that not only had minerals created our planets, moons, and stars, but they were also the materials used to create and sustain life. The calcium and magnesium found in our bones, the copper and iron in our blood, and the zinc and potassium in our cells were all part of the cosmic nebula that exploded and blasted material throughout the universe to eventually create all of the celestial objects in our solar system. The iron circulating in our blood today was once lodged in the center of Earth millions of years ago, and the phosphorus that strengthens our bones today originally came from one of over 22,000 meteorites that have been catalogued to have crashed into Earth. The largest bodies of matter in the universe are comprised of the same elements we find in our bodies, and I found it ironic that atoms, the smallest particles of matter, happen to be the only particles small enough to pass through cell membranes to reach the interior of a plant or animal cell. Indeed, minerals permeate every facet of our existence.

WHY THIS EXPLORATION NOW

The 20th century was a time of discovering new elements and identifying which minerals were essential to the growth and vigor of both plants and animal cells. During the first half of the century, minerals were being recognized as paramount in human nutrition. As early as 1936, a United States Senate document explained: "Our physical well-being is more directly dependent upon minerals we take into our systems than upon calories or vitamins, whereupon the precise proportion of starch, protein, or carbohydrates we consume." The document continues to stress the overall importance of minerals by saying: "It is bad news to learn from our leading authorities that 99 percent of the American people are deficient in these minerals, and a marked deficiency in any one of the more important minerals actually results in disease. Any upset of the balance, any considerable lack of one or another element, however microscopic the body requirement may be, and we sicken, suffer, and shorten our lives."

Over the next few decades research continued to discover new and exciting characteristics of each mineral that revealed how they affect the growth and development of its living host. About halfway through the century the list of minerals that had been considered essential grew longer while many were quickly labeled as "toxic." However, by the end of the century many of those once regarded as toxic were now included on the list of "essential" or "beneficial" minerals.

From the Big Bang to your Cells: The Remarkable Story of Minerals chronicles how research in the 21st century should study which form the minerals must be in that will optimize their full potential contributions to human health. This book illustrates how every naturally-occurring element on the Periodic Table may have potential to provide some benefit to the human body but only if they are in the same form that is found in plants.

Previous literature has only mentioned which minerals are considered essential or beneficial, along with some commonly known facts about their benefits. However, what has not been mentioned was which form minerals should be in that will optimize their usefulness in the body. Never before has any book focused on this simple but universal concept. This book pioneers new ground in not just how any mineral provides benefits, but how people need to adopt a plant-based diet that includes more fruits and vegetables that will provide these minerals in their proper form.

Using an historical format, together we will take an exciting journey through space, time, and the dawn of life, and it is my hope that you will not only gain a new appreciation for the tremendous role that minerals play in our lives but you will also come to the conclusion that many of our sicknesses and diseases might be prevented once the body has the right minerals in the right form. As the human population continues to struggle with health problems, it's time to take a closer look at how the materials we were created from may provide some answers.

All of the elements in our world today have existed for billions of years and have traveled billions of miles across the universe. They eventually gathered together and formed a planet known as Earth, perfectly distanced from a sun, to participate in the construction and health of living organisms. This is that story.

Chapter 1

Where Minerals Come From

All living organisms, from plants to humans, are made from the very same stardust that formed this planet and provided the ideal circumstances for the creation of life. Earth and the entire solar system were formed from the gases and rock that were sent into disarray during the violent episode known as the Big Bang. The matter which exploded and was scattered throughout the universe carried the necessary ingredients that would eventually form suns, planets, moons, and other celestial objects. This matter was comprised of minerals. In addition, minerals helped form the first framework of amino acid structural compounds that eventually led to the development of life.

The minerals that originated in that explosive nebula can be found in our soils and plants, and more importantly they can be found today in our cells. From the Big Bang to planet Earth, minerals make life possible in nearly every possible way. Small bacterial organisms, photosynthesis, and even human growth and development all rely on these minerals for their very survival and continuation. This book tells the remarkable story of how the very same minerals that formed Earth contribute to our everyday existence and influence such things as our memory, immune system, growth, and development. Once you understand the variety of processes for which minerals are responsible in plants, it becomes easier to understand their role in our bodies.

This book is not concerned with the various mineral compounds that exist in soils or the thousands of industrial chemicals, processes, or products that are created from minerals. Instead, this book tells the story of where minerals come from, how they helped to form the Milky Way galaxy, our sun, Earth, our moon, and all the other planets and moons within our telescopic range. This book also explains how minerals are absorbed into plants, contribute to plant growth and development, end up in our food, and ultimately influence the mind and matter of man. This remarkable story conveys minerals' extreme importance in our everyday lives.

■ ■ ■

Approximately 15 billion years ago an enormous amount of dust and gases collected on the outer edge of the solar system and began to contract. Eventually, the collective gravitational power of these particles came together to create an extremely dense center of mass while a centrifugal force kept it spinning in a horizontal, but spiral, direction. The more dense the matter, the stronger its gravitational pull. After millions of years, this dense mass at the center, along with the energy created when the particles collided and compressed together, forced the mass to heat up quickly. This same process later formed our Sun.

Some particles of matter were thrown in various directions and ultimately formed the orbital pattern of the Milky Way galaxy. Over millions of years, many of these loose particles pulled together to gradually form larger lumps of matter that accumulated other particles and became even larger. Thus, some of these particles became large enough to form the planets and moons that currently rotate around our sun, while other particles became trapped and formed an asteroid belt, or got caught in the gravitation of larger particles, forming planetary rings.

During the early formation of the galaxy, the entire universe was in disarray. Matter was scattered everywhere and disorganized. After billions of years, the planets continued to increase in size with each meteorite that crashed into it, and the gravitational pull began to form structure and order as each planet became larger and larger. As Earth grew larger and larger with each new addition of matter, the strength of its gravitational pull continued to increase and attract cosmic matter. Meteorites from the asteroid belt bombarded Earth and the other planets during the first 500 million years following the Big Bang. In fact, only 5% of the original asteroid belt still exists today, because so many asteroids were dislodged by gravitation to eventually bombard a celestial object.

When a meteorite crashes into a planet, it delivers minerals such as iron, nickel, phosphorus, various silicates, and other minerals from the original nebula. Many meteorite impact sites on Earth contain extremely rare elements, such as iridium. Scientists can identify a meteorite crash site by examining the iron-nickel content as well as the heavy presence of the element iridium in the surrounding soil.

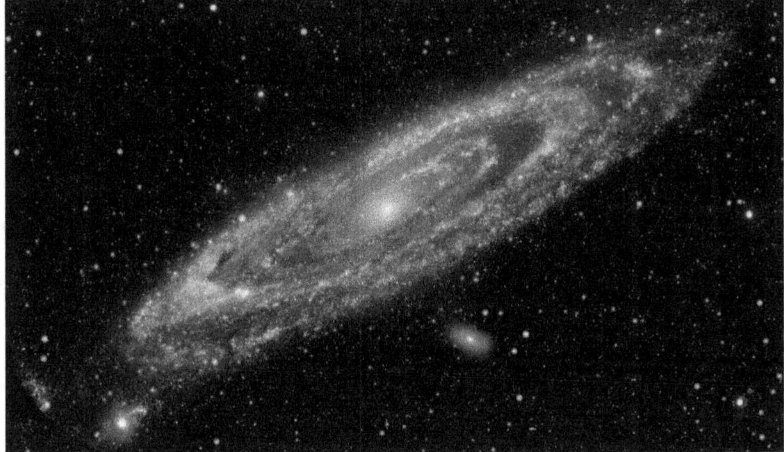

Iron-containing meteorites provided the iron that formed Earth's metallic core billions of years ago. Other types of meteorites, known as achondrites, delivered the materials that we find in Earth's mantle and crust. The surface of Earth was extremely disorganized, and over hundreds of millions of years, Earth's core became hotter and hotter and the iron and nickel melted. These heavy metals sank to the bottom of the core, which pushed the lighter elements outward, eventually forming the outer core, mantle, and crust. As the young Earth continued its rotation over hundreds of millions of years it began to take a more rounded shape. All of this geologic activity shaped the planet as it is today.

After hundreds of millions of years of planetary development and violent cosmic activity, things have relatively quieted down. Today, our planet has evolved an atmosphere, largely due in part to the rise of plants and other respiratory organisms. However, meteorites continue to strike our planet today, although the atmosphere tends to burn off most of them. In fact, as of December 1999, 22,507 meteorites have been catalogued as striking Earth, according to Monica Gray of the Natural History Museum in London, author of Catalogue of Meteorites.

■ ■ ■

During this early period of Earth, many important elements that would later prove necessary to sustain life were locked up deep inside Earth. Fortunately, some dynamic events occurred that brought many of these elements to the surface. These violent episodes involved extremely dramatic forces and sudden changes in the landscape. According to the June 3, 2004 issue of Nature, a study conducted by the Ontario Geological Society and the Geological Survey of Canada observed a meteorite impact site that struck Earth at an estimated 89,000 mph almost 2 billion years ago near what is today known as Ontario, Canada. Researchers uncovered and examined the crater that had long been concealed underground or eroded over time, although part of it was still exposed.

James Mungall, a University of Toronto geologist who worked on the project, explains that the impact was so powerful that it penetrated very deep layers of our planet, causing a massive amount of superheated rock from deep inside the planet to heave outward and settle onto Earth's crust, which almost covered the entire crater. Researchers first noticed that the area consisted of iron, nickel, and platinum, which would normally be found in deeper layers of Earth rather than on the outer crust. Upon further examination, they realized that this was the site of a large meteorite impact. The impact not only inverted the layering of the crust and brought these valuable minerals to the surface, it also delivered iridium, which is an element usually not considered native to the early formation of the planet, but is usually found around meteorite impact sites.

In the midst of all of this activity, the set was being staged for an important event that would occur: the origin of life. Most researchers believe that the dawn of life did not just consist of a biological process, but was first a chemical process. Millions of years ago, Earth's surface consisted chiefly of rock, air, and water. However, life eventually arose out of these circumstances, and experts on the subject have debated for decades how chemical activity contributed to the initial development of life. Carbon-based compounds that existed at this time were largely comprised of gases with only one atom of carbon in each molecule, such as carbon dioxide, carbon monoxide, and methane. However, the building blocks of living organisms always consist of fats, sugars, and amino acids. These substances usually contain as many as 12 carbon atoms per molecule, forming a complex "chain" that is bound together and arranged in particular orders.

Researchers at the University of Florida have shown how borax-containing minerals help transform carbon-containing molecules found in atmospheric dust clouds into a sugar known as ribose, which is a critical ingredient in the genetic material Ribonucleic acid (RNA). Ribose has a chemical structure that makes it effective in binding with mineral compounds that contain boron. Boron is essential in keeping the ribose sugar as clean as possible, while preventing it from becoming a tar-like substance. In laboratory experiments, a team of researchers were able to mimic the early Earth conditions and created ribose from boron-containing minerals. This was the first laboratory study that actually created ribose from boron mineral compounds, showing that minerals were responsible for the early creation of not only complex amino acids, but simple sugars such as ribose.

However, during the initial stages of life, the young Earth was still without an atmosphere, allowing the sun's extremely harmful radiation through. Therefore, the initial process of forming carbon molecules was difficult to achieve, as any carbon-based molecule quickly dissolved in the fierce sunlight. In order for these molecules to form and to make their chemical reactions occur they needed support and protection from the sun's rays. It is a widely-held belief that minerals provided this assistance in making these critical processes a reality.

Minerals, together with air and water, were the only materials available during Earth's early formation that could create the building blocks of a living organism. According to Dr. Robert M. Hazen, a research scientist at the Carnegie Institute of Washington's Geophysical Laboratory and Clarence Robinson and Professor of Earth Science at George Mason University, a series of chemical reactions needed to occur that would allow life to arise. In an essay titled Life's Rocky Start that was published in the April, 2001 issue of Scientific American, Dr. Hazen explained that the basic raw materials that existed at that time needed to be transformed chemically in a way that would allow carbon-based molecules to eventually replicate themselves. According to the report, "the critical transformations might not have been possible without the help of minerals acting as containers, scaffolds, templates, catalysts, and reactants."

Minerals would have acted as a container with their small holes found on weathered surfaces of compounds, which would have provided the early carbon-forming chain molecules with the necessary cover they needed from the direct sunlight. Then, the minerals could have acted as a scaffolding to catch transient organic molecules between their layers of clays. This would have provided the necessary space for the organic molecules to assemble and begin to form more complex compounds.

Dr. Hazen also explains that mineral compounds provided these organic molecules the cover, space, and time they needed to assemble and form complex chains. However, not all of the complex chains that were being formed would become significant. Research observations have revealed that amino acids are available in two different forms, one with a particular shape known as "right-handed" and the other of particular shape known as "left-handed." Through experimentation, researchers now understand that the crystal faces of various mineral compounds ideally suit the left-handed amino acid molecules. Gradually, the organization of these left-handed amino acids gave rise to a longer and longer chain of protein-like molecules which eventually began to catalyze important steps, ultimately increasing the total amount of biological processes.

Dissolved minerals played a critical role in the early development of life's origins. When these early minerals were exposed to hot water at high pressure, they dissolved and liberated their atoms, which went on to become involved in chemical processes such as enzymes. Minerals also provided a safe harbor by collecting and protecting the early carbon-based molecules, and helping to arrange them into their complex chains of amino acids. These early processes began the first replication efforts of these molecules. Soon, changes, adaptations, and mutations led to the creation of larger chains of molecules, and ultimately the competition for natural resources, which gradually developed into a process of natural selection.

■ ■ ■

From the inner core to the outer crust, the whole Earth is composed of minerals in the form of rocks and soil. All plant and animal life are dependent upon these minerals and could not function without their presence.

Understanding minerals first requires some understanding of rocks. Rocks are everywhere! In your garden, in the street, in your home, and everywhere outside. Even physical structures such as statues and everyday items we use such as chalk, pencil lead, sandpaper, concrete, and glass are all comprised of rocks. Fragments of rock are used to construct offices and homes with bricks, build automobiles and airplanes with metals such as aluminum, and form jewelry. Sand and mud are also fragments of rock.

Rocks are made up of two or more minerals that have been fused together from heat, temperature, pressure, or chemical changes inside our planet. In fact, a rock can start out as one substance and over thousands of years can be changed many times through these different natural forces. These geological changes in rocks represent what is known as a "rock cycle."

Rocks are found in three different forms. Igneous rocks form when volcanoes spew up molten rock called magma from deep inside Earth that settles on the surface and cools. Earth itself continues to form from this volcanic process today.

Sedimentary rocks form from materials that are deposited in lakes and oceans. Examples include sandstone, shale, and limestone, which are formed from compacted oceanic materials that have been pressured over time. Most ancient fossils are found in sedimentary rock since they were deposited together.

Metamorphic rocks form when either igneous or sedimentary rocks are heated or put under additional pressure. If the heat and pressure is sufficient, the original minerals will melt. As it cools, new minerals can form, depending on what mixture of elements combine to form the new compound mineral. Heat or pressure inside Earth squeezes, bakes, or folds these rocks into a new form, which can take thousands of years. In fact, metamorphic is Greek for "change of form."

Even today, rocks from deep inside Earth or from outer space continue to deliver minerals to Earth's outer surface through violent meteoric impacts, plate tectonic movement that creates mountains and hills, and volcanic eruptions.

Earth has three layers: the core at the center, a very thick mantle, and a thin crust. Rock is not always solid. Earth's center is a sphere of hot, slowly and continually moving rock that is made up of iron and nickel. The center of the core is solid while the outer core is liquid rock. This spherical core is always moving and influences the geologic forces that shape our planet.

Surrounding the core is another layer of Earth called the mantle which is made of oxygen, silicon, magnesium, aluminum, iron, and many other elements in smaller amounts. Finally, Earth's outer crust surrounds the mantle and is lighter, cooler, and more rigid than the mantle and is like a thin skin that surrounds the planet. The thickness of the crust will vary, but is very thin when compared to the mantle or core and is thought to comprise only 1% of our planet's total mass. Oxygen, silicon, aluminum, and iron contribute 96% of the total composition of the crust, while calcium, magnesium, sodium, potassium and all the other elements make up the remaining 4%. Therefore, most common minerals you are familiar with will actually be some form of chemical compound of the three most abundant elements found in the crust—oxygen, silicon, and aluminum, with smaller amounts of other elements.

The crust and outermost mantle together form a rigid layer called the lithosphere, which is separated into a dozen or so large plates that surround our planet. These lithospheric plates are thousands of miles across and are separated by large fractures. Geologic forces inside Earth keep these plates moving very slowly, sometimes rubbing past one another or colliding. If two of these plates collide, some of the rocks are pushed upward, driving up mountains and hills and creating rocky formations, and exposing pieces of the crust and mantle to the surface.

What causes these plates to move? Earth's core transfers heat by slow moving rock just below the crust. This internal heat engine is made up of a continual movement of hot rock and is responsible for distributing the plates across the surface and the movement and reshuffling of continents. According to Ron Vernon, author of Beneath Your Feet: The Rocks of Planet Earth, "Earth is a dynamic and constantly moving object, and this internal movement governs the continual change and recycling of its materials. Its large variety of rocks reflects this slow but relentless dynamic activity over the past 4.6 billion years."

■ ■ ■

A "mineral" is defined as a solid, inorganic substance created by nature. They are always crystalline solids, which mean that each individual atom is bound tightly together in regular patterns. Some minerals will have regular shapes if they are grown freely in a liquid. Minerals of this type form crystals such as the specimens you might see in museums, but if their growth is impeded by other minerals and unable to grow freely causing an irregular shape to form, or if they are fragments, they are called grains. However, the atomic structure of these minerals will remain crystalline solids, regardless of whether they create crystals or grains.

We can classify any substance two different ways: an "element" or a "compound." Elements are substances that cannot be decomposed into a simpler substance. On the contrary, a compound (such as a rock) will contain two or more elements, which means it contains two or more kinds of atoms. For example, sodium is the 11th element on the Periodic Table of Elements and when it exists by itself is an example of a single substance, or the element sodium. However, when sodium mixes with chlorine, it now comprises a new compound substance called sodium chloride—regular table salt. When one element is forced to mix with another, a compound results.

There are now 118 elements in the Periodic Table of Elements, and every so often a new element is discovered. Scientists debate about how many of them are considered "naturally-occurring;" and oddly enough the exact number is still uncertain. Most scientists recognize the first 92 elements as naturally-occurring, even though only 90 have actually been found in nature. Depending on how the term is defined, some scientists recognize 88 as naturally-occurring, while others insist there are only 83. Regardless, not all of these naturally-occurring elements are found on Earth. For example, element 43 "Technetium" (Tc) has never been found to occur naturally on earth. Rather, it is found only on very large stars.

Most minerals you are familiar with are actually combinations of two or more of these elements fused together in various geological ways. One of these elements will interact with another element to form a compound, and when a compound substance is created, the result can oftentimes be a mineral, depending on which elements are being mixed. There are an estimated 3,000-5,000 different minerals in the world. That is a lot of different compounds created from only 118 elements! Some examples of these mineral compounds include calcium carbonate, zinc chloride, and copper sulfate.

Regardless of however rocks arrive on the surface of Earth, whether through meteors, volcanoes, or other forms of activity, the forces of nature that break down these rocks into smaller pieces is known as "weathering." In general, weathering is a constant process that disintegrates and dissolves rock into smaller and smaller pieces. The breakdown of these large rock fragments into smaller pieces takes thousands of years and eventually creates Earth's outer crust and soil.

■ ■ ■

Studying minerals would be incomplete without an understanding of geology and soil science, and soil does not always receive the recognition that it deserves. A common way someone insults another person is to say that they are "lower than dirt." They may not realize that dirt is one of the most valuable commodities on Earth! Properly referred to as "soil," it is not just something we wash off our hands after working in the garden. Soil contains a geological and biological history of an incredible living world that covers the entire planet. Next time you venture outside, pick up a handful of soil and smell its earthy odor and feel its texture. Then remember that handful of soil took thousands of years to create!

I have heard people say, "You are what you eat," but what isn't said is that what you eat is usually directly related to the soil it is grown in. As we begin to understand more intimately the basics of soil composition and the complex processes that create it, we soon realize that living systems such as plants and animals are dependent upon soils that are rich in minerals.

The air we breathe is a mixture of different gases, and our soil is a mixture of solids, air space, and living organisms. Over millions of years, particles of rock are broken down into tiny fragments that make up about 97% of the solid part of soil. The remaining 3% will comprise organic materials, such as decomposed plant and animal tissues. The spaces between these particles of rock and pieces of organic matter are filled with air and water.

Soils are different from the original materials in which they were created. Soils are highly complex materials that have structural and biological elements that allow plants to grow, and are dynamic ecological systems that provide support, water, minerals, and air for the growth and development of vegetation. In fact, soils originate from various materials and rely on geologic conditions for their development.

Soil consists of weathered and loose rock, clay, or silt, and organic matter such as dead and decomposing plants. There are varieties of soils that contain varying amounts of these materials. The mineral content of the soil comes from the weathered rock and the decomposing organic material.

Soil is formed when loose materials are transported by wind, water, or gravity. They can also be carried by glaciers and deposited onto a firm landscape, or when bedrock is exposed and becomes vulnerable to weathering. Soil formation is a long, geochemical process that reduces the size of these particles, rearranges the mineral particles, changes the kinds of minerals, adds organic matter, and produces clays. Over millions of years ago, large rocks and large pieces of organic matter are broken down by erosion and weathering into smaller particles to create the sand, silt, and clay that we see in our soil today.

The original materials for soil formation must be transported and deposited to a suitable site. However, nature's way of transporting rocks is often conducted through very dynamic forces and unusually destructive methods. Across parts of Europe, storms off the Atlantic Ocean are causing waves so large and powerful they are ripping giant boulders from the top of cliffs and hurling them as much as 50 meters inland. According to Dr. James Hansom of the Glasgow University's coastal beach group, as many as 100 giant waves might hit the coast of Britain every year—large enough to overtop cliffs 20 meters high. Researchers did not originally think that it was possible Britain was being battered by waves so large they could both smash the rock and then throw it considerable distances, but have found several places where it is happening. These boulders can weigh up to 50 tons and can be up to three meters long, the size of a small truck and far heavier.

Experiments taking place in Glasgow University's wave tank show that waves are capable of snapping boulders off cliffs previously weakened by storms and carrying them inland at a speed of five meters per second. Transport of these huge boulders by the winds and ocean currents is not a modern phenomenon. Dr. Hansom's team has analyzed soil and plant samples from beneath the boulders that have washed ashore on Orkney Island and discovered that those boulders are almost 300 years old. Many of the rocks have piled up in ridges, showing that massive waves had repeated the action of hurling rocks many times since. Sometimes nature's fury is really just another form of physical weathering that marks the genesis of soil formation by depositing rocks that will eventually become soil's parent material.

Soil can only inherit the minerals found in the parent material. Its formation is a constant but slow weathering process that can take millions of years involving many different environmental processes that break down large particles into smaller and smaller pieces.

The climate of an area determines how precipitation and temperature will influence soil formation, and they will vary with latitude and elevation. The amount of precipitation—rain, snow, or both—and its distribution during the year are major factors. Increased precipitation generally results in faster rates of erosion, while rainfall intensity affects the amount of runoff, erosion, and soil destruction.

Temperature extremes through daily and seasonal fluctuations also weaken and break down large rock particles. One of the most destructive forces of weathering involves freezing. Moisture can work its way into small cracks and pits in rocks, freeze, and then expand, creating larger cracks and larger holes. The pressure that occurs can be as much as 100 times that of tire pressure. When freezing and expanding continues over and over the rock will split apart and break into smaller pieces.

Weathering can also occur in the desert environments. Wind is a strong weathering force that constantly throws sand and other debris at rocks, while hot and cold weather extremes cause large boulders to crumble.

Water is one of the most important agents in the entire soil formation process. It dissolves rocks and minerals from their original compounds into new forms, a process known as "dissolution." Water falls as precipitation and can run off the soil surface. It expands when it freezes in the cracks of rocks, causing the rocks to crack and split open.

It can also wear down rocks and grind them to smaller pieces by the slow movement of glaciers. Freezing, thawing, heating, abrasion, swelling, and shrinking are environmental extremes that break large rocks down into smaller and smaller fragments, preparing the minerals contained in rocks to be absorbed into plants.

Soil formation is also influenced by the topography of the landscape. The angle of a slope will determine the amount of water that runs off or absorbs into the soil. The slope can affect the temperature of the air and the frequency of wind. In the Northern Hemisphere, north-facing slopes will be cooler than south-facing slopes due to less sun exposure. Cooler soil has less development than warmer soil due to less fluctuation in temperature extremes. In deserts, moisture is limited so cooler temperatures and less evaporation from less sun exposure will provide a deeper soil on north-facing slopes. In Southern Hemispheres, it is the south-facing slopes that will have a different rate of soil formation.

Another important factor in soil development is its content of living organisms such as plants and insects known as "biota." These organisms come in all sizes, including some that are only visible through a microscope, as well larger organisms such as spiders and gophers. Each of these organisms creates pores in the soil and they mix organic matter with the sand, silt, and clay particles.

Plants are also involved in the formation of soil. They take atmospheric carbon and add it to the soil, and as their roots push through the soil they add organic matter through their leaves when their roots slough off and when their leaves fall to the ground. These deposit nutrients for the small microorganisms in the soil.

■ ■ ■

For centuries, humans traveled and pioneered across continents. When humans settled and developed agriculture, the food sources no longer came from a variety of soils, but were from the same acreage of land being used to grow crops year after year. Essential minerals can be depleted by intense cultivation of a single crop year after year, until eventually the soil becomes exhausted, leading to a decline in crop yield and quality. Crops today are harvested on the same soils that are used over and over, and not all farms regularly practice re-mineralization of the soils using the full spectrum of minerals. Instead, the most common fertilizer application consists of only three minerals: nitrogen, phosphorus, and potassium (NPK).

Centuries ago people prayed for annual floods that would irrigate and replenish their soils with minerals. Some of the early pioneers traveled west every 12 years because it was believed that after 12 years the soils were depleted of its mineral content. The mineral cycle involves plants absorbing minerals from soil and eventually replenishing the soil with organic matter, such as roots, leaves, flowers, fruits, which all return the minerals back to the soil to be taken up again by the next generation of plants. But as crops are harvested, the minerals are unable to return.

Fertilization is an important agricultural process that returns some of the minerals that were lost through harvesting. Some soils may be naturally deficient in phosphorus, molybdenum, or copper, while other soils may contain excessive amounts of selenium. However, over-fertilization can destroy the soil's microorganisms that are responsible for making minerals soluble or it can change the pH balance of soils to make some minerals become unavailable (solubility and availability are concepts will be discussed later).

Agriculture plays a major part in human food production. Farmers are paid on yield instead of quality, so the bare minimum fertilizer is used. It should be noted that replenishing the lost minerals using decomposed organic matter or fertilizer containing more than the basic NPK (nitrogen, phosphorus, and potassium) formula should be considered.

Flood plains are usually the site of mineral-rich land. Some of the richest agricultural land in Australia is on landscape that was flooded regularly. However, flood control has eliminated this annual deposit of fresh soil and transport of a new mineral supply. Crops yielded during these under-fertilized conditions have low growth rates and do not resist disease or pests very well. Manmade pesticides are then used to ward off the pests and increase crop yields, which furthers the problem. Living organisms with a healthy concentration of minerals are naturally able to resist pathogens. Without these minerals there will be a decline in immune system strength in both plants and animals.

The National Aeronautical Space Administration (NASA) estimates that there are 50,000 different types of soils in the United States alone! And the Ohio Department of Natural Resources has identified 400 soil types in Ohio, using physical characteristics such as texture, porosity, and acidity. Creating soil doesn't just happen. In fact, the Ohio Department of Natural Resources estimates it takes 1,000 years to create just one inch of topsoil.

Soil is responsible for many different aspects of human survival. For example, soil science aids farmers by helping select suitable farmland and creating a fertile ground for crops. It also aids construction of roads, buildings, business complexes, and other physical structures. Soil scientists conduct "soil surveys" that allow land owners to determine if their land is good for farming, or see if it can support a high-rise structure, Is the land appropriate for housing? Building roads or highways? Can it contain a landfill? Should it be used for a park or golf course? Does it drain well?

Mineral rich soil is an important commodity for many other reasons. Soil absorbs and filters chemical materials, which also prevents diseased organisms from contaminating ground water. Farmers view soil as a resource to grow crops or other types of vegetation. Engineers and construction workers view soil as the foundation for bridges, highways, roads, homes, and buildings. Homeowners view it as a source of beauty for their gardens and homes. You should view soil as a supplier of minerals for your food!

The capability of soil to provide the essential nutrients for the growth and development of vegetation is a measure of its quality and is known as "soil fertility." The soil quality allows it to produce vibrant crop yields balanced in all the essential nutrients and even some beneficial nutrients. This fertility comes from the minerals that have been locked up inside the sand, silt, and clay particles that have undergone the erosion and weathering processes.

An important feature of soil is that it is made up of sand, silt, and clay, which all have different roles in the soil. Sand is considered to be a coarse, large rock particle that range from 0.05 up to 2.00 mm in diameter. In soaks up rainfall and irrigation water, aerates the soil by providing air space, and allows drainage of water. Sand is primarily made up of silicon. Silt is much smaller rock particles that range from 0.002 to 0.05 mm in diameter. It bridges the sand and silt particles to make them compatible. Clay is even smaller rock particles that range from 0.0002 up to 0.002 mm in diameter. It absorbs and "holds" water, organic compounds, and plant nutrients. All of these particles are still rocks and their varying composition determines the soil's texture. In fact, texture has such significance to soil scientists that soils are named according to their textural classification.

You may have noticed that soil comes in a variety of colors, such as orange, brown, yellow, gray, red, white, and even blue or green. The color usually indicates a dominant presence of a mineral element. Darker soils will usually contain a strong presence of organic matter. White soils are common when salts or carbonate (limestone) exist in the soil. Red and yellow soils indicate a high iron oxide content and are usually found in highly weathered soils, usually from wind or rain. Gray, blue, or green soils are frequently saturated by water because the minerals that would originally have given them the red or yellow colors have been leached away, once again indicating the physical and chemical weathering in process.

However, inorganic rock particles are not the only ingredients in soil. Soil also consists of "organic" material. Organic is defined as a molecule of carbon that is attached to another molecule. Living matter contains carbon. Organic matter typically includes decomposed plant and animal residues that were synthesized by small bacterial and microbes in the soil. Sources of organic matter include living matter such as plant roots, leaves, and branches that fall on the ground, grass, and animal waste from microorganisms and large vertebrates. These organic materials will eventually become recycled through decomposition and decay, releasing the inorganic minerals back into the soil, eventually completing the mineral cycle.

The mineral cycle never stops.

Chapter 2

Kingdom Monera

Over thousands of years the various methods of weathering and erosion have broken down the rock particles and the minerals locked inside. By the time these rocks and minerals have finally entered the soil, they have undergone several stages of erosion since their humble beginning deep inside Earth. After thousands, even millions, of years have passed, and wind, water, and gravity have taken their toll, the stages of physical and chemical weathering are complete once the rocks and minerals have settled into the soil. Here, the last stage of weathering known as "biological weathering" represents the process that breaks the mineral particles down to their smallest unit. Biological weathering is the final process that prepares the minerals for absorption into plants.

Dr. Terry R. Roper of the University of Wisconsin-Madison Department of Horticulture says that the ability of soil to supply nutrients essential for the growth and development of plants is known as "soil fertility." However, soil is much more than just sand, silt, and clay. Biological weathering occurs when living organisms in the soil break down the minerals that are contained in it, in an effort to provide plants with the nutrients they need.

Soil crawls with all kinds of living organisms, such as worms, centipedes, grubs, termites, lice, bacteria, fungi, and more. Each of these organisms plays an integral part in soil development. Although most of the organisms found in soil are too small to be seen by the unaided eye, some worms and burrowing animals such as gophers and moles call soil their home, too. One gram of soil is home to one billion bacteria and fungi that form a complex chain that starts from the top of the soil. Large animals eat organic debris and excrete their waste into the soil, predators consume the living prey, and the smaller microorganisms feed on the decaying carcasses.

The soil population is generally made up of three classes of organisms: 1) Producers—plants and bacteria that can make their own food, either through photosynthesis or from nutrients in the soil, 2) Consumers—organisms that feed on other organisms, such as animals, insects, and smaller bacteria, and 3) Decomposers—usually bacteria and fungi that release the minerals nutrients back into the soil.

According to John Cooper of Texas A&M University, well-managed lawns typically contain more than 900 billion microbes for each pound of soil inside the root zone. In each 1,000 square feet of soil six inches deep, this amounts to 70 pounds of microbes. Ants, worms, spiders, and other larger organisms are less plentiful, but just as important. There are between one and two million (15-30 pounds) of these critters per 1,000 square feet of soil at any given time, even though they might account for less than 10% of the soil population.

The activities performed by soil organisms are extremely important. These activities include consumption, metabolism, growth, excretion, and decay of organisms, all of which break down nutrients to provide for their own energy and propagation. All of this action helps to till and aerate the soil. Their activity is highly beneficial since they excrete cementing agents that bind soil particles, which helps improve the soil structure.

■ ■ ■

One of the first processes of decomposition is the rapid colonization of bacteria and fungi. Then, larger microorganisms will chew what they can into smaller pieces and eventually defecate most of their intake back into the soil. Over time, the soil will look less like plant matter and more like a dark brown material called humus as the organic tissues disappear. Decomposing organic matter, such as leaves, grass, branches, and animal tissues, is the largest activity of the soil population.

Soil organisms are so effective at decomposition that they can decompose chemical substances and other manmade materials such as rubber, petroleum, plastic, human food, gum wrappers, and even old tires. They even decompose harmful elements such as pesticides, air pollutants, and industrial wastes that may have been deposited in the soil. Although these microorganisms spend the bulk of their activity on more natural materials, they should be appreciated for decomposing manmade waste on a daily basis.

However, soil microorganisms don't just decompose organic matter, chemical, and manmade substances. They also play a key role in breaking down inorganic minerals to eventually be taken up by roots. The inorganic minerals locked inside rocks and plant and animal tissues need to be released back into the soil in order for plants to use them again. In fact, a plant's rate of growth is largely determined by the speed at which microorganisms are able to break down these materials and release the inorganic minerals into the soil. All of this microbial activity results in a final inorganic mineral particle that is suitable for plant absorption, regardless of whether it was originally supplied from an organic or inorganic substance. A plant's health depends on the conversion and breakdown process of these nutrients into their proper form.

What is the end result of this microbial activity, and at what point is a mineral considered ready for absorption into plants? To answer that, a short chemistry lesson is needed in order to understand this process.

You should remember from science classes that the smallest possible particle, with a nucleus in the middle and electrons orbiting it, is known as an "atom." Atoms are the smallest particles that have been identified and are considered the basic building blocks of matter. They are the smallest particle of an element that still possesses the chemical identity of the element. For example, an atom of iron is the smallest possible particle of iron.

An atom has an extremely dense nucleus in the middle made up of neutrons and protons, and an atom also has electrons that orbit the nucleus. However, under certain circumstances, an atom can gain or lose one or more of its electrons (don't concern yourself with how, just know that it can). When an atom gains or loses an electron, it no longer has a neutral charge; it becomes positively charged when it loses an electron or negatively charged if it gains an electron. Charged atoms are called "ions." An ion is an atom that has gained or lost one or more of its electrons and therefore became electrically charged. This is an important concept that should be understood before you continue reading.

For example, look at the Periodic Table of Elements. Each element is given an "atomic number" that represents the number of protons in the nucleus of its atoms. Notice that sodium is the 11th atomic number. This means that each atom of sodium has 11 protons in its nucleus and has 11 electrons orbiting the nucleus. Let's say that this atom lost one of its electrons. The atom would still have its 11 protons in its nucleus, but would only have 10 electrons orbiting it. It would still be an atom of sodium, but it would have gained a positive charge.

When a sodium atom loses an electron as in this example, this ion is more specifically called a "cation" ('cat-ion') since it is now positively charged. If an atom such as chloride gained an electron, it would be called an "anion" ('an-ion') with its new negative charge. Cations arise from metal elements, such as calcium, cobalt, chromium, copper, gold, iron, magnesium, manganese, molybdenum, potassium, selenium, silver, sodium, and zinc, while anions arise from non-metallic elements such as iodine, sulfur, phosphorus, chlorine, and fluorine. To avoid too much confusion, the general term "ion" will be used throughout most of this book.

The nucleus size of each atom differs from every other depending on the number of protons the element contains. For example, look at the Periodic Table of Elements again. Notice that calcium is given an atomic number of 20. It has 20 protons in its nucleus and 20 electrons orbiting it, while in comparison magnesium only has 12. Therefore, when comparing the size of one atom of calcium to one atom of magnesium, the calcium atom will be larger. A unit of measurement used to express atomic dimensions is the angstrom (Å). Angstroms are used to measure the diameter of atoms. One angstrom is 10-10 meters, or 10 billion times smaller than one meter. Some atoms are slightly smaller than one angstrom, while some are slightly larger, depending on the size of the nucleus and how far out the electrons are orbiting it.

■ ■ ■

Physical weathering is not capable of breaking down rock particles into ions; it can only break down these particles into the compounds of sand, silt, and clay. The smallest of these particles are the clay particles, which will vary in size between 0.0002 up to 0.002 mm in diameter, much larger than ions. If a tablespoon of soil is stirred into water, the larger particles of sand will settle on the bottom very quickly. Over the course of hours, or perhaps days, if left undisturbed, the finer particles of silt will also succumb to gravity and settle on the bottom and the dirtiness of the solution will soon disappear. However, some of the very small clay particles will remain suspended in the water and will not settle out, at least within a reasonable amount of time, nor will they float to the top. These clay particles will actually remain held suspended in the water and are too small to be seen by the naked eye. The clay particles held in suspension are called "colloidal" particles. Colloids are larger than ions and vary in size from 5 up to 10,000 angstroms in diameter.

A colloidal particle is a large compound made of multiple atoms or molecules bound together. Colloids are so small that they will always disperse evenly in water and appear uniform under a microscope, but they are still large enough to scatter light. Colloids can be seen when a beam of light is directed through the colloidal solution. If a flashlight were to direct a beam of light into the colloidal solution, the large colloidal particles will scatter the light and become shiny and visible, causing a phenomenon known as the Tyndall effect. Colloidal particles can also be found in the air and are then known as an aerosol. Smoke is an example of a colloidal suspension in the air. An automobile's headlights on a dirty, dusty road piercing the dusty air is another example of the Tyndall effect.

Why are colloids in the soil important? Colloidal particles contain negative charges that attract positively charged ions. This is the single most important concept you should understand about the soil system. Here is how it works. The very fine clay particles in the soil called colloids attract positively charged ions called cations from the surrounding soil and attach them loosely to their surface (a process known as adsorption). This negatively charged surface of soil particles creates a bond that attracts positively charged ions such as calcium, magnesium, potassium, aluminum, manganese, and many other minerals. This attraction holds these particles together where they will become available for plants, and helps prevent cations from being leached away as water passes through the soil. Colloidal particles are large enough to carry many ions. In fact, since the colloidal clay particles vary in size, they can carry dozens or even thousands of ions, depending on their size and the strength of their negative charge. The ability of colloidal particles to attract and retain positively charged ions on their larger surface area is the single most important characteristic of soils.

But cations are not the only ions that exist in the soil system. Anions—negatively charged ions—are also present but are usually found in smaller quantities. They are more likely to be found loose in the soil and will not always be attracted to the soil colloids since they have the same negative charge. This allows the anions to remain loosely held in the soil and water, keeping them water-soluble and immediately available for plant absorption since they can be carried directly to the roots through water.

However, their free mobility also makes them more prone to being leached out of the soil, but at the same time more readily available to plants. In an effort to avoid leaching, plants will normally absorb whatever anions are in the area first. Eventually, as the plant quickly depletes this supply, the anions will be replaced by the cations held on the colloidal particles, and soon this supply of ions will eventually need to be replaced by the ions recently liberated by the breakdown process from microorganisms, and the mineral cycle continues. Even though the immediate source of ions for plant roots is the loosely held anions, the supply of these anions will be depleted quickly, making the primary nutrient reservoir the positively charged cations that are attached to the colloids.

Just because colloids are attracting the cations doesn't always mean that they stay attached to the colloidal surface. Cations are being continuously exchanged for one another in an active process called "cation exchange." This means that an ion of calcium can be replaced by two ions of potassium at any given millisecond. In fact, this exchange repeats itself over and over and is so rapid that the ions are actually competing for a spot on the colloid. All this exchanging and competition between ions ultimately results in a state of equilibrium between the cations and the anions. Soil is a very dynamic and active system, with ions constantly being exchanged for one another between the colloidal particles with those in water. Fortunately, the strong attraction to the colloids helps keep many ions available for absorption into the roots.

At this point it should be remembered that since the finer clay particles have a negative charge, and all the clay particles totaled together will comprise a larger surface area than the sand or rocks, the soil's ability to supply a sufficient amount of nutrients is greatly enhanced. Thus, clay-dominated soils will retain more water, organic matter, and nutrients than sand-dominated soils. However, other materials such as pesticides also tend to be retained longer as well.

Decomposed organic matter also contributes to the soil's ion-supplying capabilities since it breaks down into very small particles that mix with sand and clay. And by its very nature, organic matter contains many plant nutrients that are released into the soil as ions through microbial activity. Soils with a good supply of sand, silt, clay, organic matter, and microbes represent an optimal mixture.

■ ■ ■

Organic and inorganic nutrition are the two ingredients that provide plants their nutritional requirements, with organic matter usually providing most of the requirements needed for the growth and development of plants. When microorganisms decompose organic material, this long breakdown process is called "ionization." Ionization is the process where mineral ions are liberated and released into a medium. Heavy metal minerals, such as iron and nickel, require ionization in order to be available to plants as ions.

Water also plays a key role in the ionization process. To understand ionization, consider common table salt: sodium chloride. Sodium and chlorine are two of the 13 required elements for plants. When the compound sodium chloride is dissolved in water, it separates into sodium ions and chloride ions. If the water evaporates, these two elements will once again join together to form the white powder, sodium chloride. Plants cannot absorb the compound sodium chloride, but they can absorb the individual sodium ions and chloride ions.

Let's assume your soil lacks two minerals, potassium and nitrogen, so you decide to add the fertilizer potassium nitrate to make up for this deficiency. The potassium nitrate compound is unable to be absorbed by the plant until the soil microbes dissolve it into potassium ions and nitrate ions. Therefore, nature liberates the ions that are held in organic matter or inside inorganic compounds to make them available for absorption into plants.

Another example of soil's ability to break down large inorganic compounds is if you were to take an iron nail and bury it in the soil. If you came back in 10 years, you would find a rusty nail going through early stages of ionization. Some of it would have broken down into very small particles of iron that you wouldn't be able to see with the naked eye. The water and microbes in the soil would have been busy breaking it down and releasing the iron ions into the soil.

Ions can be released from a large compound not only through ionization, but also through the action of water. "Dissolution" is a process that specifically refers to a large compound that dissolves in the presence of water. During this process, ions will disassociate themselves from the surface of a solid and dissolve into water. However, the opposite of dissolution is "precipitation." If the water were to evaporate, the dissolved ions would come out of solution and once again form the solid.

Imagine a glass of perfectly clean water that is saturated with millions of independent magnesium ions. As the water evaporates, the amount of water in the glass declines, forcing the magnesium ions to bunch together and eventually bind into larger magnesium particles. When this occurs, the solution of water is no longer filled with water soluble ions, but rather large magnesium particles. The ions would have precipitated into larger particles (forming a magnesium crystal) since there was not enough water to keep them dissolved and independent from one another. The glass of water containing magnesium ions would have precipitated out of solution.

In the soil, precipitation occurs regularly. Heavy rainfall or irrigation provides water to the soil and keeps ions in their ionic state. However, if the soil dries, ions will begin to precipitate and start forming compounds with one another, making them no longer available to the roots. Another example of precipitation can easily be seen in household showers. The water from the showerhead may be filled with water soluble minerals ions, but as the water dries, discoloration can occur, caused by the mineral deposits, which results when the water dries and forces the ions to bind together once again. Water is able to dissolve some mineral particles into water soluble ions, but if the water evaporates, the dissolved minerals will precipitate back to their large particles once again. This shows not only the dissolving power of water, but how water ions remain in their ionic state.

■ ■ ■

By this time, it should be clear that whether the source of the minerals was organic decomposed matter or inorganic materials such as rocks and sand, the microorganisms will liberate the ions and release them into the soil. Plants will then be able to absorb these minerals back into their roots once again, and the cycle continues.

A plant's mineral nutrition is dependent on several chemical processes that occur in soils, most of which have been mentioned so far. But there is still one more important step in the journey of minerals through soil. There are two different ways ions are transported to the roots. On one hand we have the cations that are attached to colloidal particles, and on the other hand we have the anions found loosely in the water that are available for immediate absorption. Both types of ions are delivered to the roots differently.

Ions move through soil either through mass flow or diffusion. Mass flow more aptly refers to ions that are carried by water to within close proximity of roots or leaches them out of the soil. Elements that dissolve in water will be absorbed when the roots absorb the water. Therefore, mass flow is an effortless process.

Diffusion, on the other hand, does not involve water, but involves a more complex process that explains the movement of ions from an area of high concentration to an area of low concentration. If you dropped a tablespoon of soil into a glass of water and watched it separate and spread across the surface and throughout the volume of water, you would witness diffusion in action. Diffusion is simply the spreading of one substance through another equally. Similarly, ions that are liberated through ionization will spread throughout the soil system through the principle of diffusion.

Mass flow is dependent upon the rate of water movement through the soil. Mass flow from water should provide enough transport of ions to satisfy the root's demand. However, mass flow can fall short in its nutrient delivery, and a deficiency will develop around the root zone. When this occurs, the lower concentration area of the root zone will be quickly resupplied with new ions through diffusion. Diffusion complements mass flow. It involves the movement of ions from soil particle to soil particle because of their charge. Mineral ions in high demand by the plants, such as nitrogen, chlorine, calcium, and potassium, diffuse quickly through soil when compared to minerals in lower demand, such as phosphorus, zinc, and copper.

Diffusion is a slow process. Ions can only move short distances that can involve millimeters and take several minutes. For example, the movement of a nutrient across the diameter of a plant cell takes approximately 2.5 seconds. At this rate, mineral nutrients traveling the length of one meter would take over 30 years! Clay particles that creep from the topsoil down to deeper subsoil can take thousands of years.

When ions diffuse to the roots, it is their positive charge that moves them into the root system. This will be examined closer in the next chapter.

■ ■ ■

Soil fertility means more than having the right minerals in the soil. The minerals also need to be available for absorption. The soil's pH level controls this factor of mineral availability. First, understand that pH stands for "parts hydrogen" and is used to measure the alkalinity or acidity of soil. The pH scale ranges from 1 to 14, where 1 is very acidic, 14 is extremely alkaline, and 7 is considered neutral. Each number represents a tenfold increase in acidity or alkalinity. For example, a pH level of 9 is ten times more alkaline than a pH level of 8.

The pH levels in virgin soils are largely determined by its parent material, texture, and presence of salts such as calcium carbonate. The pH level of the soil is a serious concern for farmers. Farmers know that minerals must be in their water soluble state before they can be absorbed into plant cells. Therefore, farmers try to control the soil's pH level that will maximize the solubility of most minerals, which maximizes growth rates.

Having improper pH levels affects the availability of minerals in different ways. Extreme pH levels will force the minerals into different compounds, causing the minerals to lose their solubility. When minerals lose their solubility, they begin to form compounds. When this occurs, they will no longer be available for plant absorption. For example, management of phosphorus, iron, and zinc becomes much more difficult in a high soil pH level because it causes these minerals to become insoluble.

Calcium carbonate is a compound that forms when the elements carbon and calcium exist in soils. This compound is very alkaline and is purposely added to fertilizer to raise the pH level of the soil if it was determined to be too acidic. Limestone is an example of calcium carbonate that forms naturally when calcium binds to carbon. When farmers add calcium carbonate to acidic soils, it is expected that the soil pH will rise back to neutral and it will eventually break down into calcium ions.

Ammonium nitrate, on the other hand, is mixed into fertilizers in an effort to neutralize alkaline soils containing too much calcium carbonate. Ammonium nitrate is water-soluble and gets carried deep into the soil quickly from irrigation or rainfall. When conditions in the soil favor microbial activity, such as warm, moist conditions with proper pH, ammonium nitrate breaks down within a few weeks, releasing hydrogen ions into the soil, a process that results in lowered pH levels. In fact, one pound of ammonium nitrate added to the soil can neutralize 1.8 pounds of calcium carbonate. For severe cases, farmers can also use one pound of ammonium sulfate to create enough acidity to neutralize 5.3 pounds of calcium carbonate. All of this effort is to bring the pH back to a neutral range by adding either acidic or alkaline materials to neutralize the soil. Some soils do not require pH management. They naturally have pH levels anywhere between 5.5 and 8.5, which allows for most minerals to remain in their available form.

Generally, various crops require different levels of soil pH. Dr. Robert L. Stevens explains that the pH of farmland soil "can affect vigor, nitrogen cycling, calcium and magnesium relationships, phosphorus availability, manganese levels, and pesticide activities. Although fruit trees will produce over a wide range in soil pH, management will be much easier if pH is maintained in the 6.2 to 7.0 range." Adult trees can tolerate pH levels below 5.2, but younger trees require 6.0 pH levels in order to grow optimally.

Other problems arise when the soil's pH level becomes too alkaline or too acidic. Under optimal pH conditions, small areas on the colloidal clay particles can have their own positive charge capable of absorbing anions. However, if soils become too acidic, for example, this positively charged surface area can increase, potentially disrupting the original process where a negatively charged area dominated the colloidal particles.

The pH level of water can even influence the downward movement of minerals through the soil. At a neutral level between 6.5 and 7.5, both positively and negatively charged ions will dissolve in proper proportions to each other. If the pH level gradually becomes more alkaline or more acidic, ions in the soil will be out of balance and could create mineral deficiencies. At lower pH levels, water has a stronger leaching power.

This is why farmers often try to neutralize the pH of their soil. They try to lower very high soil pH levels when it becomes too alkaline, or increase the soil's pH level when it becomes too acidic. Minerals that lose their solubility in a lower pH range include phosphorus, calcium, and magnesium. However, iron and manganese, for example, will lose their solubility in alkaline soils.

When the pH level is between 6.5 and 7.0, most minerals are generally considered soluble and most vegetation and microorganisms will flourish in a neutral pH range. However, research shows that not all plants require a neutral pH level—blueberries tend to grow well in acidic soils around 4.5 to 5.5, and cabbage grows best in higher alkaline soils.

It is important that minerals not only be within close proximity for the roots to reach them, they must also be in an easy to absorb form. In order for plants to absorb minerals, they must first be dissolved into their ionic state in order to be carried to the plants through mass flow or diffusion. Plants cannot absorb any insoluble compounds, and ions are always considered water-soluble. For a list of mineral ions that can be found in soils, see Appendix A.

Nature's gradual geologic process of weathering parent material into smaller and smaller fragments is only the beginning of a process that is further carried out by microorganisms in the soil into even smaller particles for eventual plant absorption and human consumption. It should be clear that water, microorganisms, and a proper soil pH level are all required to dissolve minerals into water-soluble ions in order to be ready for absorption into the plant roots. Now that the ions have been transported to the roots for absorption, they will begin an incredible long distance journey through the plant…

Chapter 3

Through the Ion Channels

Plants are considered to be autotrophic organisms, which means they create their own food. They are at the bottom of the food chain; mineral nutrients absorbed by plants will eventually create the foods that animals, including people, depend on. Plants must constantly seek out and absorb minerals in the soil in order to continue their own survival, including growth, metabolism, and development. The nutrients that make this happen are the minerals, and the means to collect them is through the roots.

Photosynthesis occurs in the leaves and creates organic carbohydrates, sugars, amino acids, and vitamins for the plant's growth and development. However, photosynthesis is unable to complete its processes without the water and minerals that roots provide.

A major responsibility of the root system is to anchor the plant in the ground. Very rarely do people see large trees being uprooted during a storm. The trunks may get snapped like toothpicks but the roots usually remain steadfast in the ground. They also prevent landslides and soil erosion. But the main purpose of roots is to rapidly spread out underground to seek out water and minerals.

Root systems are constantly mining the soil for minerals and some have been measured growing to phenomenal depths and lengths. The root system of the common grass plant, for example, has been measured at 375 total miles with 14 million individual roots, measuring 2,500 square feet of surface area. The root system of rye plants has totaled 387 miles, and corn plants have drilled to depths of more than 20 feet. Typically, the plant's height will determine the horizontal span the root system will extend.

Fortunately, roots are not dependent upon themselves for this responsibility to continually dig and mine the Earth. In fact, plants are not very efficient at nutrient absorption by themselves, so they rely heavily on a type of soil fungi called mycorrhizae. These special fungi, which look like long, thin hairs, live on root cells and extend out of the roots up to four centimeters. Their job is to increase the plant's total surface area for absorption. In fact, the total mass of the mycorrhizae can increase this surface area by up to 100,000 times, helping plants secure more water and nutrient absorption by exerting less energy. For example, plant biologists have measured mineral content of plants with and without mycorrhizae working for them. They found that plants with these special fungi had mineral levels 36-118% higher.

Minerals in the soil do not move passively by themselves. There are certain characteristics of ions, such as their electrical charge, that make them capable of being transported from one place to another. Therefore, ions must be actively transported to within close range of the roots which requires special energy from the plant. Some of this energy is called adenosine triphosphate (ATP), and is a substance used in many processes in the cells.

The absorption process is known as "mineral uptake." Absorbing minerals into roots requires two different processes—one where the ions are transported through the soil and delivered within close proximity to the roots and another process where they are absorbed into the cells. These two processes are dramatically affected by the negative and positive charge of the ions.

Another important factor that influences mineral uptake is water. The water in the soil plays an important role in the absorption process because many of the mineral elements absorbed by the plant are first dissolved in water, which is a characteristic of an ion. The negatively charged ions (anions) can usually be found in the water that is in the soil. They are loosely held and are readily available for easy transport and quick access to the roots. As roots grow and push their way through the soil, the water will easily carry the anions toward the roots.

■ ■ ■

Somewhere along the way, ions are going to be faced with an insurmountable task of entering the tissues of roots. Since most of the ions that arrive are attached to colloidal clay particles, getting into position is the first step. The next step is to be carried through the various cell membranes and eventually into the cell.

However, plant cells have protective layers and walls that surround them to protect against parasites, viruses, and toxins such as particles larger than ions. The first obstacle ions encounter is a protective barrier known as the "plasma membrane." This important membrane is the first port of entry the ions must pass through in order to reach the inside of the cell. The plasma membrane surrounds the cell and regulates the traffic of substances that move into or out of the cell. This membrane is actually two layers: one layer is protein, and the other layer is lipids (oily or fatty molecules), with protein molecules sandwiched in between. These proteins help transport substances across the membrane and assist in the communication between the cells. Together, these layers form a tight seal and are very strong for their size.

The plasma membrane gets its strength and integrity from the internally supplied nutrients rather than from externally supplied compounds such as antibiotics. Research indicates that antibiotics such as nystatin cause leakage, higher permeability, and weak membrane strength. Monocarboxylic acids such as acetic acid and butyric acid can also weaken membranes by changing the fatty acid composition of membranes, and decreasing the proportion of polyunsaturated fatty acids such as linolenic acid. These types of cellular damage expose the cells to an influx of infectious pathogens from the outside, and they can also leak ions and solutes out of the cell. Interestingly, research shows that some plants experiencing an increase in permeability of this membrane have indicated deficiencies in zinc and phosphorus.

A major responsibility of the plasma membrane is to regulate the flow of ions that are allowed to pass through. In order for ions that have arrived via colloidal clay particles to pass through, they must first detach from the colloid. As stated in the previous chapter, soils contain extremely small colloidal particles that are negatively charged. This charged particle attracts hundreds of positively charged ions and attaches them to their surface. As the roots push their way through the soil, they get closer and closer to these colloidal particles, eventually close enough to absorb the ions they have on their surface.

Because the interior of most cells is negatively charged and carry a much stronger charge than the smaller colloid, the positively charged ions ferried by the colloids are attracted to this stronger negative charge and will detach when they get in range, putting them just outside the membrane. After the ions detach from the colloid, the colloids return back to the soil and the ferry process begins again. Because of their size, colloidal particles might be able to pass through normal filters, but they are simply too large to be able to pass through the extremely small ion channels of a plasma membrane.

During this ferry process, large numbers of ions can gather on the outskirts of the plasma membrane, ready to enter inside and participate in various cellular processes. Once the ions have detached from the colloid, they are attracted to the negative charge of the cell's interior. The ions first pass through a porous membrane known as the cell wall, which is simple since this wall is porous.

However, passage through the next layer, the plasma membrane, is much more difficult. Due to its tough, resilient strength, ions are unable to pass from one side of the plasma membrane to the other without some assistance. Fortunately, the plasma membrane contains certain methods of transport that allow ions to pass through, since both positively and negatively charged ions are transported differently. Dr. Curt Rom, a horticulturalist at the University of Arkansas, explains that soluble ions in the soil move through this membrane by two processes, either through small channels inside the plasma membrane called "ion channels" or by being ferried across the membrane by protein carriers.

Inside the plasma membrane are very small channels that are designed to transport ions across the membrane. These ion channels are ion-selective, and passage through this membrane is the first filtering process the plant uses to prevent unwanted materials, such as viruses, fungi, parasites, colloidal sized particles, and any other materials from entering the cell. The strong permeability of the plasma membrane is extremely important for this responsibility.

Ion channels are either open or closed, and open only under certain conditions, such as the presence of hormones, changes in membrane potential, mechanical stress, or the ion itself. Most of the time, however, ion channels are closed, but when they do open they allow a swift penetration of cations to cross the membrane. In fact, research shows that as many as 10 million to one billion ions scurry across the ion channels per second, so it doesn't take large numbers of channels to fill the need of each cell.

The total number of ion channels per cell seems to be rather small, although they contain specific ion channels for each mineral element. Channels can be identified by the species of ion that they allow to pass through. The number of identified ion channels has increased, and there is evidence of specific ion channels for potassium, chlorine, hydrogen, and calcium, and research insists that channels exist for other ions, too.

At the start of the absorption process, ions that are already inside the roots contain an opposite electrical charge. This is important because a state of equilibrium must remain between the plant and the soil. Since cations are positively charged, the root will send out a negatively charged ion in exchange for the incoming positively charged ions, resulting in an ion exchange. Eventually, the concentration of ions inside the roots can accumulate more than the concentration of ions in the soil by as much as 10,000 times. Overall, the passage of ions through ion channels is a passive process, requiring little to no energy from the plant, other than emitting negatively charged hydrogen ions in exchange, although any ions can be released, not just hydrogen.

However, some ions have certain characteristics that make it difficult for them to easily diffuse across the membrane, such as either being negatively charged or a higher concentration of the element may exist inside the cell than outside in the soil. Since these ions cannot pass through the ion channels, a different process has to occur for them to enter the cell's interior. In such cases, a process that requires energy is needed to absorb these elements. On the outer edge of the plasma membrane, the other transport method, the "carrier proteins," meet the particular ion species for which they have an affinity. These small protein molecules will attach the ions to their surface and ferry them across the membrane, drop them off inside the cell, and then return back to their original position. They will repeat the process and carry more ions of that same mineral across the membrane.

Carrier proteins actually "pump" ions from outside the cell walls into the cells. This pumping process is an active process that requires energy from the plant. This process uses the plant's energy by exchanging hydrogen ions that come from root respiration or various other processes. These hydrogen ions are released into the soil to maintain a state of equilibrium with the soil. Although carrier proteins are primarily responsible for transporting anions, they are less selective between cations and anions and are thought to be the most likely method that will transport both across the membrane.

While ion channels are more involved in large numbers of ions transported per second, carrier proteins are slower than ion channels but pay more attention to selectivity, although they can still transport anywhere from 100,000 to 1 million ions per second—a large number, but not when compared to ion channels. Not all ions, molecules, or organic solutes are selected to be transported across the plasma membrane. Carrier proteins are very choosy about what gets transported across the membrane and deposited inside the cell. Eventually, the accumulation of ions inside the cell will surpass the number of ions available outside the cell, sometimes reaching thousands of times more concentrated. When this occurs, these transport methods stop.

■ ■ ■

Some mineral ions resemble each other quite similarly. For example, when ions of potassium and rubidium are present together in the soil, the radius and the number and orbit of electrons of these two ions can be so similar that the plant will absorb both elements. Since the plasma membrane is not always able to distinguish between these two ions, uptake for both can occur, even though only one of them is essential and one cannot replace the other in their roles of plant metabolism.

Competition between ions can also occur between magnesium ions and potassium and calcium ions. In fact magnesium deficiencies can occur because of strong competition for uptake when high concentrations of potassium and calcium exist in the soil. Therefore, competition between ions is not always caused by the plant's nutritional requirements being selective, but can be due to similarities between ions that are beneficial and those that have little to no function in the plant. Therefore, plants are not always able to exclude unneeded ions from uptake.

When the outside of the cell accumulates more cations than the number that are found inside, an imbalance occurs, signaling the ion channels to open. The transport of cations across the plasma membrane is a result of the electrical properties of the cell, called the "electrochemical gradient." Because ions carry either a positive or negative electrical charge, their movement creates an electrical current. The ions will move across the ion channels in response to the positive and negative charges they carry. For example, potassium ions with a positive charge will be attracted to a region of negative charge; consequently, the inside of the cell.

The electrochemical gradient results in cations flowing into the cell. Cations are positively charged and flow into the negatively charged interior of the cell, resulting in millions of ions per second flowing in. Anions, however, must rely on the carrier proteins, or they may be carried by water into the free space of the roots in between the cells. This explains why anions will reach the interior of a cell in far less abundance than the cations. To make room for the incoming flow of anions, the cell will emit a hydrogen ion for every anion it carries across.

■ ■ ■

So how does water enter the plant? Plant cells require a large amount of water to maintain pressure and to carry some ions, as well as products manufactured during photosynthesis, such as carbohydrates, proteins, and vitamins. The cellular framework of plant tissues is not always tight. There are small, open-air spaces between the cells that allow water and the anions it carries into the roots. Water can enter roots by seeping into the free, open space between the root cells, or it can enter the cells directly through "osmosis," neither of which require any energy from the plant.

Osmosis is how water can pass from cell to cell. It occurs when a high concentration of water enters an area that has a low concentration of water. As water enters the root cells, the cell will expand and pressure inside the cells will increase, but only if the cell walls are strong enough to sustain this pressure. As the pressure continues to build, the overall osmotic potential becomes more balanced and eventually the water stops entering. This pressure is known as "turgor pressure," and plants depend on turgor pressure for much of their strength and integrity. When plants become wilted, their cells have weakened and have become unable to hold this pressure, and have leaked valuable water and mineral ions out of their cells.

If two cells are next to each other and one cell contains more water than the other, using pressure the water will move into the lesser cell, making the water levels between the two equal. Osmosis is the primary means of how water enters the roots, and just like the cations and anions, water traverses from cell to cell until it reaches the interior of the root and gets carried up to the leaves. Most importantly, osmosis is considered a passive process because it doesn't require energy. It is a free and automatic process that provides nutrients into the cells without any energy being spent by the plant.

Over time the mineral supply that surrounds the roots could become exhausted if nature didn't have ways of replenishing the supply. As water is absorbed into the root system, water from other areas will replace the lost water and will bring in a fresh supply of ions. Even if water were scarce, cations would still be able to diffuse toward the root to replace those that were absorbed. Meanwhile, roots will also continue to dig and mine the Earth in search of new minerals throughout the life of the plant.

These processes ensure that plants have a continuous flow of minerals and water available for absorption.

■ ■ ■

Reaching the interior of a root cell is one thing, but traveling through the maze of organs, water, enzymes, and other products inside the cell is another. At this stage of their journey, the ions have now entered the cells of roots and must navigate through the vast interior of a cell. Navigating through the inside of the cell can be tricky; there are several stops along the way. Ions must pass through several regions and membranes. First the ion must be transported through the outer cell wall. According to Daniel Branton of the University of California at Berkeley, ions then must pass through other membranes, such as the plasmalemma, that might contain proteins, sugars, pectin, fatty oils, and other polymers that all protect the cell and participate in various processes. Finally, after the ion has moved through these membranes, it has gone through all filtering processes and has reached the vast interior of the cell, generally known as the cytoplasm.

The cytoplasm refers to the overall interior of a cell and all of its "organs," and is surrounded by the plasmalemma membrane. The interior of the cell is safe from the external environment due to the tough structural layers the ions have just passed through. These layers also provide an effective seal that prevent the cellular organs, ions, and other important organic substances from accidentally leaking out of the cell.

However, once they reach this point, their journey is still not through. The ions then travel across the immense interior of the cell where they will penetrate one last membrane—the "tonoplast," which is the membrane that surrounds the storage vacuole. Vacuoles are cavities inside the cell that are filled with a watery solution of ions, organic substances, and some enzymes. Some ions will remain in the vacuole and participate in various cellular processes, although most of the ions will continue their journey across the cell.

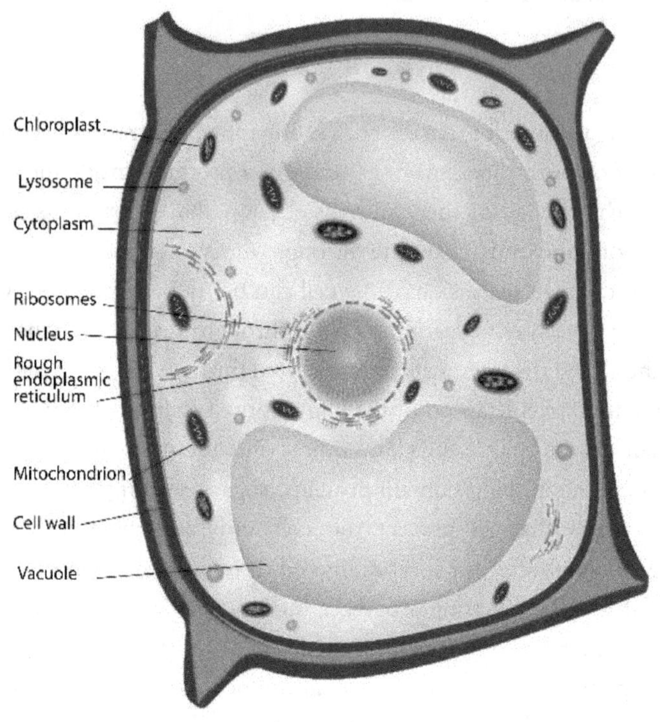

Storage vacuoles accumulate and store ions, water, and other substances such as carbohydrates and vitamins manufactured during photosynthesis. Vacuoles are storage units that occupy as much as 80-90% of the cell's volume, and exist only in plant cells—not in animal cells. The plasma membrane and the outer wall of the vacuole, called the tonoplast, both share and exchange ions such as calcium and potassium. In fact most of the calcium that enters through the plasma membrane is still available for exchange with the tonoplast within the first 30 minutes. However, during this time the faster moving potassium ions have already been exchanged and transported across the cytoplasm and entered into the vacuole.

In seeds, some proteins can be stored for years in vacuoles. Later, when the seeds germinate, the preserved proteins become hydrolyzed and the resulting amino acid becomes a nutrient supply for the budding embryo. The ions that are stored in vacuoles will remain either until the plant requires them, or they will be recycled throughout the plant in case of future soil deficiencies. Vacuoles play a very important role in the long-term survival of a plant.

As ions continue to move through the interior of a cell, some ions will enter the ion channels of other organelles of the cell and participate in their cellular processes, such as mitochondria. The mitochondria are small sacs that are responsible for the cell's respiration, and are the sites where organic substances are broken down into carbon dioxide and water, releasing the energy that is needed to create a molecule called Adenosphine triphosphate (ATP). ATP is the most prominent molecule required to power important chemical reactions in the cell, and requires sodium and potassium ions.

Other ions will participate in the cellular functions of other organs inside the cell. For example, ribosomes are extremely small, dense bodies 15-25 nanometers in diameter that are responsible for synthesizing proteins and are themselves made of ribosomal RNA and other special proteins. Ions from the mineral boron, for example, play a key role in the ribosomal production and synthesis of these proteins.

■ ■ ■

After participating in most of the activities of the cell, ions are ready to continue their movement by exiting out of the cell. The ions and water must continue to travel through the remainder of the root cells, and there are two pathways that they will follow. One pathway is through the open space between the plasma membrane and the outer cell wall, called the "apoplast," and the other pathway is through a bridge-like formation known as the "symplast."

The apoplast refers to the open, free space between cells that exists just outside the plasma membrane, but inside the porous cell wall.

Research indicates that some metabolic activity takes place here. This is a free space inside roots where both water and ions can reside. The water and ions located in this space are inside the root, but not inside any cells. This area is known as the "apoplastic pathway" and transports primarily water, anions, and other solutes. When water and ions enter a plant through this route, they are only able to seep their way in between cells, although they are traveling deeper and deeper into the root system. However, when this watery solution reaches a certain point, it will be redirected into a region of the root cells where it will be filtered.

The other pathway that ions follow when exiting a cell is a very unusual formation inside the plasma membrane that connects two cells together. Where these two cells touch, the plasma membrane of one cell is connected to the plasma membrane of its neighbor cell through a bridge-like formation called the "symplast." A part of the plasma membrane actually extends outward, forming a tube that connects to the plasma membrane of neighboring cells. This forms a passageway that allows only ions and organic substances such as glucose to pass out of one cell and into another. When ions enter this pathway, they will be able to continue moving from cell to cell and bypass any further vacuoles or filtering membranes on their way to the inner regions of the root system. This pathway acts like a large freeway system by allowing these molecules to travel from cell to cell as much as 1,000 times faster versus going through stop-and-go traffic by traversing through hundreds of individual cell membranes. This interconnecting system from cell to cell is sometimes called the "symplastic pathway" and is so unique that an entire plant could easily be considered one giant cell due to the efficiency of this sharing and movement of molecules.

But the symplast is not necessarily a hollow tube that conveniently allows anything to pass through. The plant strictly regulates the substances that flow through it, and the symplast is no exception. The symplast can act as another filtering step in the transport of molecules through a plant because it restricts any particles larger than 10 nm (one angstrom) to pass through. Small molecules, such as ions and glucose, pass easily, while larger molecules such as proteins, fulvic acids, toxins, viruses, pathogens, or ions that have been chelated (bound to a protein or an amino acid) inside the cell are restricted and even prevented from entering this pathway. Recent research indicates that if some plant viruses that have invaded the plant are too large to pass through, they can force their way through by inflaming and expanding the diameter of the symplast so they, too, can continue their passage through the plant and spreading their infection from cell to cell.

Another impediment that can cause restriction in the amount of flow in the symplastic pathway is an excessively high amount of calcium. Also, an oxygen deficiency, as well as phosphorus and nitrogen deficiencies, can reduce the hydraulic conductivity that moves the solutes through this pathway. Unfortunately, if the flow of ions through the symplastic pathway slows down, the plant will experience limited growth and depressed metabolic rates.

■ ■ ■

The ions still have a long way to go. They still need to travel across the entire diameter of the root to reach the center. Roots are comprised of four main sections that surround the circumference of the root. The outer layer, which supports the mycorrhizae hairs and is externally exposed to the soil, is called the epidermis. This epidermal layer is only one cell thick. Moving inward, the next layer is called the cortex, which is several cells thick. Closer towards the center of the root is another layer called the endodermis, which has a Casparian strip that runs through it and is also one celled thick. And finally, the innermost part of a root is the vascular system that carries the water and ions upward to the tops of the plant. This vessel is known as the xylem, and it transports ions and water upward. Once an ion is absorbed into the root, it must travel across each of these root layers to finally reach the xylem.

Once ions begin moving from cell to cell, they will travel across the diameter of the root to reach the xylem vessel, which is a very unique transport system that carries ions upward to the rest of the plant. As the ions begin their movement through the symplastic pathway they quickly move into the next layer of cells called the cortex. The cortex, unlike the epidermis, is comprised of several layers of cells. Once the ions pass through this series of cells they will move into the last layer known as the endodermis. The endodermis is the innermost layer of cells where ions will accumulate. It is here that a strong, impermeable layer called a Casparian strip, made from a waxy substance, surrounds the cells in the endodermis.

Water and ions that travel toward the xylem through the free, open space will arrive at a dead end when they reach the epidermis. This marks the end of the road for the water and ions that travel through the apoplastic pathway. The watertight seal of the Casparian strip is designed to prevent anything from entering the xylem, including water, ions, and even infectious microorganisms and viruses, which have not been redirected through the endodermal cells to be filtered.

The Casparian strip forces water and ions to pass through the endodermal cells before they can continue their journey. The water and ions traveling in the free space must be redirected into the cytoplasm of the endodermal cells if they are to proceed any further. Here they will pass through these cells and eventually enter into the symplastic pathway where they will meet up with ions that have already been on that path since they first entered the root. Here the ions from the symplastic pathway and the water and ions from the apoplastic pathway come together during the last leg of their journey. This is an extremely important step during the long journey of mineral ions.

Without the Casparian strip, substances traveling along the free space between cells—the apoplastic pathway—could enter the root's vascular system without being filtered. This could create problems if viruses were present. Nutrients must pass through at least one membrane before they are allowed to enter the plant's vascular system. This is extremely important; it keeps the plant in total control of what is allowed to pass into the plant's vascular system. The apoplastic pathway goes through porous cell walls but the Casparian strip forces the water and ions into the endodermal cells where they get filtered and end up in the symplastic pathway.

Together, all of the ions will eventually reach the inner layer of the root once they complete the last leg of the symplastic pathway. After they reach the center of the root, the ions will reach two very important and large transport vessels known as the "xylem" and "phloem." Here they will be loaded into the vascular system through pumps that pump them into the xylem. These vessels act similar to blood veins in humans by carrying mineral ions, water, and other solutes upward toward the plant's stems and leaves.

■ ■ ■

Ions travel the same path as water—through the epidermis, across the cortex, and into the xylem. The overall movement of water from the soil and into the roots is caused by the evaporation of water through the plant's leaves. Roots are constantly drawing on water from the soil because water inside the plant is constantly evaporating. More than 90% of water that enters a plant will evaporate. A common red maple tree will lose 200 liters of water per day, while a birch tree with an average of 200,000 leaves can lose as much as 1,000 gallons per day during peak growing season. This evaporation process inside plants is called transpiration, which acts as a cooling process and is responsible for the movement of water through the plant.

Mineral uptake by the roots is regulated by other factors such as the nutritional status of the plant. As the internal concentration of the minerals increases and the plant's demand for nutrients declines, the rate of uptake will fluctuate. Occasionally, when soil conditions permit, the plant will absorb very high amounts of nutrients during periods of high availability and store them in the vacuoles. This allows the plant to survive during periods of drought or when root supply is interrupted. It also holds true when unfavorable weather conditions flush nutrients out of the soil.

Inside the roots, most minerals will remain in their ionic form. However, some of the minerals may be used to form various compounds that plants will use. In spite of this, it should be understood that minerals are always absorbed as ions—any change of ions into a compound or some other molecule is minimal and is the sole discretion of the plant.

Water, nutrients, and other assimilated compounds will move from roots up to the branches and outer leaves through transport vessels to be explained in the next chapter. The entry of water and ions into the root system is just the first step in their remarkable journey through the plant. Once the ions and water have traveled across the symplastic and apoplastic pathways through all the layers of the root, and have made it through the tough screening and filtering processes, they will be loaded into the vascular system and carried upward toward the leaves.

Chapter 4

Pathways, Pumps, and Photosynthesis

Minerals have come a long way so far. They traveled across the universe for billions of years, have been lodged deep inside Earth for millions of years, spent a few thousand years being mixed and dissolved in the soil, and in the past few days have traveled through networks of underground roots. Eventually, however, the time comes when minerals contribute to one of Earth's most important living organisms: the plant. Now, one of the most exciting stages of minerals' voyage involves a long-distance journey through a plant where they will eventually participate in photosynthesis.

After the ions and water have traveled across the diameter of the roots and reached the vascular system, they are ready to be loaded into the xylem vessel, a process known as "xylem loading." This point marks the end of the journey for the ions that have either traveled cell to cell through the symplast or weaved their way through the apoplast.

Somehow the ions need to be pumped out of the root system and into the xylem. According to M.G. Pitman (1972), there are ion pumps strategically located so that ions traveling through the symplastic pathway will be pumped into the xylem. The pumps are located in positions where they will greet the ions arriving from the symplastic pathway. At this point inside a plant, ions have not had to travel very far. Moving across the diameter of a root is a very short distance when compared to the next leg of their journey. After they are pumped into the xylem, the long-distance stage of their journey begins.

The xylem is like a pipeline that extends from the bottom tip of roots and all the way up to the tallest part of the plant, and extends out to the branches and leaves. The xylem works similarly to blood vessels in humans. It is the plant's transport vessel for delivering the water and nutrients absorbed through the soil that will be distributed throughout the plant. This solution travels up to the leaves, where the water will evaporate and the ions will contribute to photosynthesis.

The xylem's ability to transfer water from the roots upward to the leaves requires a force not entirely understood by plant physiologists. Imagine a large tree such as a Redwood in California. How can a tree that is hundreds of feet tall carry water upward from deep inside the Earth against gravity all the way to the top and to the outermost branches and leaves? This phenomenon is best explained through the cohesion-transpiration theory.

The xylem is part of a pressurized system that carries water upward in response to water that evaporates in the leaves. When sunlight strikes the surface of the leaves it initiates photosynthesis and warms up the leaves. Water will gradually drip out of the leaf or it will evaporate. The loss of this water is known as "transpiration," which causes tension (negative pressure) to pull the water inside the xylem upward to replace the water that is being lost. On warm days, as much as 99% of a plant's water is lost through this process; the remaining 1% is used during photosynthesis. Water continues to be replaced as it evaporates, filling the plant with fresh water and keeping ions constantly on the move, which is critical during the growing season. Most researchers agree that the water is chiefly pulled through the plant, rather than being pushed from the root system.

The liquid inside the xylem is known as xylem sap, and is extremely clean because it has undergone several filtering processes as it traveled through the roots. Xylem sap contains critical life-giving nutrients, including ions, phytohormones, and enzymes such as peroxidases, as well as organic substances like sugars that were manufactured during photosynthesis that have leaked over from other vessels. The rate of transport of the xylem sap has been recorded to be between 10-15 meters per hour, or 1-30 inches per minute, depending on the rate of transpiration. Sunny and hot days will generate faster rates of transport than cold or humid days.

There are several factors that allow xylem sap to flow smoothly through a plant. Water molecules in the xylem act like an adhesive to the xylem walls by sticking together through hydrogen bonds during transport, which prevents the fluid from sliding back down due to if there was a loss of pressure. This helps to counteract the effects of gravity, while a slight amount of pressure from the roots helps to push water upward.

Besides carrying ions and water, the xylem can benefit the plant in other ways. It also provides some structural support for the plant and its cells can provide some storage for ions. The hollow and tubular structure of the xylem walls serves two critical functions. First, it allows large amounts of water to be transported at a time. Second, it allows ions to occasionally enter and exit the xylem as the needs of the plant dictate.

Occasionally, the plant may need some of these ions that are in transit in the xylem sap for various functions. The plant will allow ions to pass through the xylem walls to participate in other necessary functions. It is very important for ions to be able to move into developing organs such as fruits, or into areas of critical need such as responding to an infectious attack. The translocation of ions out of the xylem and into other organs can sometimes be necessary for metabolic functions in certain plant species. For example, molybdenum accumulation in the xylem inside roots is quite high in sunflower plants, while a low level of molybdenum transport occurs in tomatoes.

Transpiration is a very critical process for a plant, in that it keeps water and ions constantly moving. The delivery of water and nutrients allows photosynthesis to occur, supporting the growth and development of a plant. During periods of very high transpiration rates, such as on hot, sunny days, the loss of evaporated water can exceed the amount of water absorbed in the roots, causing drought-like symptoms to occur. Also, under these dry conditions there may not be enough water in the xylem for the nutrients to reach external sites such as fruits and flowers, causing abnormal growth.

The late Emanuel Epstein of the University of California-Davis stated, "Transpiration is a wasteful process, the result of an evolutionary compromise between two conflicting requirements—the need for exposure of moist, green cells to light, and that for open pathways for gas exchange between these cells and the atmosphere. It does, however, serve the function of conducting mineral nutrients from the roots to the tissues of the shoot, and that of cooling the leaves."

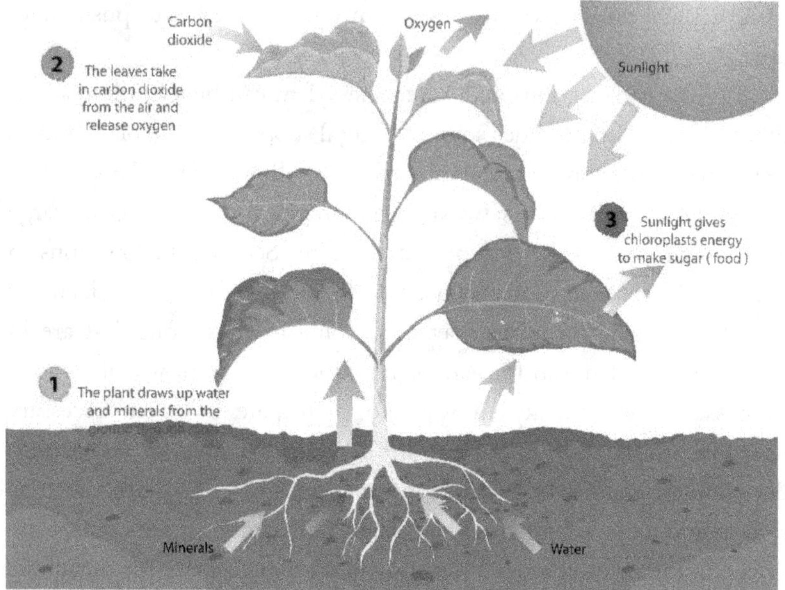

Generally, tissues with high transpiration rates such as leaves will dominate the delivery of water and ions. Manganese is one mineral that tends to accumulate in leaves during periods of high sunlight and transpiration rates than in cooler, shadier areas. Some plant organs, including fruits, also depend largely on transpiration and require an accumulation of certain mineral elements for their development. However, fruits tend to have slower transpiration rates, making them unable to compete with the leaves and other vegetative tissues for nutrients.

■ ■ ■

After the water and ions traveling through the xylem have reached their respective destinations, they will eventually exit the xylem. According to Epstein, plants transport the essential and even some of the beneficial minerals in a highly selective manner. Although some ions may have exited prematurely out of the xylem, most of the ions remain and will reach the leaves, causing the xylem sap that reaches the leaves to be of a different composition than what was originally absorbed by the roots. Xylem unloading is a process that moves ions out of the xylem and into small veins inside the leaves, which will distribute the ions throughout the surface of the leaf.

We need to take a closer look at the physical structure of a leaf in order to understand where ions and water will flow. The anatomy of a leaf consists of an upper and lower layer of cells called the epidermis, which are the large green surfaces you see when you look at a leaf. Both of these layers contain small epidermal cells and a waxy layer inside them called a cuticle, which is made of long-chain alcohols and fatty acids. This waxy coating is important because it protects the flow of ions and water from leaking out of the plant to prevent excess transpiration and leaching. It also helps keep the inside of the leaf from drying out and protects against infectious pathogens from entering. This barrier acts similarly to the Casparian strip in root cells by keeping the ions in the leaves and preventing too much water from transpiring. It performs its roles so effectively that it can inadvertently prevent external mineral ions from entering.

The primary function of leaves is to capture sunlight and transform it into sugars, carbohydrates, vitamins, amino acids, and other organic substances through photosynthesis. Most of the leaf space is composed of parenchyma cells that contain chloroplasts that manufacture these substances. These cells collectively make up the mesophyll, which is the interior of the leaf sandwiched between the upper and lower layer of epidermal cells. The mesophyll contains thin, moist cells and is the site where water evaporates.

The mesophyll cells obtain their nutrients from the delivery of ions through the veins. Even before the ions can participate in metabolic processes in the leaves, they are delivered to the outer edge of the leaves where they will bathe the mesophyll cells in their solution. The network of veins inside a leaf is so efficient and spread out that it is able to bring the water and ions so close to the cells that the furthest distance the ions will have to travel to their conducting tissues amounts to just the diameter of a few cells.

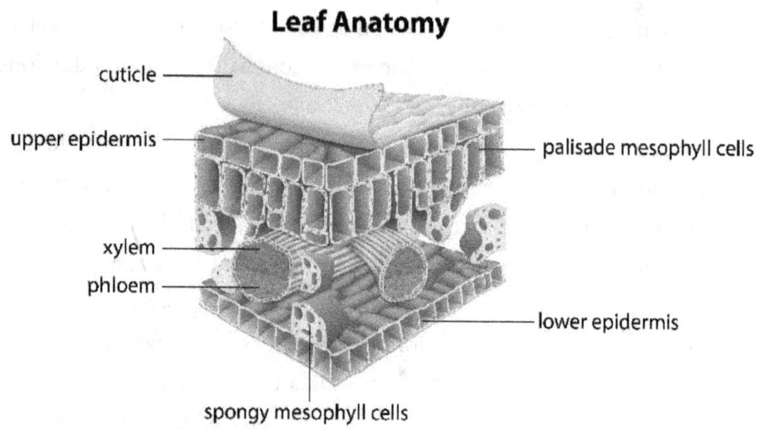

The ions traveling through the xylem and into the small network of veins in the leaves will soon exit and become accumulated inside the free space between cells—the apoplastic pathway. Fortunately, the waxy cuticle layer is there to protect the supply of ions from being leached out by rain or being lost through transpiration. At this point the ions have exited the xylem piping and have been deposited in the free space between cells in the leaves. However, the ions have not yet had a chance to pass through any cellular membranes or enter the symplastic pathway, and in order for them to become useful to the leaf cells and participate in metabolic processes, they will need to get inside the cells through the normal process of absorption.

However, according to Epstein, most ions must be absorbed twice by cellular transport mechanisms, first when they enter a root cell, and again when they enter leaf cells, before they reach the interior of a leaf cell to participate in photosynthesis. In order to enter the interior of these cells and participate in cellular processes, they have to be transported again through ion channels in much the same way as other plant cells. The water and ions will be transported across the membranes of the mesophyll cells, where the water will evaporate, leaving behind the rich supply of minerals. Once they are transported across these membranes and have entered the mesophyll cells of leaves, they will begin their passage through a symplastic pathway from cell to cell and become distributed across the surface of the leaf. In this position the ions are ready to assist in the important biochemical process known as photosynthesis.

Photosynthesis occurs primarily in leaves. Each leaf contains thousands of mesophyll cells, and inside each of these cells are 20-60 chloroplasts, although several hundred chloroplasts have been found in some plant species. Although all green parts of a plant contain chloroplasts where photosynthesis occurs, but the primary site for this process is in the leaves. Photosynthesis is the process that absorbs sunlight and uses it to convert carbon dioxide and water into the simple sugar glucose. Photosynthesis occurs when light touches a chloroplast, which then stores some of the light energy in its chlorophyll pigment. As a result, electrons become excited and are then ejected.

Nitrogen is a large component of the photosynthetic process. Since four atoms of nitrogen are required during the production of a green chlorophyll pigment molecule, nitrogen is moved into areas of high metabolic activity and high light exposure such as leaves. When sunlight touches these leaves, these chlorophyll molecules absorb the sunlight and release the electrons that provide the energy to activate the entire photosynthetic process.

An important phase of photosynthesis involves the splitting of water (H2O) into oxygen and hydrogen. The hydrogen molecules are used to produce organic substances such as NADPH, which is a critical coenzyme used in many plant processes. These hydrogen ions are also exchanged in the original uptake of minerals into the roots, and the exchange of ions that are transported across cell membranes. Although water, a compound of hydrogen and oxygen, is taken up through the soil, this water-splitting phase is used in many metabolic activities.

Sunlight initiates photosynthesis by exciting the flow of electrons inside the chloroplasts. Although there are many colors in the spectrum, green plants make use of red and blue wavelengths the most since they have the right amount of energy to start the process. Yellow and orange wavelengths are also absorbed and help enhance the light absorption capacity of red and blue. Wavelengths that are absorbed disappear. If something absorbs all wavelengths it appears black; white pigments reflect almost all wavelengths. However, none of the photosynthetic pigments absorb green wavelengths, which results in the color green being reflected in the appearance of the plant.

Undoubtedly photosynthesis is the most important process to sustain life on the face of the Earth. It is a very complex process that is not entirely understood, is still being researched, and is well beyond the scope of this book. To summarize, leaves absorb sunlight and the organic solutes created during this process are converted to sugars and carbohydrates such as disaccharides, polysaccharides, and other forms of carbohydrates. The sugars are then involved in the creation of amino acids, proteins, vitamins, and other types of substances that will be used as food for the plant. Anything manufactured during this process is assimilated; therefore, byproducts of photosynthesis can sometimes be referred to as "photoassimilates." Photosynthesis is responsible for 94% of the dry weight of green plants—the remaining 6% comes from the soil.

Since the process of photosynthesis is a dynamic and complex process, it is beyond the scope of this book to identify every stage of the process or even try to provide details, but it should be understood that some mineral ions play a role in this process.

During photosynthesis, magnesium ions found in chloroplasts initiate the flow of electrons, while iron and proteins that contain copper help to regulate the flow of electrons. Research shows that chloride and manganese are two other minerals that are necessary in the water-splitting stage. Chloroplasts maintain high amounts of chloride during photosynthesis, although some researchers argue that calcium plays a stronger role than chloride.

■ ■ ■

The mesophyll cells at the outer edges of leaves are the farthest reaching stations that ions will reach. However, this does not mark the end of their extraordinary journey through a plant, rather they are only halfway finished. Now they must take one of two possible routes. They can either exit the plant through leaching, guttation, or leaf fall, or they can travel back through the plant where they will be stored or used in various other metabolic processes to continue to benefit the plant.

If the ions exit the plant, there are several methods by which they become separated. When the solution of water and ions bathe the mesophyll cells, they can be exposed to the outer space of the cell walls and thus the outside air if the cuticles are thin. Therefore, ions can sometimes be subject to being leached by rainfall, irrigation, or other forces that can wash them away from the plant, which is common in rainforests. Occasional freezing can damage some of the cell's tissues, making ions even more prone to being leached away.

Leaching is a term that describes the removal of ions and organic substances from plants by rain, irrigation, wind, and other types of weathering. The amount of ions that are prone to leaching varies based on the intensity of rainfall or irrigation. According to Marschner, a decreased pH level between 5.5 and 3.0 increases the leaching potential of calcium, magnesium, potassium, manganese and zinc by a factor between 2 and 10. However, it should be understood that leaching is part of the regeneration of soil minerals that replenish the soil, which happens constantly in the tropics and rainforests, but can be a serious limitation to plant growth and development during heavy irrigation or sprinkler spraying.

Guttation is another force that removes water and ions from the plant. When soil is very wet, the excess water entering the roots can act like a pump by forcing extra water up through the xylem. The plant forces this excess water out through special openings in the leaves called hydathodes, causing droplets of water to form on the tips of leaves, and is not to be confused with dew. This condition of guttation occurs during humid weather where transpiration is low and the soil moisture is high.

Although most of the mineral nutrients that arrive in the leaves come from the soil, some growers will use fertilizer applications to spray the plants directly, a practice known of foliar application. This application provides the plant leaves with a quick supply of minerals faster than soil applications. However, several problems with foliar applications can result. Some plants have thick cuticles that cause low penetration rates of ions from the outside, and there is a high chance that run-off will occur before they can be absorbed. Rain and rapid drying of water can also cause low penetration rates. However, foliar applications can be a great alternative when the nutrient availability in the soil is low.

The ions that are not leached will continue their remarkable journey through the plant. At the conclusion of photosynthesis, the ions and the organic substances created in this process are transported from the leaves so they can benefit the rest of the plant. Once again, the method of transport is the vascular system. However, since the xylem is already filled with substances flowing upward, another vessel will be used to transport these materials in a downward direction. This vessel, known as the phloem, runs alongside the xylem; the two vessels are separated by only a few cells. However, the phloem is not hollow like the xylem. Rather, it is comprised of hundreds of small, individual tubes that carry the materials. The phloem carries the ions and the organic products that were assimilated during photosynthesis, such as sucrose, carbohydrates, and amino acids, away from the leaves and in a downward direction to various organs where they are consumed, stored, or utilized.

Phloem loading closely resembles xylem loading. The distance that these photoassimilates need to travel from the site of photosynthesis to the port of entry into the phloem is very short. In fact, most mesophyll cells are no further than a few tenths of a millimeter, or three or four cells distance, from a small vein ending where they will be loaded. Although there is still some disagreement among researchers as to what path is followed, most researchers believe that photoassimilates move by diffusion through the symplastic pathway from cell to cell. However, organic substances are also thought to be carried through the mesophyll cell membranes and deposited in the apoplastic pathway.

One of the most important photoassimilates that needs to be transported are the carbohydrates that are created from photosynthesis. Carbohydrates can be found in the form of sucrose and serve as a source of carbon that helps synthesize all other organic substances. About one half of the carbohydrates that are manufactured are immediately available to exit the leaf and enter the phloem, because some plants may store a portion along the translocation path.

Carbohydrates are also used as energy when they are converted to Adenosine triphosphate (ATP), which is the metabolic energy used during cellular processes. Carbohydrates are sometimes stored as starch in the chloroplasts and later exported out of the leaf as common sugar—sucrose. Generally, these sugars make up about 80-90% of the total volume of phloem sap exported from the leaves.

■ ■ ■

Once everything is loaded into the phloem, the ions' long-distance journey continues once again. Most of the substances that enter the phloem consist of the ions and products manufactured during photosynthesis. However, during phloem loading, foreign particles along the way can inadvertently be swept up by the flow of photoassimilates that are entering the phloem. These other products may include nitrogen compounds, viruses, and synthetic compounds such as herbicides.

Phloem loading occurs through a process introduced earlier as the pressure-flow hypothesis. As stated before, when substances are loaded and water is sucked into the phloem, an internal pressure is created. Since sugars and carbohydrates are the majority of substances that are loaded, the phloem's flow rate equals the rate at which these substances are loaded.

Research shows that phloem loading is influenced by the amount of potassium that is present. Potassium is frequently the most concentrated ion in the phloem sap. Plants with high potassium concentrations experience higher osmotic potential and rate of volume flow, which does not adversely affect the concentration of sugars or carbohydrates. What has not been confirmed is whether it directly affects the loading process or indirectly increases the osmotic potential of the phloem sap that will increase the volume flow. In fact, high potassium concentrations can almost double the rate of volume flow.

Some experiments have measured the phloem's rate of flow to be anywhere between 10-100 centimeters per hour, which is much slower than xylem flow, likely due to less water content. According to Marschner, not only does potassium help regulate the phloem loading process, but it also helps regulate the flow of the sap as it travels through the phloem. Some researchers have tried to explain this phenomenon by reasoning that higher potassium concentrations result in either faster rates of phloem loading, sucrose synthesis, or controlled rates of osmosis in the phloem tubes.

The concentration of ions in the phloem that are "beneficial" but not necessarily "essential" to the plant's survival is usually low. It is possible that the plant used its supply of beneficial minerals elsewhere since they are not usually found into the phloem. However, one exception is boron since it has been found in broccoli stems.

Phloem normally have a high pH range of 7-8.0 and is comprised of water and photoassimilated products. Around 90% of the solid material found in phloem consists of carbohydrates and amino acids such as glutamine and asparagines. Other organic products such as vitamins, proteins, ATP, and hormones have also been found in various samples of phloem sap. Although water makes up the largest percentage, all of these organic products make up as high as 15-25% of its dry matter.

The walls of the phloem contain small, hollow tubes that can actually flow upward in their own in a bi-directional pattern. Depending on the nutritional needs of the plant, a small percentage of the phloem sap can actually be transported through these small tubes in an upward direction. And in some cases, some nutrients flowing in phloem sap can pass through the walls of the phloem and traverse across the membranes, and again enter into other tissues.

However, most substances inside the phloem travel downward. During transport, the concentration of organic substances found inside the phloem can change for various reasons. Some of the photoassimilates that leak out of the phloem will either be put into storage cells or they will benefit the plant by providing nutrients to various tissues. Transporting photoassimilates through the phloem helps to recycle mineral nutrients and provides the plant with a chance to use the ions once again.

The total rate of flow tends to slow down during winter and increase during spring. Common examples of phloem sap include maple syrup and sugarcane. The leaves are considered the main factories of photosynthesis, but the plant organs that will consume and store the sap, such as roots, fruits, flowers, and seeds, are known as "sinks."

The nutrients in the phloem sap are traveling away from the sites of photosynthesis and toward important plant organs that need to consume them. Flowing in a downward direction, the ions will eventually reach the sinks where they will be deposited, a process known as "phloem unloading." Phloem unloading involves releasing the nutrients into the tissues of sinks. Some sinks may be young, developing sinks, such as fruits, flowers, or buds, while others may be long-term storage sinks, such as seeds. The storage sinks all have their own nutritional requirements, and different metabolic activities.

The regulation of organic substances in the phloem is still being researched. Experiments have not been able to definitely explain how the plant determines how material in the phloem sap will be distributed throughout the plant. How does a plant determine which areas will receive the most nutrients? Most researchers suggest that the needs of the plant, such as genetically controlled programs, growth, and development, are ranked. Young and growing leaves tend to import a high percentage of the phloem nutrients, but as they mature and become more self-sufficient they will be able to import less and export more and more, allowing the plant to redirect its nutrients towards younger sinks.

The unloading process is very similar to the loading process, only now the organic photoassimilates exit the phloem and enter sites of consumption. Here, they will follow symplastic or apoplastic pathways once again as they enter various sites of consumption. Some nutrients that follow the symplastic pathway will end up in the younger, developing leaves, while those that travel through the apoplastic pathway will be distributed into flowers and fruits. For example, the sugar known as sucrose traverses through the symplastic pathway and into sinks where it will be utilized.

■ ■ ■

An interesting characteristic about minerals is that some have shown to be more mobile than others, whether they are in the soil, water, or being transported through a plant. Researchers Mason and Maskell found in their investigations that some elements could be transported easier and farther than others. By studying plants, phosphorus and potassium, for example, were found in high concentrations and evenly distributed throughout plants, proving it was transported very easily, while minerals such as manganese and calcium were not. In fact, the amount of calcium found in phloem sap is very low when compared to more mobile minerals.

Many researchers have used radioisotopes to determine which minerals are mobile and which are less mobile in plants. The radioisotopes allow the researchers to trace the elements as they move through the plant to reveal circulation patterns. They can follow the minerals as they are absorbed through the roots, transferred into the xylem, traverse upward toward leaves, deposit in the leaves, and are loaded into the phloem.

However, observations also show that not all minerals get loaded into the phloem equally. Although loaded elements will be redistributed through the phloem, the low mobility of some elements makes them less able to get loaded into the sieve tubes of phloem. Researchers reason that minerals that are usually missing in high concentrations from phloem sap struggle to enter the small sieve tubes during phloem loading.

Observations by researchers Bukovac and Wittwer (1957) used radioisotopes to trace the path of mineral elements through the leaves using bean plants. They classified the mobility of some major elements:

Mobile	Intermediate	Immobile
Potassium	Iron	Lithium
Rubidium	Boron	Calcium
Sodium	Zinc	Strontium
Magnesium	Copper	Barium
Phosphorus	Molybdenum	Manganese
Sulfur		
Chlorine		

Note that lithium and boron are two of the elements considered "immobile." However, the chemical resemblance of lithium is strikingly similar to calcium, which might help to explain its low mobility. Also note that the Intermediate mobility group tends to contain the heavy metal elements. These elements are more mobile and are more likely to get transported through phloem than the immobile elements, but not as likely as the Mobile group. Although some mineral elements are considered immobile, that doesn't necessarily mean they are never found in sap. In fact, all mineral elements have been found, except molybdenum and nickel, which are still being investigated.

There is a close correlation between the low mobility of calcium and the transpiration rate of plant organs such as flowers, fruit, etc. When comparing the amount of calcium concentrated in fleshy fruits with leaves that experience high transpiration, the leaves can have as much as 10-20 times the amount of calcium ions present in their tissues. Thus, plant organs that experience low transpiration rates, such as fruits, will tend to have a low concentration of minerals with low mobility, such as calcium. However, minerals such as potassium and magnesium have high mobility; their concentration in fruits and throughout the plant is usually consistent.

Studies determining the mobility of elements have found a correlation between the mobility of elements and deficiency symptoms in plants. Peanuts, for example, grow underground, and are therefore not likely to be subject to the transpiration flow or the phloem transport of elements. Harris (1949) observed that when calcium was provided to the roots only, most of the peanuts failed to grow, but when calcium was sprayed directly onto their flowers above the ground, they were able to resume development. This example shows how calcium mobility in phloem sap is low, which illustrates that some flowers and fruits require fertilization.

By tracing its route through the phloem and into developing fruits using boron isotopes, boron is recognized as having intermediate mobility. It is unmistakable that boron has intermediate mobility, with only a moderate amount of boron eventually reaching the sinks. All nutrients that are considered absolutely essential to the growth and development of plants, except calcium, are mobile, while nutrients considered beneficial to plant development are intermediate, manganese being the only exception.

Not all minerals that are transported up through the xylem have the same mobility in the phloem. Observations have shown some mobility of manganese and calcium; however this mobility is very low. In fact, some observations have found unusually high amounts of these elements in some sap samples. However, most growing sinks that require calcium and manganese are only receiving 10-20% of their requirements. Therefore, these two nutrients remain on the list of immobile elements, even though some of the sinks' demand for calcium and manganese can be met when these elements are transported through xylem. Potassium, however, sees more than one half of its transport occurring in the phloem, while magnesium, another mobile element, experiences 25-40% of its transport in the phloem.

Fruits require a high amount of calcium for their growth, development, and even flavor. Because calcium's mobility in the phloem is so low, fruits usually have to rely on the calcium that is present in phloem. Since fruits tend to have low transpiration rates when compared to the leaves, they can still experience low calcium flow, even from the xylem. Ultimately, most growers realize that adding calcium through foliar sprays is usually the best way to add calcium to the crop.

■ ■ ■

Photosynthesis produces nutrients and carbohydrates that provide necessary ingredients for the plant's growth and development, such as the growth of leaves, expansion of the roots and trunk, development of fruits, and formation of flowers. However, the plant must determine areas of priority for which developing area is experiencing the highest demand for nutrients. Therefore, a balancing act is in place that regulates the flow of nutrients during certain seasons that influence the plant's various metabolic activities

The nutrient demand of a fruit tree, for example, closely resembles its growth pattern. During the spring, much of the nutrient supply comes from the storage cells in the roots and other storage tissues from nutrients that were assimilated during the previous year. However, various plant organs will also be demanding these nutrients, and competition will ensue. These organs compete to different degrees and at different times of the year.

Dr. Curt Rom of the University of Arkansas has explained that when growth patterns of the various organs of fruit trees, for example, are evaluated together, a harmonic pattern is observed in their seasonal growth rate. For instance, roots begin to grow early in the spring. As they provide the water that is necessary for cell expansion, and absorb the soluble nutrients that produce its metabolic activities, leaves emerge producing new carbohydrates. Soon the external organs such as the flowers and fruit begin to form during the spring and summer. These newly developing organs experience high demand for the plant's nutrients, which in turn causes root growth to slow down. Eventually, during the summer months, their growth will also begin to slow down, causing the second cycle of root growth to occur. Managing trees to cause vigorous or stunted growth of the organs and/or roots will negatively affect fruit development because of this harmonic timing of competition.

During autumn leaves will change color from green to different shades of red, brown, and yellow. Leaves and fruits drop to the ground and flower petals wither away. This occurs when the highly mobile elements are retranslocated from these older leaves back inside the plant and into other organs and younger leaves, causing the discoloration of the autumn leaves.

Dr. Rom explains that some nutrients are being remobilized back into the mother tree before they separate; they don't all become part of decaying material for future use. Nitrogen, potassium, phosphorus, and zinc are examples of highly mobile minerals that will be remobilized and loaded back into the phloem, while less mobile nutrients such as calcium, iron, boron, and manganese continue to accumulate in the leaves until the leaf drops.

When the leaves begin to turn from green into rustic colors, they are being separated from the tree through a process known as abscission, or separation. The abscission zone of the tree senses a drop in temperature and shorter days, signaling the end of summer and the start of autumn. The abscission zone will weaken and the area will be plugged up to keep out infections, until the leaf eventually falls to the ground. After the leaves and fruits fall to the ground, decompose, and return their minerals back to the soil, they will be taken up again by the plant. Some of the discoloration of leaves during autumn can be either the result of mineral deficiencies that result when highly mobile nutrients exit the leaves, or excess mineral toxicity that results when less mobile nutrients accumulate until the leaf finally falls to the ground.

Nutrients are also lost when fruit is harvested. Ripe apples have high concentrations of potassium, and when they are harvested, these and other nutrients are removed from the orchard. As a consequence, it is common for soils to experience a gradual decline in potassium content and other nutrients if fertilizers are not applied.

Common yard waste such as freshly cut grass, weeds, flowers, pruned branches, and other organic waste can be mulched and recycled into the soil, which allows the minerals it contains to return and benefit the soil. These items could also be mixed into vegetable gardens or used as compost to provide organic fertilizer. Too much inorganic fertilizer can burn plants, but organic waste cannot. You could even use organic compost as the sole potting soil for vegetables and other garden plants.

Gardeners cannot produce more compost than what they can use as a fertilizer. The natural cycle involves fallen leaves, branches, fruits, and other organic material to sit under a blanket of snow during the winter months, decomposing and returning their mineral ions back into the soil. This provides a fresh, green, fertilized lawn for the spring. Rather, people seem more willing to discard these rich mineral sources during autumn as they rake up their leaves, only to hire a professional lawn care service during the spring to bring their dying lawn back to life.

Chapter 5

The Macrominerals in Plants

All plant cells needs minerals in order to carry out their functions. Mineral ions are assimilated into the cell—not just absorbed—and participate in each of the cell's processes. A lack of essential minerals will stunt a plant's growth, weaken its immune system, cause a breakdown in cellular structures and weaken it, and even prevent metabolic and biochemical reactions from taking place.

Mineral nutrition is a very important subject in plant physiology. There can be as many as one hundred different elements available in the soil at any given time, and concentrations are generally considered to be either deficient, sufficient, or toxic.

Each mineral has its own unique responsibilities and distinct role in plant metabolism. Some minerals are more essential than others and needed in larger amounts. However, current research is still trying to evaluate the contribution of each mineral to determine which are absolutely essential to the health of a plant, and which play a more supplementary role. It is generally accepted among plant physiologists that three criteria must be met in order for a mineral to be considered "essential." They are:

1. The plant must be unable to complete its life cycle in the absence of the mineral.
2. The function of the mineral cannot be substituted by another mineral.
3. The mineral must be directly involved in plant metabolism.

Minerals that do not fit these strict criteria but still provide some unique and helpful benefit to a plant are placed in a separate category called "beneficial." Beneficial minerals may not necessarily be critical to the life of the plant, but they do provide many less specific functions. If they are left out of agricultural fertilizers or are not naturally found in the soil, the optimal growth potential of the crop is compromised.

There are a total of 17 essential elements that are absolutely essential to the health of a plant. Three of these—hydrogen, carbon, and oxygen—are obtained through air and water. The dry tissue of most plants is comprised of 94% or more of these three elements. The remaining 6% consists of the 14 remaining elements.

The most up to date research available on plant nutrition now lists 14 elements derived from the soil that are essential to most plants. Within this group of 14 essential elements, some are needed in much larger quantities than others. Therefore, two categories were developed: macronutrients and micronutrients. Macronutrients are essential minerals that are needed in larger amounts, usually anywhere from .5-3.0% of the dry weight of a plant. Micronutrients are minerals that are still considered essential, but needed in lesser amounts, comprising between 1-1,000 parts per million (ppm) of the plant's dry weight. This chapter will discuss the different roles and responsibilities of these elements and their individual impact on the growth and development of the plant.

This table lists the essential elements, their atomic symbol, and their average concentration in dry matter:

Element	Symbol	Concentration (mg/kg)
NUTRIENTS FROM AIR AND WATER		
Macronutrients:		
Oxygen	O	450,000
Carbon	C	450,000
Hydrogen	H	60,000
NUTRIENTS FROM SOIL AND WATER		
1. Nitrogen	N	15,000
2. Potassium	K	10,000
3. Calcium	Ca	5,000
4. Magnesium	Mg	2,000

5. Phosphorus	P	2,000
6. Sulfur	S	1,000

Micronutrients:

7. Chlorine	Cl	100
8. Iron	Fe	100
9. Manganese	Mn	50
10. Boron	B	20
11. Zinc	Zn	20
12. Copper	Cu	6
13. Nickel	Ni	?
14. Molybdenum	Mo	0.00001

These 14 elements derived from the soil may be found in varying concentrations in plant tissues, but that does not imply that they are of ranking importance over one another. Rather, they are of equal importance and all fit into the category of "essential." These elements are so critical to the survival of the plant that research has established minimum amounts for each of them that will still provide the necessary benefits. Studies have shown that gradual increases in these amounts results in a proportional increase in growth and development. If any of the essential elements were to drop below that minimum threshold, the plant's overall development and metabolic processes would noticeably decline, even if the remaining elements were maintained at healthy levels. Likewise, research has also dictated maximum levels of these elements. If plant uptake goes beyond this maximum threshold, toxicity can result, resulting in impaired development of the plant.

■ ■ ■

One of the most exciting things about studying plants and minerals is determining which minerals are present in the tissues and understanding what benefits the plant receives from each mineral. In addition to this list of essential minerals, there are still other minerals that are not considered essential, but still provide many exciting benefits. This category of minerals is known as "beneficial", which usually includes such minerals as sodium, silicon, selenium, vanadium, arsenic, mercury, aluminum, and cobalt. It has always been an industry understanding that if any of the beneficial elements are ever discovered to provide essentiality to the health and vigor of higher plants, they may be moved up to the list of essential.

In 1860, two German researchers, Julius Sachs and W. Knop, proved that plants do not necessarily need soil to grow. They dissolved mineral ions in distilled water in order to discover which minerals were needed by plants and to uncover the required amounts. This type of experimentation is known as "hydroponics," and vegetables such as tomatoes, spinach and others are grown in hydroponic greenhouses every year.

In 1905, Gabriel Bertrand, a French researcher, discovered that manganese was required for plant nutrition. Subsequent research studies have validated this finding and show that the amount of manganese required is much lower than most other micronutrients. Epstein explains that in the 1920's, Katherine Warington of Oxford, England first examined the role of boron and realized its essential need in legumes. Researchers A. L. Sommer and C. B. Lipman of the University of California have shown plants' requirement for boron to be essential in nonlegumes also. In Kentucky, J.S. McHargue gave us our first experimental glimpse at manganese, and Lipman and his associates then added zinc and copper to the list of essential micronutrients in 1931. A few years later, P. R. Stout and D. I. Arnon performed experiments removing certain elements from solutions and documented conclusively that molybdenum was essential to the tomato plant, which added this element to the list as well. It wasn't until 1954 that T. C. Broyer discovered chlorine as an essential mineral by experimenting with tomatoes and other plants at the University of California. And in 1988, nickel was moved from the beneficial category to the essential category, due to consistent research showing how essential it is.

Some plants, grasses, and trees still require other mineral elements besides those listed so far, while other plants may not necessarily require all of these, or even in such great amounts. But for the most part, all species of plants will require the "essential" minerals, while the "beneficial" minerals will sometimes vary. For example, certain grasses need ample amounts of sodium, but most plants and trees do not need as much. Some plants have shown a need for selenium, while the friendly bacteria that provide nitrogen for legumes require cobalt. Even though silicon is found in many soils, it has not yet been found essential for the growth and development of plants, except in certain cases, so it remains listed as a beneficial element.

■ ■ ■

The mineral content of soils varies dramatically, making any tissue sample of a plant yield quite an unexpected list of elements. But that does not necessarily mean that every element is absolutely essential to its nutritional health. A plant growing in soil could easily contain traces of 40-90 different elements. However, not all plants absorb everything in the soil. There are many plants that have evolved unique methods of mineral absorption. It is widely known that some plants are unable to differentiate and will absorb any and all minerals that are found in the soil, whether they are useful to them or not, while other plants are selective in which minerals they will absorb. According to Marschner, certain mineral elements are taken up preferentially, while others are discriminated against or are almost completely excluded.

The minerals that are found in soil are managed by different forms of farming activities. Farm managers will determine not only what crops will be grown, but also what type of soil, fertilizer, and pest management policies will be used. There is a difference in soil activity between conventional farming methods and organic farming methods. Organic farming, as defined by the US Department of Agriculture (USDA), involves stringent farming methods. "Feed the soil, not the plant" is one of the mottos of organic farming.

Instead of relying on chemicals and synthetic pesticides for the growth and development of the crop, organic farmers focus on building healthy soil that is rich in minerals and becomes pest and disease resistant. Organic farmers rotate crops instead of repeated plantings of the same crop year after year, which leaves soil unbalanced and depleted of those minerals. They also cover crops to protect soil from erosion and use beneficial insects and companion planting to utilize the plant's own defenses against pests. Organic farmers also carefully choose a variety of plant selection for hardiness and suitability to the site.

Organic farming also recognizes soil as a biological system and uses traditional techniques that prolong the soil's fertility for long-term production. In 1980 the USDA compiled a report on organic farming that found little evidence of soil erosion and documented that most of the soil practices were highly recommended by the USDA. The Swiss Research Institute of Organic Agriculture conducted a 21-year study that observed organic farming and discovered that the population of soil organisms was twice that of conventional farm production.

A study found that organically-grown wheat contained about three times as much potassium and calcium and twice as much iron and manganese. Although conventional farming practices have produced higher crop yields than organic farming practices, clearly the suppression of biological activity in the soil has resulted in mineral deficiencies in the harvested crops, for both macronutrients and micronutrients. Observations show a documented reduction in the amount of minerals in both fruits and vegetables since conventional farming practices became standard procedure. A study in the United Kingdom discovered that levels of potassium have declined 16%, magnesium 24%, iron 27%, calcium 46%, and copper has declined 76%, between 1940 and 1991.

A reduction in soil mineral content will result in a loss of plant health, including its growth, development, vigor, and ability to resist infections and diseases. The Consultation on Draft Soil Study for England, 2001, determined that a high use of pesticides may be partially a function of this loss in plant vigor and health already. It is a concern for the longer term if nutrient levels continue to fall. Even if these trends are not yet affecting plant health or this can be addressed in other ways, this definitely carries major implications for human health because of our reliance on crops for our own nutrition.

It is important that fertilizers contain as many of the macrominerals and microminerals as possible. However, the most common fertilizer that is used, known as "NPK," contains only nitrate, phosphorus, and potassium. According to Dr. William A. Albrecht, Chairman of the Department of Soils at the University of Missouri, "NPK formulas, as legislated and enforced by State Departments of Agriculture, mean malnutrition, attack by insects, bacteria and fungi, weed takeover, crop loss in dry weather, and general loss of mental acuity in the population, leading to degenerative metabolic disease and early death." Without a wide range of essential and beneficial minerals, plant growth and development is impaired.

The rest of this chapter will discuss the role of the macronutrients, and the next chapter will discuss the micronutrients.

The Macronutrients

Nitrogen

Nitrogen is one of the most common elements found in plants. On average, it is the fourth most abundant element behind oxygen, carbon, and hydrogen. Nitrogen comprises about 1% of the total mineral content found in soil, although it is usually tied up in organic matter. Through decay, nitrogen ions are slowly released into the soil where they are either taken up by the roots or easily washed out of the soil. When nitrogen is found as an ion in the soil, it will either be in the form of "nitrate" (NO_3) or "ammonium" (NH_4). Estimates of agricultural crops have found that as much as 100 pounds of nitrogen can be absorbed per acre every year.

Nitrogen in the soil (nitrate) is readily available and provides a plant with plenty of benefits. According to Dr. Warren Stiles, fruit trees are impacted heavily by nitrogen. The presence of nitrogen influences the tree's growth, flowering, fruit set, fruit growth and development, and fruit quality. Homeowners and gardeners who fertilize their gardens and lawns will realize the quick effect nitrogen provides plants by giving them a deep green color and stimulating vigorous growth.

Nitrogen's high mobility allows it to be distributed throughout the plant where some areas may demand it more than others. One of nitrogen's roles is to provide balance so that plant organs can receive an efflux of nutrients. As new leaves develop, their demand for nutrients such as nitrogen exceeds the need to keep these nutrients in the older leaves. Plants transport these nutrients to the younger generation of developing leaves, where need is much higher. This is one way plants manage the available content of nutrients by prioritizing the needs of its growth and development stages and transferring nutrients to sites of critical demand, leaving the older leaves yellow and falling off. Thus, some nitrogen deficiency symptoms will appear in the older, lower level leaves first, and symptoms will not appear in younger, developing leaves unless deficiency is extreme.

The role of nitrogen is profound. In fact, it is found in almost every cell and participates in almost every cellular activity. All proteins, enzymes and metabolic processes in plants require the presence of nitrogen in order to carry out their functions, and it is essential for the plant's ability to synthesize and transfer energy. In the absence of nitrogen, certain enzymatic processes fail to activate. One enzyme, nitrate reductase, is initiated by both nitrogen ions and molybdenum. When either nitrogen or molybdenum are absent, this enzyme fails to perform its critical functions. Vitamins, enzymes, hormones, and proteins that plants manufacture all contain a lot of nitrogen. In fact, nitrogen makes up about 18% of the proteins found in plants and is a building block of amino acids and most enzymes.

Dr. Stiles explains that fruit development is one area of concern with regard to nitrogen deficiency. Nitrogen stimulates the growth of growing sinks, such as fruits, since their demand for nutrients is very high during this stage of development. A deficiency of nitrogen can throw off the plant's timing leading to premature flowering or insufficient fruit firmness. Oversupply or late supply of nitrogen can lead to reduced fruit color or even delayed development. Nitrogen also provides other functions for the plant, such as increasing the seed and fruit yield, determining the size of fruit, and stimulating other vegetative development.

Nitrogen is contained in some of the most important areas of plants. Chlorophyll, the green substance that activates photosynthesis, relies heavily on nitrogen. A healthy plant will contain around 70% of its total amount of nitrogen in the chloroplasts. Four nitrogen atoms are required to produce each chlorophyll molecule, which is eventually used to absorb light and produce energy during photosynthesis. Also, the leaves of plants where photosynthesis occurs grow and expand rapidly when nitrogen is plentiful.

Pale green or yellow discoloration in leaves is called "chlorosis" and is one of the most common visual signs of nitrogen deficiency, especially in older leaves. Leaves can become discolored when nitrogen is lacking, which causes chlorophyll synthesis to decline. Like a chain reaction, photosynthesis eventually slows down, resulting in a lack of amino acids and loss of the products that synthesize carbohydrates and other organic substances.

Research shows that a low concentration of nitrogen results in plants that are stunted, grow poorly, are discolored in the leaves, and experience premature defoliation in the fall. Low nitrogen status also jeopardizes the plant's tolerance to low temperature stress. Research suggests that these conditions are a result of a lack of carbohydrates, which results from a low nitrogen status. A lack of carbohydrates can be characterized by a decline in surface area of leaves or premature loss of leaves, either of which eventually results in depressed rates of photosynthesis. With all of these important metabolic and biochemical processes relying on nitrogen, it should be easy to understand why there are so many symptoms when nitrogen is deficient.

Sometimes too much nitrogen can result in just as many problems as not enough. In some plants, excess nitrogen can cause too much leafy growth in flowers or fruits, although this may not always be a problem with crops such as spinach. High nitrogen content can also delay flowering or fruit development. Taller plants with excess nitrogen usually form fragile stems, making them more likely to host infections.

Potassium

Potassium is highly mobile and is found all over the plant. It is used in very large quantities and plays such an important role that only nitrogen is used more than potassium. Although it may not get as much attention as the other nutrients, plants actually use potassium almost four times as much as phosphorus. Potassium is the only monovalent cation ($K+$) that plants will absorb; its positive charge is attracted to the negatively charged surfaces of clay particles. According to Dr. A.E. Ludwick, this bond is strong enough to prevent leaching from excess irrigation, flooding, or rainwater, but still weak enough to exchange with other cations in the soil. The potassium that is found bound to the negatively charged clay particles represents the largest reservoir of available potassium in the soil.

The high mobility of potassium ions allows it to be easily distributed through the phloem and other transport vessels. It is found in almost all cells and tissues, and it is easily transported from older leaves to younger, growing leaves and organs. Overall, fruit crops tend to use a lot of potassium for development and growth.

One of the chief responsibilities of potassium is to activate a large number of enzymes by helping to stabilize pH levels between 7 and 8, the ideal range for most enzymes. Researchers Evans and Sorger documented 46 enzymes in plants, animals, and even microorganisms that rely on potassium to be activated because it brings about changes in the enzyme protein that activates them. Some of the enzymes regulated by potassium include those involved in photosynthesis and respiration, as well as processes involving proteins and carbohydrates. However, some researchers suggest that potassium is needed more for protein synthesis than enzyme activation. Although there may be other minerals that can be substituted in enzyme activation, such as rubidium and ammonium, they are not as effective as potassium. Observations have concluded that potassium is undoubtedly one of the most functioning elements in most enzymatic reactions in plants.

Potassium is used during various stages of photosynthesis, including the development of photoassimilates such as sugars, amino acids, vitamins, proteins, and carbohydrates. Even the loading of these products into the phloem and their overall transport requires potassium. For example, after photosynthesis has occurred and produced carbohydrates and sugars, potassium regulates their transport from the leaves to the roots, where they will be converted into starches, benefiting vegetables that grow deep in the soil, such as potatoes and other tubers. When the plant has enough potassium, about half of the photoassimilates will travel through the phloem and will be deposited in areas where they will be consumed, including developing fruits, within 90 minutes. Therefore, potassium not only participates in photosynthesis, but is also critical for the quick export of photoassimilated products out of the leaves and into the phloem to maintain high rates of photosynthesis. These photosynthetic responsibilities of potassium occur due to its high mobility and its ability to maintain a high pH level inside the plant.

Another responsibility of potassium is to help magnesium enter the cells. Potassium helps transport magnesium ions across the plasma membrane by activating the magnesium ion pumps that bring these ions from the soil into the roots, where together they will help sucrose travel quickly through the cell and deposit in storage vacuoles. If potassium is deficient, this transport time slows down and can increase to well over four hours, resulting in an accumulation of substances in the leaves that can cause photosynthesis to slow down.

Potassium plays a key role in cellular integrity and stability by promoting thicker cell walls, which in turn strengthens tissues that increase the plant's structural firmness and helps protect against infections. Other physiological benefits of potassium include strengthening stems and branches, promoting sturdy root formation, preventing wilting, and protecting against water loss by thickening the waxy cuticle layer found in leaves. During periods of cell expansion and growth, potassium is the main element found in the cell's storage vacuoles, indicating heavy responsibility during this process.

Fruits require large amounts of potassium for their growth and development, including the fruit's size, color, firmness, and quality, as well as overall fruit production. Observations show that fruits, vegetative parts, and other organs contain potassium ranging from 2-5% of their dry weight. It enhances the flavor and color of vegetative crops, increases the amount of oil found in fruits, and is important for the development of leafy vegetables. When fruits are lacking potassium, they tend to be smaller, irregularly shaped, have a dull color, and poor flavor, all of which are a result of excess acidity. Potassium also helps prevent nitrogen from causing too much leafy growth or phosphorus' tendency to overripen fruits. Although potassium is not used in any organic compound in fruits, it does help to regulate the fruit's water balance and helps to activate various fruit enzymes that are involved in photosynthesis and respiration.

Potassium is responsible for movement, balance and timing, which are three critical features. It plays a role in plant movements, such as the opening and closing of the stomatal guard cells, which open and close during the day to release gases into the atmosphere. Leaves also need potassium to help orient them towards sunlight to maximize the rate of photosynthesis. The plant's proper sleep movements during the night also require sufficient potassium levels. It can even determine how nitrogen, calcium, and sodium are absorbed and utilized.

The movement and balance of water in plants are both influenced by potassium levels. Potassium helps to adjust water balance during times of drought or heavy rains, and helps to improve the salt balance in the cells. Osmosis occurs when water evaporates from the plant or diffuses through cellular membranes, leaving behind an accumulation of salts inside the cells, which, if left uncontrolled, can reach toxic levels and damage enzymes. However, an accumulation of amino acids and sugars can help relieve some of this water stress, otherwise known as osmotic potential. Potassium's influence in helping balance the water-to-salt levels is a phenomenon known as osmoregulation.

When potassium is deficient, the symptoms a plant experiences tend to coincide with potassium's benefits. Enzymatic processes begin to flounder, thus making plants susceptible to many deteriorating circumstances and exposing the plant's defenses to infections and diseases. When potassium is deficient, toxic accumulations of starches, proteins, sugars, and other photoassimilates will often appear since they will be unable to be loaded into the phloem. These accumulations slow down the rate of photosynthesis, which in many instances becomes unable to complete its biochemical processes altogether.

The growth of the plant—the leaves, roots, stems, and other organs—also show signs of deterioration or slowdown during periods of potassium deficiency. Growth of the limbs and outer extremities becomes retarded, or in severe cases become completely stunted. Leaves become chlorotic or necrotic (discolored and wilted). A study on bean plants experiencing low potassium levels resulted in loss of rigidity, cell size, and leaf surface areas when compared to leaves that had sufficient potassium. The same study also showed similar results for potassium quantities in carrot crops. Other symptoms of potassium deficiency can include irregular fruit development and reduced seed formation.

When potassium is lacking, yellow patches can appear on leaves, and in severe cases they will look dry and burned. Mature leaves will have to sacrifice their potassium ions which will be relocated to the younger, growing leaves. This sudden discharge of potassium from older leaves can result in mottled chlorosis (yellow spots) or necrotic (dead) brown spots. The leaf tips and leaves that curl downward are visual signs that this is taking place. Obviously, the exit of potassium will affect the rate of photosynthesis in these older leaves as well. Therefore, symptoms of potassium deficiency will usually be found in the older leaves first. However, visual results such as these are not always potassium deficiencies. Similar problems can also result when some parasitic organisms such as multi-cellular nematodes (worms) penetrate the tissues of a plant.

Environmental circumstances such as drought can cause the chloroplasts in leaves to break down and lose large amounts of water and potassium, which slows down the rate of photosynthesis. When water is lacking, the uptake of water soluble ions such as potassium from the soil become restricted. However, this can be reversed when potassium is resupplied to the plant in extra high quantities, alleviating some of the effects of the drought. Also, during periods of potassium deficiency, fruit trees become more susceptible to cold temperature stress.

Too much potassium can affect the plant negatively by affecting the levels of other minerals. Although some plants can substitute sodium when potassium levels are low, if there is too much potassium in the soil deficiencies in magnesium and possibly calcium can result.

Due to potassium's large role in the nutritional health of a plant and its high mobility, potassium is largely included in most fertilizers and may have to be supplied frequently. The large volume of potassium in lawn and garden waste can be recycled back into the soil with proper care, rather than sending it all to the trash bin. During decomposition, potassium ions are released into the water or soil and can easily be washed out. However, if the clippings are used as mulch, this important nutrient can eventually find its way back into new plants.

Calcium

Calcium is available for absorption from the soil into a plant only when it is found in its ionic form, a divalent cation (Ca++). It is immediately put to good use in the plant, either remaining in its ionic state to carry out various processes, or used to bind with other elements or organic products created during photosynthesis, depending on the needs of the plant. Calcium ions are not very mobile, which makes them move slowly through the plant's vessels. However, its ionic strength allows it to adhere to cell walls during transport.

There is usually plenty of calcium available in soils and is rarely deficient under natural conditions. It is well-known for its ability to strengthen the cell and cell membranes, which is where most of the calcium found in plant cells is concentrated. According to Marschner, calcium strengthens membranes by bridging carboxyl and phosphate groups of phospholipids and proteins, usually at the membrane surfaces.

Although calcium's low mobility hinders it from being transported into the storage vacuoles, it builds up within the membranes where it is absolutely critical for their physical integrity and healthy functioning. Calcium has such low mobility that once it is deposited and established in plant tissues, it tends to remain there, causing the plant to require a steady flow of calcium for other purposes.

Calcium's role in cell walls and membranes also includes regulating which molecules will be transported across the membrane. Calcium is crucial to providing the plant with highly selective ions into the cells or into the symplastic pathway. Plant tissues with an appropriate level of calcium will transport ions across the cellular membranes in only one direction—into the cell. Very rarely will high-calcium membranes leak solutes such as those found in vacuoles back across the membrane and out into the open space between cells. This protection also includes preventing leakage into the symplastic pathway. When calcium is absent, cells break down and there results almost an immediate attempt among competing ions and unwanted material to penetrate the membranes.

Since tissues that are lacking calcium tend to show signs of leakage into and out of the cells, this also affects cellular respiration by increasing the storage vacuole's membrane permeability, allowing respiratory solutes to leak out of the storage vacuole and into the respiratory enzymes in the center of the cell. This causes an unusual amount of high and unnecessary respiration to occur. When calcium is added to the plant, these respiratory rates begin to slow down and adjust back to healthy rates.

Calcium is a major ingredient in a substance known as pectate, which is a material that protects the cell walls from fungi and bacteria that try to attack and dissolve the cells, such as the fungus Rhizoctonia solani. Cells with a good supply of pectate around the cell walls provide rigidity, which fortifies the entire plant, since calcium cross-links the pectic chain that gives the cell its shape and structure.

Some calcium deficiencies have shown a deterioration and collapse of the plant tissues. Calcium's role in cellular membranes provides a defense against bacterial and fungal infections, provides assistance in developing fruits, and minimizes damage to the cell during periods of freezing and thawing pressure. Therefore, the role of calcium in cellular membranes is clear—it prevents diffusion of solutes across the cell membranes by strengthening and protecting the cell walls, and it assists the cells in their selection of ions that will transport across the membranes.

Calcium is a very important, but stubborn, mineral. It is not easily absorbed by the roots of fruit trees, especially if there is competition with other minerals. Inside the plant, there is strong competition between the plant's organs for calcium. Vegetative parts are constantly stealing what little calcium is available that would otherwise be deposited into the developing fruit. Also, the small amount of calcium that does get absorbed moves very slowly through the plant. Some studies indicate that it can take 2-4 years for calcium ions to travel from the root tips and eventually be deposited in fruits, justifying the need to supplement calcium by using foliar applications. Some growers will even supplement additional calcium to fruit even after it is harvested, with great results. Overall, calcium aids the development and appearance of fruit.

In fruits, calcium concentration is generally low in the flesh, but it can be found in the core, outer skin, and seeds. In fact, an interesting characteristic of calcium involves seeds. Research shows that the higher the number of seeds in fruits, the higher the amount of calcium that will be found. Research suggests that seeds may help to direct the flow of calcium into the fruit. However, when calcium is deficient, fruit tends to ripen prematurely, be low in quality and stores poorly. Low calcium fruit softens faster and tends to develop various forms of rotting disorders. If the outer skin of fruits are firm, this is a good indicator that its cellular membranes have been strengthened by calcium.

Calcium also plays a critical role in the growth and development of roots. According to Emanuel Epstein, roots of germinating seeds grow well for a few days, even though calcium's presence is low due to its low mobility through the phloem. However, when roots of germinating seeds are exposed to a solution that lacks calcium, they stop growing immediately. If soils are lacking calcium for a short period of time, roots become discolored and can have a slippery feel if the middle lamella, a thin layer comprised largely of pectin that cements the walls of two adjacent cells together, has broken down. After a prolonged period of deficiency, roots become stunted and appear deformed. When soils are severely lacking calcium, root expansion stops within just a few hours and completely fails to grow.

Some researchers conclude that minerals become toxic or unavailable when calcium is lacking. Many plants require calcium to be present in order to absorb nitrogen, while the absorption of most other minerals will decline if calcium is lacking in the roots. These examples illustrate how calcium helps the plant to absorb other minerals.

A study conducted by J.B. Hanson at the University of Illinois in 1960 investigated the root growth of maize and soybean plants when they were treated with ethylenediamine tetraacetic acid. His observations showed that these plants were thereafter unable to absorb the surrounding elements in the soil because this acid removed calcium from the roots. He concluded that the permeability of the root tissues was increased when calcium was lacking, causing the cells to leak, making the ions being absorbed follow their own path, rather than being able to enter the cells.

Some enzymes are only activated when calcium is present, including amylase, an enzyme that has a metal component, otherwise known as a metalloenzyme. Calcium can also increase pH levels in the soil, which helps prevent disease by furthering cell growth.

A calcium deficient plant will exhibit many different signs of deterioration. Low calcium in apples oftentimes results in diseases such as bitter pit or cork spot, which are characterized by soft dimples or dried pits of collapsed tissue in the fruit, both of which are worldwide concerns due to the commercial losses. Since calcium is required for cell expansions during periods of growth, deficiency symptoms usually appear in areas where new cells are trying to develop. Due to calcium's low mobility through the phloem, younger leaves are usually the first sites of deficiency, making them deformed and discolored. The tips of leaves hook back, yellow spots form along the edges, become dry, and finally fall to the ground. Some leaf margins will display brown scorching and in extreme cases the mesophyll tissues will disintegrate. Leaves such as these lack the physical integrity and cellular strength that calcium provides.

Other parts of a plant are also affected if calcium is deficient. Some stems can become hard while the roots become stubby and dark brown in color. A common symptom of calcium deficiency in tomatoes and peppers is called "blossom end rot," which occurs when the bottom of a fruit becomes discolored, usually brown or black.

Some general problems with uptake of calcium can result because it is easily leached from the soil. It is an absolutely critical mineral for healthy growth and development, so there should be a constant supply of calcium from either the soil, fertilizers, or from foliar sprays. Since adding calcium to the soils is probably the least effective way to increase the calcium concentration in developing fruits, it should be applied directly to the fruit so it can be quickly absorbed through the skin. Foliar application is a common practice. Although this method is susceptible to leaching from wind and rain, it does provide the quickest and surest application. Calcium can even be applied to fruits after they are harvested and sitting in storage. The calcium will migrate around in the fruit where it will increase the fruit's firmness and protect it from invasive attack and rotting diseases.

Magnesium

Magnesium is absorbed as a divalent cation (Mg^{++}), and can be found either tightly bound to clay particles in the soil, being exchanged with other mineral ions, or loosely held in the soil moisture. Magnesium's rate of uptake is largely determined by the concentration of calcium, potassium, and nitrogen already present in the soils. It is a highly mobile element that has many different functions in plants, including development and quality. Magnesium is the central atom in the green chlorophyll molecule, activates many important enzymes, and it is the essential activator of ATP. According to Dr. Stiles, magnesium is also a component of carbohydrate production, energy transfer, and protein synthesis.

Magnesium is responsible for several important roles that allow a plant to grow and develop. One of these is to activate more enzymes than all other minerals. The long list of enzymes that requires magnesium includes glutathione synthase and PEP carboxylase. According to Epstein, magnesium is a component of almost all enzymes that have an effect on the transfer of phosphorus, which makes magnesium the preeminent activator of enzymes concerned with the plant's energy metabolism. Magnesium is also responsible for enzymes that concern the production of carbohydrates, sugars, and fats during photosynthesis. However, activation of these enzymes does not rely solely upon magnesium; manganese can sometimes be substituted.

Overall, magnesium can be found in large concentrations in chlorophyll molecules. Each chlorophyll molecule contains one magnesium ion as a permanent fixture. Marschner explains that between 6% and 25% of the total magnesium in leaves is bound to chlorophyll. Another 5-10% is bound to pectate (one of the few times ions become bound to protein, known as chelation) in the cell walls or inside the storage vacuoles as soluble salts, while the remaining 60-90% is usually found in water. However, if magnesium levels were to exceed 25% in the chlorophylls, leaf growth can become stunted and visual symptoms similar to deficiencies can occur.

Visual symptoms of magnesium deficiencies tend to appear in older tissues first, since magnesium will gravitate toward maturing tissues and seeds. Fortunately, this makes it unlikely that growing fruits and other newly-forming organs and tissues will experience magnesium deficiencies provided there is sufficient magnesium in the plant to begin with.

Magnesium is needed to form fruits and nuts, and is required for the germination of seeds. Fruit's high requirement for magnesium, coupled with magnesium's high mobility, helps to explain why magnesium deficiencies in fruits are rare. However, if fruit are lacking magnesium, poor fruit development and production will result. Visual symptoms of magnesium deficiencies usually occur late in the season, since its high mobility causes it to be leached from the older leaves and moved to the younger, growing leaves, or other areas of need.

One of the first visual signs of a magnesium deficiency occurs when there is a breakdown in the chlorophylls. As a result, a deformation in the leaves known as chlorosis occurs, which is characterized by leaves that curl upward, grow brittle, droop, or become pale in color and have dark green veins. Following chlorosis, like a domino effect the rate of photosynthesis will slow down since magnesium is a primary component in chlorophylls and an activator of enzymes that have a role in photosynthesis. The enzymes that are activated by magnesium affect every facet of the plant's metabolism. Overall, a magnesium deficiency affects the structure, size, and the metabolic function of chloroplasts, as well as the relocation of magnesium ions and proteins from the mature leaves to the younger, growing leaves. Photoassimilates are unable to move into younger tissues when magnesium is lacking, which makes chlorophylls deteriorate even further. When magnesium levels are low, the entire plant and all of its processes suffer.

Plants usually tolerate high concentrations of magnesium. However, when imbalances in the soil occur, the uptake of other minerals and how they're utilized are affected. Researchers have confirmed certain "antagonisms" that result between magnesium and calcium, and between magnesium and potassium. An imbalance of either of these minerals can often result in diminished uptake of the other, causing an imbalance in the plant. These observations seem to be most pronounced in fruit crops. These antagonistic effects have shown that heavy concentrations of one element can result in a deficiency of the other. For example, an imbalance between magnesium and potassium can slow down the plant's rate of growth.

Phosphorus

Phosphorus can be found in several different forms in the soil, such as phosphate ions, attached to other minerals, or inside organic compounds or decomposing matter. It is a highly mobile element that is absorbed into the roots in its ionic form, simply known as "phosphate." Once absorbed, phosphorus is used for various energy reactions, or incorporated into some organic compounds, depending on the needs of the plant.

Phosphorus plays a key role in contributing to biochemical processes such as photosynthesis. This nutrient must be present in the leaves in order for photosynthesis to occur. For the most part, phosphorus can be present in the soil in small quantities, even as small as a few parts per million, and still be able to carry out its critical functions. In fact, acceptable amounts of phosphorus for plant growth can reach small quantities such as .001 parts per million, and just like nitrogen, phosphorus exits the older leaves and enters the newer generation of leaves. When plants mature during the growing season, phosphorus makes its way into the budding flowers and growing fruits and other areas of high metabolic activity, where it assists in fruit formation and development.

On the molecular level, phosphorus is responsible for the utilization of starch and sugars in the cells, the utilization of energy transfer, the formation of the nucleus, the transfer of the cell's genetic identity during multiplication and division during periods of growth, cell organization throughout the plant, and is a component of nucleic acids. Phosphorus aids the plant in synthesizing adenosine triphosphate (ATP), which is involved in almost every metabolic process in the plant. All of these cellular functions also help make phosphorus critical to the cell's vitality and defense against infectious pathogens.

Most plants require high amounts of phosphorus since it is involved in more than the general growth of the plant. Phosphorus is used for flowering, fruit production, and seed development. Roots are unable to grow and develop unless phosphorus is present. The plant's stems become stronger, which improves the quality of the developing vegetables, when there is sufficient phosphorus. Phosphorus can counterbalance excess amounts of nitrogen, while also acting as a component of phospholipids and phytic acid. It also activates some enzymes, while regulating and acting as a coenzyme in others.

Deficiency symptoms usually include visual signs such as reduced or delayed growth. Stunted or deformed leaves and other exterior limbs can also result, as well as discoloration, resulting in a dull, blue-ish green or purplish color followed by bronzing. Some leaves may display burning effects, and some buds may appear dormant or dead. Most of these visual symptoms are the same as nitrogen; although the first signs of deficiency are purple or dark green, instead of yellow. Inside the leaves, the chloroplasts appear deformed and display abnormalities in most, but not all, plants.

Flowers and fruit formation benefit from an influx of phosphorus. Phosphorus plays an active role in the metabolic processes that concern both energy and the growth of the plant, including seed germination, root growth, and cellular expansion. The structural integrity of the plant will be compromised during periods of phosphorus deficiency. Root growth becomes stunted, stems become brittle and thin, leaves and fruit will drop prematurely, and the yield of fruits and flowers will be poor or deformed.

Other nutrients depend on phosphorus for their utilization. Phosphorus enhances the absorption and utilization of molybdenum. Zinc and iron may not experience full absorption unless phosphorus is present, although zinc deficiencies can result when phosphorus is deficient or is found in toxic amounts in the soil. A lack of phosphorus reduces the absorption of nitrogen, while soils with high aluminum content can create a phosphorus deficiency. In general, a lack of one mineral is usually accompanied by a lack of or excess uptake of another.

The external environment plays a key role in the successful absorption of phosphorus. The solubility of phosphorus, along with all other elements, is largely dependent upon the pH of the soil. Like most other nutrients, extremely alkaline or acidic soils can make a mineral become insoluble. Phosphorus becomes insoluble and unavailable in both acidic and alkaline environments. As the soil becomes more alkaline, phosphates tend to become attached to the alkaline minerals, namely calcium and/or magnesium, forming compounds such as calcium phosphate. However, if the pH level drops below 4.0, phosphates tend to bind with the acidic minerals, such as iron, aluminum, or manganese to form compounds such as aluminum phosphate, or remain locked up inside organic matter. Therefore, phosphorus is more soluble and readily available for absorption at a neutral pH range of 6.0-7.0. How the pH balance of the soil affects minerals will be discussed further in later chapters.

During cold weather, the activity of microorganisms responsible for decomposition slows down, making the soil less concentrated with nutrients such as phosphorus. Although phosphorus may be highly mobile, fertilizers containing phosphorus should be applied close to the roots of the plant.

Sulfur

When sulfur is found in its ionic form in soils, it is known as sulfate. Sulfur is an essential macronutrient that tends to play an important part in the manufacture of many substances that are created in the plant. Some amino acids can trace their genetic makeup to sulfur. It acts as a structural component for proteins, amino acids, and vitamins such as thiamin and bioimin. Sulfur activates some enzymes and it provides a building block for many proteins that build plant tissues. Some of sulfur's biggest responsibilities include the synthesis of proteins and amino acids, and helping with electron transport during photosynthesis.

When sulfur is deficient in a plant, the protein content in the plant will suffer. However, amino acids that require higher concentrations of other nutrients besides sulfur will continue to get synthesized and benefit the plant, but the proteins that require sulfur will not. Interestingly, a lack of protein synthesis can often prevent some amino acids from being synthesized. Eventually, a chain-reaction of deficiencies can result from restrictions in protein synthesis, resembling deficiency symptoms found in nitrogen and phosphorus deficient plants. Low levels of carbohydrates can result from low photosynthesis rates, as well as an accumulation of nitrogen, since some of the nitrogen is not able to be used in the synthesis of proteins. Starch can begin to accumulate inside the plant if carbohydrate synthesis is restricted.

Sulfur is a constituent of coenzyme A, which is an important element in the plant's respiration process and helps metabolize fatty acids. Sulfur activates other enzymes and can sometimes be substituted for phosphorus deficiencies. It is also a necessary ingredient in the creation of chlorophyll, is a component of the cell's protoplasm, and adds flavor to many vegetables.

Sulfur is rarely deficient in soils, although some small parts of the United States along the east and west coasts and even small areas in the Midwest could contain low levels of sulfur. It is usually found in sufficient quantities since there are many soil organisms that are capable of dissolving sulfur from compounds found in organic matter. Sulfur can be deficient in soils that lack decomposing matter or in soils that do not have a lot of fine, clay particles. It can also be deficient in shallow soils or in soils where the topsoil has been removed due to industrial development. Simply adding decomposing organic material to the area of concern is usually enough to provide plenty of sulfur compounds that will be broken down to sulfate. Therefore, the availability of sulfur is largely determined by the activities of the soil organisms and their ability to decompose organic matter. Although organic matter provides most of the sulfur presently found in soils, some water supplies can also provide this mineral.

Although sulfur deficiencies are uncommon, visual symptoms can be similar to those found in nitrogen deficient soils. This can include general chlorosis of leaves and stems, impaired protein synthesis resulting in discoloration, and impairment of chlorophyll synthesis. Sulfur deficient plants experience stunted growth and pale color. Sometimes leaves will appear light green when the deficiency creates a lack of chlorophyll content, which will also affect photosynthesis. Sulfur-deficient plants can also have small leaves, rolled ends, and become hard and brittle.

Sulfur is not remobilized very well inside the plant, making deficiency symptoms more likely in younger, newly-developing leaves. Plants grown in sulfur-deficient soil experience impaired growth of developing organs even more than the roots, which occurs more common in nitrogen deficiencies. Overall, the plant's growth and development suffers when there is a lack of sulfur in the soil.

Chapter 6

Microminerals in Plants

Iron

Among all the micronutrients, iron is the most required, and in such large amounts that some consider it to be a macronutrient. There is usually plenty of iron in soils and it has many important functions.

One of the most important responsibilities of iron in plants is to activate enzymes. Some of these enzymes are involved in important metabolic processes, such as respiration and photosynthesis, as well as nitrogen fixation, which is the process by which nitrogen is taken from the atmosphere and converted into useful compounds for other chemical processes. Iron is also an important component in oxidase enzymes, such as catalase and peroxidase.

Iron is necessary for chlorophyll formation, and a major portion of iron can be found inside chloroplasts where it is required for photosynthesis. In fact, there is a strong correlation between the amount of chlorophyll and the amount of iron if the level of iron fluctuates. With its high involvement in chlorophyll and photosynthesis, an iron deficiency results in an impairment of chloroplast development. This includes a loss of chlorophylls and deterioration of the entire chloroplast framework.

Iron is necessary for the young developing parts of plants. If the amount of available iron in the soil is low, the cell's ability to divide is impaired, which will stunt the growth of leaves. The effects of iron deficiencies have more impact on the size and protein content of the chloroplasts than on leaf growth or number of chlorophylls per cell or cells per area.

There are several other responsibilities of iron. It provides the plant with the ability to help synthesize proteins, and during periods of iron deficiencies, the number of ribosomes (the sites for protein synthesis) usually decline. Iron also has responsibility in the oxidation and respiration systems of plants. During respiration, for example, iron becomes part of some molecules in the electron transport chain.

Visual symptoms of iron deficiencies include chlorosis, which is the discoloration of leaves and veins. Chlorosis usually involves the leaves turning dark green or yellow, followed by a scorching, or burning appearance, of the leaf tips. Since iron has low mobility and is slow to be withdrawn from the older leaves, chlorosis will usually appear first in the interveinal areas of the younger, growing leaves. In fact, when deficiencies are severe, some leaves will turn white.

In order for a mineral to be ready for absorption into a plant, it must be soluble. The solubility of minerals is largely determined by the pH level of the soil. If the soil's pH level is too alkaline, iron forms insoluble iron hydroxides and calcium complexes. However, if the soil is too acidic, iron tends to react with aluminum. In either case, iron would become prone to precipitating out of the soil, resulting in deficiencies.

Iron's sensitivity to the pH levels of the soil can cause it to be unavailable for absorption when pH levels are unfavorable. As a result, the soil's pH level should be in a neutral range that would allow iron to remain soluble. And since iron is not very mobile, it can easily be leached out of the soil. Therefore, iron is often applied during agricultural fertilization.

Boron

Like any other element, boron requires ionization in order to be released as ions into the soil. Boron is known as "borate" when referring to its ionic form that is found in plants. Microorganisms release boron from the decomposing organic matter as borate ions into the soil, where it is found attached to clay particles and loosely held in water. When boron is absorbed into a plant, it is usually absorbed through active, rather than passive, transport.

Once boron is absorbed into the plant, it moves passively through the plant's transport vessels. Along with most other minerals, boron's movement depends largely on warm temperatures since it flows through the plant's transpiration stream, which is the evaporation process that causes the water to move upward through the plant. However, boron has low mobility and can be easily leached from the soil.

Boron was first recognized in the 1920s as having essential benefits in a plant, although the exact role of boron is still being researched since it is the least understood of all the microminerals. Although some argue how boron even made it to the list of micronutrients, researchers have studied boron's effect on plants by withholding it from the plant, or resupplying it after a lengthy deficiency, to determine what role it has as a nutrient. Research has observed that in order for the plant to benefit from boron, it should be available for uptake throughout the life of the plant. Boron doesn't have to be available in heavy concentrations. However, too much boron can be toxic to the plant, but amounts even as small as one part per million is usually enough.

Researchers have listed 16 functions of boron so far, including roles in flowering, male fertility, pollen germination, fruit development and growth, root development, and even helping plants move hormones. Boron is also useful for cell division, reproduction, and it helps regulate water intake through the cell membranes. Other functions of boron include RNA metabolism, phenol metabolism, and carbohydrate metabolism. Although boron may not be required in high amounts, it makes a definite impact on the development of fruits, flowers, and other external organs of the plant, and the general physical strength of cell walls. Although boron has not yet been found to activate enzymes or even participate in enzymatic activities, this long list of important responsibilities puts boron on the list of microminerals.

Most boron is found in the cell walls where it helps to form stable organic compounds with other components of the cell walls (although glucose, fructose, and galactose are sugars that do not normally participate in this binding). When boron is withheld from the cell walls, abnormalities usually result, which implies that it is a necessary element to the physical integrity of the cell.

Plants rely on boron for many other responsibilities. Boron is used to make proteins and participate in carbohydrate metabolism. This makes it a constituent in cell growth, although how boron affects cell growth in this manner is still being researched. Some researchers think it may be due to boron's ability to help nucleic acid and hormone metabolism. Boron also acts as a catalyst by moving sugars and starches throughout the plant. This mineral even helps calcium remain soluble for uptake in the soil and helps to keep calcium soluble throughout its useful life in the plant.

As is common with most other mineral elements, a lack of boron results in chlorosis. One of the plant's first visual symptoms of boron deficiency is when the branches and roots appear stubby or become stunted altogether. The cells slow down their process of expansion and if the deficiency is severe enough, the roots and outer limbs will become chlorotic and die. Boron deficiency seems to be more common among the newer, younger developing leaves and branches, which is likely due to its low mobility.

Periods of boron deficiency can also include the disintegration of internal tissues and cellular membranes, resulting in abnormal water relations and weak membranes surrounding the cell, ultimately collapsing the entire tissue. Eventually deficiencies kill terminal buds, causing a rosette effect, which is characterized by the leaves becoming thick, brittle, and curling inward. According to Epstein, in some herbaceous plants the leaves and stems develop a stiff, woody feel. Some vegetable crops such as lettuce develop water-soaked areas and chlorosis of the leaves, such as brown or black discolorations.

If a boron deficiency is severe enough, flowering can become impaired or prevented completely. Fleshy fruits, such as strawberries and peaches, experience very poor growth and impaired development. Fleshy fruits, such as strawberries and peaches, experience very poor growth and impaired development, while citrus fruits experience a decrease in the pulp to peel ration. Overall, fruits become discolored, cracked, and peppered with brown spots, becoming useless. Eventually, early rotting and infectious pathogens gain entry due to the breakdown in cellular integrity. Dr. Frank J. Peryea has cited some dramatic effects of boron deficiency that include impairment of various growth factors, such as production of auxins (plant hormones), lignification, (hardening of cellular walls), and inhibited sucrose transport.

During harvest, apple growers have observed boron deficiencies in their crops being characterized by irregularly shaped fruits, spots, cracking, premature ripening, increased fruit drop, and low seed count. The apple trees also experienced symptoms, such as dwarfed, brittle leaves, discolored bark, and dead buds. Apricot growers have noticed similar symptoms, including cracking, shriveling, browning, deformed apricots, and increased fruit drop. Fruit and flower blossoms are more likely to experience deficiency symptoms than the vegetative parts of a fruit tree. Interestingly, research shows that pears tend to require more boron than other fruits during spring.

When the supply of boron is removed from the soil, root growth becomes impaired within three hours, and severely impaired after six hours. After 24 hours, root growth completely stops. However, observations show that after 12 hours of boron being reintroduced, root growth was able to resume its normal rate. Studies involving fruit trees have shown that boron is critical to the absorption of potassium, which occurs due to boron's support of root development. A boron deficiency can also occur in the soil during periods of excess potassium or unusually high pH levels.

Jim Barrow, author of the article "Understanding Soils and Nutrients," explains that boron comes to us naturally through sea spray. Therefore, a boron deficiency is more likely to occur in areas that are far inland, making this element most likely to be deficient in the Midwestern United States.

Dr. Peryea has stated that the availability of boron in the soil declines during periods of heavy rains, very dry climates, when the pH level is above 6.5, cold soil temperatures, or excess decomposition of organic matter. Boron can be added to crops through foliar applications, and even if rainfall carries it quickly into the soil, it can be absorbed through the roots of the tree.

Copper

Like other minerals, copper regulates and activates many different enzymes. Observations have even shown that copper is used to manufacture enzymes and chlorophyll. Copper also activates some oxidative enzymes, which are an important part of photosynthesis. Such enzymes include plastocyanin, which transports electrons during photosynthesis, cytochrome oxidase, an enzyme used during respiration, and ascorbic acid oxidase. Other enzymes activated by copper include phenolase, lactase, diamine oxidase, ascorbate oxidase, and the free radical destroyer known as Superoxide dismutase (SOD). During periods of copper deficiency, enzymatic activity decreases quickly, which affects some metabolic processes, including photosynthesis and development of chloroplasts, and a deficiency will slow the plant's rate of growth enzymes. Copper's influence on enzymes helps to explain its role in protein and carbohydrate synthesis.

After copper ions are absorbed from the soil, 98-99% of the ions are used to form various organic compounds, such as proteins. Some proteins in plants require a metal component in order to be a complete, functional protein. Copper happens to be a component of three different proteins, one of which requires four copper atoms per protein molecule in order for it to be useful to the plant.

Iron can bind with copper to form a protein known as cytochromes oxidase that is involved with oxidation inside the mitochondria. Copper is also a constituent in nitrogen metabolism. In fact, without enough copper protein synthesis becomes impaired and can result in a buildup of nitrogen compounds, as well as changes in metabolic activity and impaired plant growth.

A large concentration of copper can be found in the roots, where it participates in the root's elongation and the plant's reproductive stages of growth. Copper also participates in the development of fruits, seeds, and grains, and has some participation in the growth of vegetables.

According to researchers Frank Salisbury and Cleon Ross, plants are rarely deficient in copper since it is a micromineral and they need so little of it. Deficiency symptoms of copper tend to resemble those of iron.

Stunted growth and disorders in young leaves are common. Citrus trees experience a condition known as "die-back," where young leaves die quickly. Some exterior growth organs also experience die-back when copper levels are low.

Chlorosis is another common symptom of copper deficiency. Leaves can develop bluish-green discoloration, and in severe cases leaves can form speckled brown spots. Wilting is common and the edges of the leaves can show rosetting. Younger leaves tend to experience the most from copper deficiencies, in that they may wither and become discolored in their tips.

Copper is usually found tightly bound inside organic matter. It has intermediate mobility so it may not be easily leached from the soil, but it tends to be deficient in soils that have high nitrogen, phosphorus, and zinc content. Copper can become toxic to plants if levels in the soil are too high, and too much copper can create an iron deficiency.

Zinc

Zinc can be found in several different forms in the soil, including water soluble ions, attached to clay particles and exchangeable with other ions, or extractable from chelates, all considered readily available for absorption. It is absorbed as a divalent cation (Zn^{++}), most commonly broken down from zinc chelates. Zinc can also be found in the soil as secondary and primary clay mineral-associated compounds that are unavailable and insoluble.

More than 80 enzymes found in plants require zinc in order to function. According to Epstein, zinc is the metal component of many metalloenzymes, as well as the enzymes dehydrogenases, alcohol dehydrogenase, and lactic dehydrogenase, and it helps build auxins (plant growth hormones). Some of zinc's enzymatic activities assist in the metabolism of carbohydrates, such as the carbonic anyhydrase reaction. Two zinc-dependent enzymes are found in the chloroplasts and the cytoplasm.

Zinc makes up part of the physical integrity of ribosomes and when its levels are decreased, the ribosomes can actually disintegrate over time, but can rebuild their cellular strength when zinc levels are increased. Zinc also influences the activity of the enzyme ribonuclease, which suggests that zinc is also heavily involved in the regulation of protein synthesis in many fruit trees. When zinc is deficient, protein synthesis slows down and results in an accumulation of amino acids. However, when zinc is resupplied to the plant, protein synthesis resumes to normal levels.

Zinc's role in regulating protein synthesis means it is a critical element for the maturity and growth of plants. Plant growth is also influenced by indoleacetic acid, which is another substance regulated by zinc. According to Marschner, zinc also strengthens the physical integrity of some cellular membranes, which protects them from oxidative damage by hindering the oxidation of NADPH, which prevents toxic oxygen radicals from forming. Dr. D. Neilsen has observed that zinc also appears to help cells regulate their pH level as well as synthesizing RNA and tryptophan, which influences the growth of plant stems.

When zinc is deficient, the physical integrity of plasma membranes is in jeopardy; an increase in permeability will likely occur. Also, unsaturated fatty acids in membranes and the cell's phospholipid content both decline when zinc levels are low. However, when zinc is resupplied, the cellular integrity returns within 12 hours.

While being transported inside the plant, zinc travels through the xylem as either the divalent cation or bound to various organic acids. Inside the phloem, zinc concentrations are fairly high, as it has likely been used to produce organic products that were manufactured during photosynthesis. During reproductive periods of the season, zinc's intermediate mobility causes it to move out of the older leaves and tissues and into newer, developing tissues, causing common discoloration and deficiency symptoms in the older tissues.

Other minerals such as nitrogen, copper, and aluminum, when found in excess quantities, can impair the absorption of zinc. When zinc reaches minimum levels, it can lead to iron deficiencies because zinc is more readily available at pH levels below 5.5, which happens to be the minimum pH level where iron retains its solubility. Zinc is easily leached out of the soil, but is found soluble and available in acidic soils. If the pH level continues to decrease and becomes more and more acidic, it can result in too much zinc, which can be toxic to a plant.

Zinc is critical to carbohydrate metabolism and stem growth, a lack of which results in visual symptoms that include stunted growth and chlorosis. All minerals contribute to the growth of the leaves, but the impact of zinc is so severe that terms such as "little leaf" and "rosetting" were coined. Rosetting is the failure of stems to expand, which results in the leaves lying close together like a flat plane. Leaves may look mottled and will curl along the edges. These visual symptoms usually result from the inability of the plant to metabolize auxins, due to the lack of zinc.

Some discoloration such as scorching, bronzing, or purpling occurs in leaves when zinc is removed from the soil. Newer leaves appear smaller and deformed and fruit development is impaired. Growers usually add zinc by using sprays directly on the crop, a common practice for improving fruit trees.

Manganese

Manganese appears to have an effect on several different processes and it metabolizes different organic products. It is responsible for activating 35 different enzymes, including decarboxylase and dehydrgenase, but is actually found inside only two enzymes—the manganese-protein found in photosynthesis and the free radical destroyer Superoxide dismutase (SOD). Manganese is heavily involved in synthesizing vitamins and chlorophyll, and helps the plants utilize nitrogen and carbon. Sometimes manganese can be substituted for magnesium, including activating enzymes and reactions that involve ATP, and it can compete or substitute for calcium in various reactions.

Manganese is best known for its role in respiration and other photosynthetic oxygen processes. According to Dr. Curt Rom, it is critical to the chloroplast membrane, which is the structure that contains the light-absorbing chlorophyll pigment. Epstein explains that manganese also plays a heavy role in many of the reactions of the Krebs or tricarboxylic acid cycle. This cycle has such importance to other metabolic processes that an impairment can result in a decline of other metabolic processes, including the evolution of oxygen and the structural integrity of the chloroplasts.

During periods of manganese deficiency, photosynthesis begins to slow down. The amount of chlorophylls will begin to decline since manganese is needed to construct its membranes. Also, a process known as photosynthetic O2 evolution drops by more than half. However, after the leaves are supplemented with the proper amount of manganese, the photosynthetic O2 evolution process is restored within one day to the appropriate levels. Most of the fatty acids that are usually found in photosynthetic cells will decline because manganese is needed for their synthesis.

Severe manganese deficiencies can often result in severe consequences and overall impairment of many of the plant's metabolic processes. Studies show that low concentrations of manganese result in impaired plant growth, specifically in the roots, which is usually due to a lack of carbohydrate metabolism, which dependents on manganese. This domino effect is not just a manganese phenomenon. Most minerals can set off a chain reaction of deficiency symptoms.

Chlorosis is a common symptom of a manganese deficiency, which is usually displayed as greenish-gray spots on the leaves of cereal grains. In legumes, as well as other types of plants, low manganese levels can result in extreme discoloration and deformation between the leaf veins. Other symptoms include depressed growth in buds, twigs that die back, and deformed leaves.

Some heavy metal ions, such as manganese, when found in high levels, are known to compete with iron and can create an iron deficiency. Epstein explains that this phenomenon occurs between competitive effects in the uptake of iron and competitive effects by the inhibitory heavy metals for functioning sites of iron binding.

Most soils around the world, including highly leached tropical soils, derive manganese from parent material that contains this heavy metal. Manganese becomes insoluble in soils that have either high pH levels or high levels of carbon material such as organic matter. Most agricultural applications of manganese involve soil fertilizers or foliar sprays.

Application of manganese directly into seeds can help the plant sustain healthy growth. Interestingly, some observations also show that manganese deficient plants are more prone to freezing damage.

Molybdenum

Molybdenum is the lowest required element of all the microminerals, except nickel. It is found largely in the soil as the molybdate anion, but most plants require such small amounts of this element that deficiencies are rare. It is a highly mobile element during transport through the xylem and phloem. Molybdenum is found in some enzymes, and shares similarities with vanadium and tungsten, as well as sulfur and phosphorus.

Only a small number of enzymes have shown to be truly dependent upon molybdenum. According to Marschner, these enzymes are dinitrogenase, nitrate reductase, xanthine oxidase/dehydrogenase, and sulfite reductase, which all have different roles in the plant's metabolic processes. For example, dinitrogenase is the enzyme responsible for reducing atmospheric nitrogen, while nitrate reductase is usually found in roots and leaves where it reduces nitrate to nitrite, which prepares nitrogen ions for amino acids and other organic substances. Epstein explains that molybdenum functions mainly as a component of metalloenzymes rather than an enzyme activator. Overall, the role of molybdenum is so closely matched chemically to nitrogen that nitrogen fixation (a process where nitrogen is taken from the atmosphere, converted into compounds, and used for chemical reactions in the plant) is a strong byproduct of molybdenum.

A well-known symptom of molybdenum deficiency is an effect on the size of pollen formation in some plants. One study showed that flowers failed to open and the capacity of the anther for pollen production was reduced. The pollen grains that were produced were smaller, lacked starch, and had impaired germination, all of which affect fruit formation. Another study showed that seeds that contained high amounts of molybdenum were able to grow and produce high yields even though the soil had very low molybdenum concentrations. The researchers concluded that molybdenum's effects on plant growth were related to the content of molybdenum in the seeds and in the fertilizer.

Deficiency symptoms of molybdenum usually involve interveinal chlorosis in older leaves and tissues, since molybdenum is relocated to younger, newer tissues. Another sign of molybdenum deficiency is called "whiptail," characterized by young leaves being twisted and deformed. Molybdenum deficient plants also experience lower levels of sugars, ascorbic acid, and amino acids. Other symptoms resemble a nitrogen deficiency, since molybdenum is instrumental in nitrogen fixation. These symptoms include impaired growth and chlorosis, deformed leaf blades, and discoloration along the veins of mature leaves.

Chlorine

Chlorine is distributed throughout the world through many different methods, including irrigation water, rain, air pollution, fertilizers, and other soil reserves, making chlorine readily available in most soils, so deficiencies are rare. Because chlorine is plentiful, concerns over chlorine tend to focus on toxicity rather than deficiency.

Chlorine is a highly mobile element and can be found in large concentrations throughout the soil. Chlorine's high mobility allows it to be absorbed by roots and be transported both short and long distances inside the plant with ease. It plays a part in the ionic balance, which helps roots absorb other minerals. It is usually delivered to the roots after it has broken down into ions, then known as "chloride." Chloride dissolves easily in water, but can also be leached from the soil rapidly. The difference between chlorine and chloride is so significant that the term chloride, which more appropriately refers to the form that is found in plants, will be used throughout the remained of this chapter.

Chlorine is required in surprisingly high concentrations by most plants, and it is absolutely essential for many biochemical reactions. In 1946, researchers Warburg and Luttgens first identified the critical role of chloride in photosynthesis, an important role that has been confirmed and accepted since then. During photosynthesis, chloride is required for oxygen evolution. The water-splitting stage of photosynthesis also needs chloride to bridge ligand—a waxy polymer—to stabilize oxidized manganese and to provide physical strength to other polymers. Recent investigations into chloride and its role in oxygen evolution have duplicated this finding using sugar beets.

Inside cells, chloride helps transport products across membranes while maintaining their neutrality. While other mineral elements assist the plant in proton pumping ATPases and Ppases, inside the cell chloride is more specifically responsible for the proton pumping ATPase at the tonoplast (the membrane surrounding the storage vacuole). Chloride also plays an active role in the storage vacuoles.

Although research has not shown a direct role for chloride in activating, regulating, or even as a necessary constituent of enzymes, chloride can sometimes act in conjunction with enzymes that are concerned with photosynthesis. However, it does stimulate some growth in the roots and tops of the plant, and is needed for cellular division in leaves and other exterior limbs.

Marschner has explained that chloride aids the plant's ability to control and regulate the opening and closing of the stomata, which is the organ concerned with releasing atmospheric gases into the air. Potassium and chloride both regulate this process of stomatal functioning. The opening of the stomata is impaired when chloride is deficient. Certain families of plants, such as coconut and palm trees, which contain chloroplasts that contain starch in their guard cells, tend to need chloride for correct stomatal operation. When chloride is deficient in palm trees, stomatal opening is delayed by around 3 hours, which helps to explain why these trees suffer abnormal growth and wilting symptoms when chloride is lacking.

Chloride deficient plants have a tendency to wilt, which implies some problem with transpiration or respiration, but is most likely the result of impaired stomatal functioning. Young leaves tend to curl and shrivel, suggesting chloride's role in osmosis (the movement of water in cells).

Plants that lack chloride can show other visual symptoms such as stunted growth and chlorosis. Coconut trees experiencing a chloride deficiency experience fractures and cracking of the stems. Amino acids can accumulate in plants that lack chloride, but it remains unclear if this means chloride has some responsibility in amino acid synthesis.

Chloride deficient plants experience low overall dry weight and reduced leaf sizes, resulting in discoloration and chlorosis in mature leaves. The reduction in leaf surface area is usually the result of cells being unable to divide and expand in the leaves and roots. Chloride deficient plants also experience swelling and stubby formation in the roots.

Various plant species have different minimum level requirements before showing chloride deficiencies. Squash has little response when chloride levels are low. However, lettuce experiences stunted growth until the chloride is resupplied. Kiwifruit tends to require an unusually high level of chloride, although researching explaining this phenomenon is lacking.

Nickel

Nickel was recently added to the list of essential micronutrients according to the Agricultural Research Service Plant, Soil, and Nutrition Laboratory in Ithaca, New York. It is usually plentiful in the soil and highly absorbable by roots. Nickel may have taken so long to be added to this list because of the difficult role in establishing it as a necessary nutrient due to being the least required out of all the micronutrients. Researchers estimate that the amount of nickel necessary for a plant to complete its life cycle is only 200 nanograms (ng), an amount so small that the tiny amount found in seeds is usually enough to suffice. This mineral is required for iron absorption and it chemically resembles iron and cobalt.

Seeds are highly dependent on nickel to initiate the germination process. During seed germination, the presence of nickel in the seed helps the plant mobilize nitrogen and begin to grow. When plants are lacking nickel in the seeds, deficiency symptoms are usually noticed once the plant matures and starts to reproduce; if there was not enough nickel during the growth of the plant, many plants will not produce reproductive seeds to carry on the next generation.

The essentiality of nickel was established after it was shown that an enzyme known as urease that contained nickel was shown to be absolutely critical to the life of a plant. Research has now identified two enzymes that need nickel in order to function: urease and hydrogenase. Both enzymes are found in many different plants and are distributed throughout the plant kingdom. Urease is an enzyme that breaks down urea and frees the nitrogen into a soluble form. Hydrogenase is responsible for recovering hydrogen to be used in the nitrogen-fixation process, which slows down when nickel is deficient.

However, most all enzymes require a metal component in order to carry out their functions, and there are several other enzymes in which nickel is found to be that metal component. Marschner explains that inside these enzymes nickel is coordinated either to N-and O-ligands, S-ligands, or N-ligands of tetrapyrrol structures. From what is known so far, the only enzyme that actually contains nickel is urease. Its presence appears critical for this enzyme's overall structure and catalytic function. It appears reasonable to conclude that probably all plants need the urease enzyme and nickel.

In plants that lack nickel, the enzymatic activity of urease declines and results in an accumulation of urea, causing necrosis in leaves. However, when nickel is added to plant fertilizers, the rate of urease activity resumes to normal levels and any necrosis or urea accumulation is reduced.

Research studies have shown that soybeans that were lacking nickel experienced impaired growth and a decline in urease enzymatic activity. However, observations have confirmed that when nickel was resupplied to the soybeans, growth increased dramatically and urease activity was enhanced to more than five times its current rate. It was concluded that in these plants that were deficient in nickel, utilization of the urease form of nitrogen was depressed, which resulted in toxic levels of urea and severe necrosis in the leaves. Interestingly, the plants also suffered impaired growth of the roots and external organs, experienced pale green discoloration, and some leaves were not able to unfold.

Originally, nickel was known to have a primary role in growth and development of legumes, but it wasn't until 1975 that nickel was first demonstrated by Dixon to have an influence on plant growth and development. Later studies have found nickel to be a requirement in non-legumes as well. These investigations have identified some of the functions of nickel and proven that plants require this mineral in order to complete their life cycles, ultimately adding nickel to the list of essential micronutrients.

The remaining naturally-occurring elements listed on the Periodic Table of Elements are usually found in such scant amounts that they can go undetected or are rendered nonessential. Some of these trace minerals can still be beneficial and help stimulate growth but may not necessarily be essential to the survival of the plant, or if they are essential, may be only for a few select plant species. This group of minerals is called "beneficial elements," and they play a more supplementary role in plant nutrition. The most common minerals cited in this group are sodium, silicon, and cobalt.

Sodium

Most plants do not require sodium, although researchers Brownell and Crossland have found some scant requirement for sodium in a few plants that have a certain photosynthetic pathway that is unlike most other plant species. They hypothesized that a trace amount of sodium can affect the transport of pyruvate between cells. However, plants that grow frequently in salty soils show some need for sodium and have a strong tolerance for the high levels of salt and sodium. Interestingly, research has shown that certain plant species known as monocots, such as sugarcane, corn, and range grasses, operate with a peculiar photosynthetic process now known as C-4. Sodium has shown to be an essential element in plants known as C-4 species.

Some investigations have identified sodium's role in cell division and expansion, such as increasing the leaf's surface area and the number of stomata per unit of surface area. However, this can also create lower chlorophyll content, thus decreasing the rate of photosynthesis.

Sodium can sometimes be used by the plant to substitute for potassium in the storage vacuoles. In fact, sodium can accumulate more readily than potassium in the vacuoles, helping the plant carry out cell expansion and growth. When water supply is limited, sodium can assist the plant in the water balance by helping to regulate respiration in the stomata. Under drought conditions, sodium can influence the stomatal regulation differently than potassium by delaying their opening and closing the stomata faster. This causes the leaves to retain a higher amount of water when sodium is acting on behalf of potassium under drought conditions.

Overall, plants lacking in sodium can be characterized by leaves, stems, and roots that have chlorosis (yellowing) and necrosis (dead tissue), while experiencing a slower growth rate.

Silicon

Silicon is plentiful in the soil—it is the second most abundant element found in Earth's crust. Plants generally have no problem finding silicon, although investigations into silicon have not shown this element to be a requirement for most plants. In fact, most plants can take up and accumulate appreciable amounts of silicon, and it may have an important role in certain plants, such as wetland grasses.

Grasses have a tendency to absorb and utilize silicon and store it in cell membranes, especially the epidermal cells of the roots, where it can have some influence in fighting off infectious pathogens. Wetland rice that lack silicon suffers vegetative growth impairment, grain production, and necrosis of older leaves. Although this may suggest a role of silicon in these grasses, it has not been observed that plants require silicon in order to complete their life cycles.

For the rest of the plant kingdom, however, silicon is easily mobile but only transported through the xylem, where it can be found accumulating in the walls of the xylem and adding structural integrity and strength during periods of high transpiration, protecting against compression and stress. In the epidermal cells of roots, silicon combines with other minerals to provide a thick, protective barrier inside the walls to help prevent water loss and to protect against infectious bacteria and fungi, such as powdery mildew, which enters the root system by penetrating unprotected cell membranes.

Marschner cites investigations into silicon that show over and over a strong correlation between the presence of silicon and cellular strength, while allowing elasticity during periods of growth and expansion. This rigidity and integrity is crucial to the long-term health and vigor of a plant. Overall, silicon does have a small role in combining with other elements to create tougher walls that provide a strong barrier against infections and everyday pests. In fact, research studies show that some plants will transport silicon toward areas of infection to combat the attacking pathogen trying to penetrate the cell walls. The strengthened walls also provide protection against environmental stresses, such as intense heat and drought conditions. Silicon may not be on the list of essential or beneficial elements, but if we add disease prevention as a fourth criteria in determining essentiality, silicon should then be considered.

In addition, silicon also increases the surface area of leaves and provides proper leaf erectness. Silicon's presence in the epidermal cells of leaves allows for increased light interception and it can counteract the negative effects that high nitrogen can have on leaf erectness. Furthermore, silicon also protects against iron and manganese toxicities, and it plays a supplementary role in most plants, but is essential in only a few.

Cobalt

Cobalt has not been found to provide any function that directly affects any of a plant's metabolic processes. However, a few species of plants, such as legumes, play host to nitrogen-fixing bacteria that need cobalt in order to supply nitrogen to the plant. In other words, without these bacteria present in the root system, the plant would not be able to absorb sufficient nitrogen to carry out its growth and development, and could result in symptoms of nitrogen deficiency. The plant itself may not need cobalt, but the bacteria supplying the plant's nitrogen do.

This special case makes cobalt an important requirement for legumes. However, researchers Wilson and Nicholas (1967) discovered that the legume subterranean clover and the non-legume wheat both need ample amounts of cobalt but do not need bacteria for their nitrogen supply. This documents that there seem to be a few species of plants that require cobalt to carry out their metabolic processes, but don't necessarily need cobalt to support nitrogen fixing bacteria. If studies continue to document findings that support a strong case for cobalt and can show how cobalt is required for a plant to complete its life cycle, cobalt could eventually be added to the list of essential microminerals.

Selenium

Selenium is chemically related to sulfur (which can suppress selenium's absorption) and can both compete for their positions involving enzymes. Ions of selenium in the soil are known as selenate, and two well-known plants known for their selenium absorption are broccoli and black mustard.

Research is lacking that shows a requirement for selenium; there are no documented cases where selenium provided any benefit to plants. However, some plants frequently found in selenium-rich soils appear to have high accumulations and have developed high tolerance for selenium, and they may even have some small use for it. Some research into this suggests that selenium provides these few plants some defense against infections. However, it is possible that these plants may have some other needs for selenium nutrition. It is true that selenium is required for human nutrition, but for the majority of plants selenium is not known to be beneficial.

Some researchers theorize that any growth-promoting effects of selenium in plants are a result of selenium's ability to control the absorption of phosphate, which would normally be absorbed in excessive amounts.

Aluminum

Most people are unaware of the high aluminum content of Earth's surface. It is estimated that 8% of the surface of Earth is comprised of aluminum, so there is a good chance that aluminum ions (Al+++) will be found in plant tissues of fruits and vegetables.

Research has failed to reveal plants' need for aluminum in their growth and development. In fact, most of the research into aluminum involves trying to understand a plant's high tolerance for this element and documenting toxic effects of severe aluminum content.

Marschner explains that research has found that small amounts of aluminum can provide some benefit. However, the benefits of aluminum on plants are not necessarily the direct effect of aluminum, but rather the tendency of aluminum to alleviate some toxic effects of excess copper and phosphorus. This secondary effect on plant nutrition is usually in small amounts and in highly specific circumstances in plants that have a high tolerance for aluminum, such as wheat, barley, corn, and sorghum.

Other minerals

The task of defining what is considered beneficial and essential can prove daunting, especially in the case of trace minerals. Technological developments in laboratory research may yet add new elements to the list of "essential" nutrients in the future as research continues to try to identify new mineral requirements, as was the case recently with nickel, which was the first element to be added to the list of essential micronutrients since chlorine was added in 1954.

With all the other elements in existence, it is expected that many of them could appear in tissue analyses of plants at any time. These extremely rare elements are found in such trace amounts that research indicating any real nutritional need for these elements is lacking. However, Epstein explains that calling these elements "nonessential" would be inappropriate. Rather, using terms such as "apparently nonessential" or even "not known to be essential" would be better expressions. Even in highly purified tissue samples, some trace elements may still exist and could provide some benefit to the plant.

The elements vanadium and iodine provide benefit to certain lower plants such as algae and fungi. However, Marschner explains that research has failed to show a role for these elements in higher plants, although vanadium does provide some benefit in tomatoes, and in certain crops titanium provides some growth stimulation, as well as photosynthetic and enzymatic processes.

Chromium, mercury, lead, and cadmium are heavy metals that have been found in plant tissue samples. However, plant physiologists remain unconvinced that they provide any significant nutritional benefits. In China, the elements lanthanum and cerium have shown to provide some growth benefits when they are mixed in trace amounts with agricultural fertilizers. The Chinese have reported increases in plant metabolic processes with these elements, but more research is required in order to further understand if these elements provide any other benefits.

■ ■ ■

With all of the health benefits that plants receive from both the macrominerals and the microminerals, it should come as no surprise that minerals strengthen plants structurally, biologically, and against infections. Minerals play an extremely important role in protecting a plant from invasion of pests, as well as minimizing pest damage once they gain entry. Plants are susceptible to infections from bacteria, viruses, fungi, and parasites at any time, either through the roots, leaves, stems, flowers, fruit, or any other vegetative parts. The primary goal of an infectious agent is to get inside the plant by invading and attacking the cell so it can multiply and further its advancement. The cell is usually the primary victim of an infectious invasion, and it is here that a fierce battle begins…

Chapter 7

Minerals and Plant Diseases

In the deficiency or absence of minerals, metabolic processes, including those responsible for the absorption and transport of minerals, cellular expansion, and photosynthesis, slow down. Performance declines and health deteriorates. When one metabolic process is impaired, a chain of events eventually results that will disrupt other processes, since each metabolic process is part of an interconnected system of metabolism. Inevitably, if one process suffers, every other process will unavoidably suffer, until every metabolic process in the plant is affected. Eventually, the entire plant can become unbalanced and even take on a deranged and unrecognizable appearance, so that toxic levels of unassimilated materials can accumulate in the plant and its growth and development diminishes.

Similarly, diseases can wreak havoc on plants. Plant pathology is the study of diseases in plants, which are recognized as being either infectious or noninfectious. Infectious diseases are comprised of organisms that invade the plant tissues, such as bacteria, fungi, parasites, viruses, and even other plants. Noninfectious diseases, on the other hand, stem from environmental elements, such as mineral deficiencies, mineral toxicities, temperature, severe weather, drought, and even over-watering.

Just about anything can affect the growth and yield of plants, but plant growth and production is also concerned with protection from parasitic infection. Dr. George Agrios, a retired plant pathologist at the University of Massachusetts, explains, "Plants suffer from diseases whose causes are similar to those affecting animals and man. Although there is no evidence that plants feel pain or discomfort, the development of disease follows the same steps and is usually as complex in plants as it is in animals and man."

A plant is considered diseased when a disturbance interrupts normal plant metabolism and growth rates and interferes with the manufacture, translocation, or utilization of food, mineral nutrients, and water so that the affected plant changes in appearance and/or yields less than a normal, healthy plant of the same variety. Infectious diseases with visual symptoms can easily be misinterpreted as mineral deficiencies, when it's really a plant playing host to a nutrient-consuming parasite.

When the term "parasitism" is used in conjunction with plants, the plant in reference is playing host to various types of organisms that benefit at the plant's expense. These parasites that attack plants belong to the same group as those that cause disease in animals and humans, although they may not necessarily be the same ones. These infectious pathogens grow and multiply rapidly and can spread between infected and healthy plants, causing disease symptoms to spread. Infectious pathogens cause disease in plants either by 1) consuming the contents of the plant's cell upon contact, 2) killing or disturbing the metabolism of the plant's cells by excreting toxins, enzymes, or other growth-inhibiting substances, 3) weakening the plant by stealing its nutrients for its own gain, or 4) blocking the transport of food, water, or nutrients that travel through the plant's transport vessels.

When diagnosing a crop, there are usually many different potential reasons that a crop has failed, or will. An entomologist will look for infectious pests. A plant pathologist will look for small bacterial infestations, and a horticulturalist will look for a mineral deficiency. A particular mineral deficiency usually appears when that particular mineral is in highest demand. For example, symptoms of iron, boron, and zinc deficiencies appear before bloom, while potassium and magnesium deficiencies appear in late summer. In agriculture, most problems are mineral deficiencies and can be reversed by changing the fertilizer or adding foliar sprays.

Plants that lack minerals not only experience stunted growth and impaired metabolic processes, but also become weakened, which makes them prone to invasion from other insects, parasitic infections, and environmental stresses such as drought and temperature extremes.

Resistance is usually characterized by the plant's ability to restrict penetration, development, and reproduction, or hinder the nutritional consumption of the microbes. Tolerance is defined as the plant's ability to maintain its rates of growth and development in spite of the presence of the microbes.

Resistance and tolerance are both genetic responsibilities, but the plant is unable to perform these functions unless certain conditions are in order; the plant's overall nutritional status determines their effectiveness. This nutritional status determines whether or not the plant possesses the appropriate minerals necessary in order for these two genetically controlled responses to infections to occur. Minerals are responsible for the plant's resistance to infections and tolerance, and they may either increase or decrease depending on circumstances.

Infectious pathogens invade plant tissues because their evolutionary development requires them to exist on the tissues and manufactured substances that are found in plants for their continued survival. Since these required substances are usually found inside the plant's cells, these pathogens will try every trick in their arsenal to get inside.

Fungi are microscopic plants that lack conductive tissues and are unable to make their own food using chlorophyll and photosynthesis, such as higher plants. They are parasitic in nature; meaning they have to feed off of higher plants for their survival. Approximately 100,000 species of fungi have been identified, and most of these are busy decomposing organic matter. Fungi such as mycorrhizae provide benefits to the soil system by living off of dead organic matter, thus decomposing and releasing the ions into the soil. Around 50 species of fungi cause disease in humans and animals such as external diseases of the skin.

However, as many as 8,000 species of fungi cause various diseases in plants, and most estimates state that fungi are responsible for as much as 80% of all infectious diseases found in plants. While penetrating the cells and reproducing and spreading across the tissues, infectious fungi feed on living plants and release toxins. The results of fungal infections can be either cosmetic, such as powdery mildew, or death, such as root rot.

According to Dr. Agrios, in order for parasites, fungi, and bacteria to penetrate the tissues and cause infection, they must pierce the many layers of cellular membranes, steal its nutrients, and neutralize the plant's defense mechanisms. Research has shown that these pathogens are able to accomplish these acts by secreting various substances such as toxins, polysaccharides, and enzymes to damage the plant's cells. Once a parasite has penetrated the cellular membranes, one of the ways they inflict damage is by consuming nutrients that otherwise would be used by the plant, even including the same nutrients that would normally be used to defend and strengthen the plant against such organisms.

■ ■ ■

However, plants don't just sit idle and allow for easy penetration. The plant protects itself through various ways, including fortifying its cells and creating substances to repel an attack. They have evolved their own form of immune system, which includes the strengthening of various membranes and the creation of some disease-fighting substances. These substances include waxy barriers and cork layers in the cells, chemicals that are toxic to fungi and enzymes that inhibit their penetration. These defense mechanisms are genetically controlled, but rely on the presence of minerals in order to function. Many times the plant's nutritional status is overlooked and goes unrecognized as an important component of disease prevention.

Plants have also developed evolutionary responses to infectious attacks. Plants can protect themselves against infections by allowing changes in their anatomy, such as a thickening of their epidermal cells and higher degrees of lignification (strengthening of cell walls). Marschner explains that changes can also include physiological and biochemical changes, such as the production of repelling substances that will be used in case of an attack. Minerals are also used by the plant to enhance the formation of cellular barriers and the synthesis of toxins.

One element that plants use to fight off infections in several different ways is calcium. Calcium is an extremely important mineral that not only helps tissues grow, but is also used to strengthen the cellular membranes. This affects the transport of substances across the membrane, making the cell walls more selective. Calcium prevents organic substances such as amino acids and sugars from inadvertently exiting the storage vacuoles and entering the free space between cells (the apoplastic pathway).

Calcium ions are also used to strengthen the middle lamella, because fungi and bacteria can excrete destructive enzymes in an attempt to dissolve these membranes, which would allow them to enter the cells. However, the ability of these enzymes to dissolve this membrane gradually declines with the presence of calcium.

Some calcium ions will be bound to pectin to create calcium pectate, forming a glue-like substance that binds cell walls, thus strengthening the membranes against attacks from fungi such as Pythium and Fusarium. If calcium levels are low, fungal infections such as these will have an easier time entering a plant's cells, where they can invoke such conditions as seedling diseases in tomatoes, sugar beets, and peppers, and a condition in wheat known as browning rot.

Silicon is another mineral that has proven to be extremely useful. A plant's resistance to fungi appears to be related to the amount of silicon in the plant. During the growth and development of tissues, silicon becomes more and more important against fungal attack by forming an effective barrier against the invading fungus. Silicon forms deposits inside the cells that allow them to create stronger cellular barriers. Observations have shown that grasses and wetland rice require high amounts of silicon, and there is evidence of a correlation between the silicon content and the susceptibility of fungal infections such as rice blast. The physical barrier of the cell, strengthened by calcium and silicon, is critical in providing an effective protection against fungal and bacterial infections.

Unfortunately, silicon is not very mobile, so its transport through a plant can be rather slow and is usually confined to the xylem. This might explain why older, mature leaves tend to have higher amounts of silicon in its tissues than newly developing leaves. It is easy to conclude that the older leaves will have a stronger resistance than the young leaves, due to their higher concentration of silicon, however some studies have shown silicon still has some effect on resistance in younger leaves. In order for fungal infections to occur, their likelihood of success improves if they invade the younger leaves. However, some growers will use silicon in their foliar sprays to help prevent such an attack.

Microminerals affect soil-borne fungal and bacterial diseases in other ways. Manganese enhances the strength of cell walls, which increases the capacity of roots to limit the entry of fungi. Copper has also shown similar benefits. Sulfur in the soil helps to keep the soil somewhat acidic, which decreases the activities of fungi and bacteria. One catastrophic disease known as Gaeumannomyces graminis causes root rot disease in wheat and barley, and limits grain harvest in many areas of the world. Research has shown that this disease can be controlled by the presence of minerals.

Not all minerals have been studied to determine their roles in fighting infectious organisms. It may be safe to say that probably all minerals share some contribution to the plant's defenses, either by directly strengthening membranes or activating disease-fighting enzymes, or indirectly by supporting those minerals that do.

■ ■ ■

When a fungal infection attempts to invade a plant, it seeks to enter through wounds, natural openings such as the respiratory stomata, and/or directly through the cuticle or the epidermis. Once it has penetrated, it begins to steal nutrients and utilize them for its own growth and reproduction, which can cause disease-like symptoms that are characteristic of a mineral deficiency.

But plants always respond quickly by sending silicon to the site of invasion. Silicon is often the First Responder, as it can quickly build up physical barriers in cellular membranes in an attempt to slow down or stop the invasion. The plant will mobilize as much available silicon as it can to the area of infection. Studies have shown that when wheat is under attack from fungi such as powdery mildew, it responds within 20 hours by increasing the amount of silicon in the area by as much as 300-400%.

This high emergency requirement for silicon puts tremendous pressure on the root system to find and absorb as much silicon as it can for immediate transport to the site of attack. Since this great demand for silicon relies on the soil for its supply, it illustrates that the supply of silicon already inside the plant has previously been used elsewhere for deposit and polymerization processes. The current supply of silicon in the plant is therefore rendered immobile and cannot be transferred to an infected area, forcing the plant to draw on fresh sources of silicon from the soil.

One of the biggest problems with fungal infections is their production of foreign substances inside the plant, such as destructive enzymes, toxins, growth inhibitors, antibiotics, and polysaccharides. These foreign substances are extremely poisonous to the plants and can be very effective in even small quantities.

The enzymes excreted by fungi can cause cellular membranes and substances inside cells to break down, or they can artificially disrupt the plant's respiration processes by increasing its rate of respiration, thus decreasing its efficiency. Infectious activities such as these injure plants directly or they can injure plants indirectly by impairing its metabolic processes, or even making cells respond in a way that leads to other types of injuries. These toxic substances can affect all of the plant's metabolic processes in such a way as to hamper its ability to grow properly, produce yield, or reproduce. Destructive enzymes excreted by invading fungi are so damaging that they can alter the permeability of the cell's membranes. These enzymes can also block many of the plant's natural chemical reactions by acting as a chelator (binding with ions of heavy metal minerals to form compounds, rendering them useless), which would block many of the plants enzymatic processes. It is critical that plants have the mineral nutrients they need in order to protect themselves from these types of attacks.

Many times if a bacteria or fungus has successfully gained entrance into a plant by dissolving membranes, the plant's transport vessels can eventually become clogged and cause the plant to wilt. Fusarium oxysporum is one fungus that tries to dissolve this membrane in tomatoes. Marschner explains that when proper calcium levels are lacking in plant tissues, this fungus spreads and reproduces rapidly. However, when the tomato plants have as much as 500% more calcium, the plants appear healthy and resistant to attack.

Fungi can spread rapidly across the outer landscape of a plant as well as inside the plant. Water, wind, animals, birds, insects, and humans spread fungal spores that are released by fungi to reproduce, and spread across plant tissues and through the cells inside the plants. These spores can be transported hundreds of miles before germinating in a moist environment, which explains why fungi are unable to reproduce in dry weather. Recent studies in Texas have concluded that smoke drifting across the Gulf of Mexico from fires in Central America can carry fungal spores to the United States, where they colonize upon arrival.

The watery solutions inside plants are usually enough to initiate germination of spores. Research has observed that once fungi penetrate the plant's tissues, they use the flow of water and minerals in the vessels to spread and colonize the plant. Leaf spot diseases occur when bacteria penetrate the plant's stomatal openings, making the strength of the epidermal cells insignificant. Once inside the plant, the moist environment allows the bacteria to reproduce and quickly spread through the free spaces between cells.

During periods of potassium deficiencies, sugars and amino acids comprise an abnormally high concentration of the flow in leaves. The photoassimilates found in the apoplastic pathways of leaves and roots will depend on the permeability of the plasma membrane. According to observations noted by Marschner, the concentrations of sugars and amino acids along the apoplastic pathways can elevate when experiencing boron or calcium deficiencies, which increases membrane permeability and causes potassium ions to leak out of the cell, thus impairing polymer synthesis and causing hydrogen to enter the cell. This kills plant tissue (necrosis). Unusually high rates of permeability and transport inside the plant allow fungal infections to germinate and spread rapidly. However, strong potassium levels help hinder such conditions.

Seeds and fruits can illustrate potassium's effects on resistance and tolerance. During seasonal periods where potassium levels are low, the occurrence of a condition known as pod blight increases. When potassium is quickly added to the plant through the soil or through foliar application, the percentage of infected seeds have declined anywhere between 13-75%.

Farmers use potassium fertilizers to reduce fungal diseases such as Fusarium wilt (commonly found in tomatoes), rice blast, bacterial angular leaf spots in cucumbers, and stalk rot of corn. When potassium is applied alongside chlorine as potassium chloride, the incidence of stalk rots in corn decline. This decline in fungal disease is attributed to the competitive restraint of nitrogen absorption by the chloride ions. However, high concentrations of nitrogen can suppress chloride ions during competition, which results in high incidences of stalk rots.

The battle rages on. At this point, the plant can resort to producing oxygen radicals and hydrogen peroxide to fight against these parasitic attacks. This can result in hypersensitive reactions as well as strengthened membranes in an effort to damage the invading microbes. Plants need zinc, copper, iron, and manganese to produce both oxygen radicals and hydrogen peroxide, again demonstrating the need for mineral nutrition in the prevention of disease.

■ ■ ■

Bacteria are similar to fungi in that they are also very small, microscopic organisms that lack the ability to manufacture their own foods. It is estimated that over 1600 species of bacteria exist. While most are beneficial in that they decompose organic matter, some species of bacteria cause diseases in people such as tuberculosis, pneumonia, and typhoid fever. Around 180 species of bacteria are known to cause disease in plants. Bacteria are one-celled organisms that can move themselves through a medium by using their flagella, or they can transform themselves into spores for easy transport. They multiply rapidly and require warm, moist areas for their proliferation.

Potassium hinders more fungal and bacterial diseases than any other element because it is used in many cellular activities and metabolic processes. The synthesis of proteins, starches, and cellulose are all characteristic of potassium's involvement in the cell. In fact, deficiencies of potassium can result in toxic accumulations of other substances. When potassium is added to plants suffering from potassium deficiencies, growth is accelerated and toxic accumulations of these products decline until growth reaches its optimal rate. Any further increase in the potassium levels usually has little effect on the growth rate, but does provide added benefit to the plant's immune system.

Although most bacterial populations in soils are considered "friendly" bacteria, in that they release nitrogen and assist in decomposition, disease-inducing bacteria penetrate plant tissues similarly to fungi. Marschner explains that some bacteria enter a plant through its cellular membranes similarly to fungi, but some also enter through the respiratory stomata. These types of bacteria are usually transported through water, although insects and even garden tools can also play host to bacteria. Other bacteria will penetrate other openings in the plant, including wounds or stems in bark, while insects can carry bacteria and inadvertently deposit them in the plant as it feeds.

The real damage by bacteria is done after it enters the plant. Similar to fungal infections, they can clog the plant's water-carrying vessels or even absorb the supply of nutrients. Once a bacteria gains access inside a plant it is generally unable to enter through a cell membrane, but it is free to reproduce and travel throughout the free space between cells. However, there are some bacteria that will excrete destructive enzymes to break down these cellular membranes in an attempt to gain entry, which quickly results in the death of the cell. Eventually the cell collapses, releasing its water and interior contents and allowing easy access for the bacteria to enter. This process is intensified when the bacteria also releases toxins to further destroy the cell.

One of the most destructive ways bacteria afflicts a plant is when it invades the plant's vessels. Calcium's low mobility here allows for their easier reproduction and transport. Here, the bacteria can create enough slimy residues to clog this vessel, commonly known as "bacterial wilt," which is similar to human blood vessels becoming clogged. In the xylem and other vessels, they carry on their activities and continue to release destructive enzymes that break down pectic substances found throughout the vessels and neighboring tissues. When these enzymes combine with slimy polysaccharides also produced by the bacteria, together they can clog the vessels and even result in completely blocking the transport of water and minerals throughout the plant. If the bacterial disease is allowed to progress this far, it won't take long for a plant to become stunted, wilted, or die. Visual symptoms can be vaguely familiar to fungal infestation, such as chlorosis and rotting tissue.

The spread of bacteria closely resembles that of fungi, in that they also use pectolytic enzymes to dissolve membranes, but the higher the calcium content in cellular membranes, the lower the incidence of bacterial spread. The overall nutritional health of the plant plays a key role in the plant's defense mechanisms. In fact, in tissues where pectolytic enzyme activity is very high, calcium's response to infection is enhanced proportionally, until eventually the bacteria and its excreted enzymes stop functioning. When potassium and calcium are both deficient, the spread of bacteria goes unimpeded.

Experiments using tomato plants have shown an inverse relationship between the amount of calcium and the type of bacterial infection that invade and clog the vessels. These studies have concluded that without sufficient calcium, the spread of bacteria using the xylem as its mode of transport occurs uninhibited. This helps to explain the plant's natural emphasis on preventing the initial penetration through the external cellular membranes in the first place, rather than trying to deal with the infection after it has gained entry.

■ ■ ■

A virus is a microscopic organism that contains a core of nucleic acid that is surrounded by a protein coat. They can only exist and reproduce inside the tissues of a living organism, and cause many different diseases. Some viruses proliferate inside plants only, while others require the tissues of animals and humans. The number of viruses discovered is numbered in the thousands and new viruses are either discovered every year or can be hybrid creations that adapt to vaccinations. One virus can invade the tissues of many different living organisms.

A virus has a unique characteristic that separates it from other pathogens; a virus cannot be seen with a light microscope. Examining cells afflicted with a virus will not always yield virus-like particles since they are not always easy to find under electron microscopes and can go unnoticed. In fact many viruses can be pleomorphic; they can change form and shape, going unnoticed for decades.

Viruses are a major concern for plant physiologists. They do not divide or produce any type of reproductive structures such as spores, but they can multiply by forcing the host cell to create more viruses. They cause disease not by consuming any cells or tissues or creating any toxins or destructive enzymes. Rather, viruses cause diseases by upsetting and disrupting metabolic processes in cells. This can lead to the development of abnormal substances, toxic accumulations of substances, and other such conditions that create havoc with the cell's metabolism, which, in turn, leads to the abnormal development of the cell or even the manufacture of abnormal substances that can cannibalize the cell.

Plant viruses usually gain entry into a plant through wounds or punctures in tissues. They are transported through insects, such as grasshoppers, flies, mosquitoes, and aphids. These transport carriers are referred to as "vectors." Tools used in gardening and farming, and even creatures in the soil such as worms and gophers, can act as vectors.

Some research suggests that insects known as aphids spread 60% of all viruses that infect plants. Aphids insert their mouth parts into the plant, thus puncturing the tissues, and feed on the phloem sap. This allows the virus to enter the phloem without any resistance or defense from the plant. The virus that is transmitted from the aphid to the phloem is now free to roam through the plant unimpeded.

Viruses may not excrete any type of damaging substance, but they can prompt the host plant to create excessive amounts of certain substances that they may already be producing or even force it to create new substances that are completely new to the host. An example of this is when curly top virus reduces the level of starch in tomatoes by 25-30%, but induces extreme glucose and sucrose production in its leaves. This oversupply of starch is usually the result of the virus' efforts to inhibit the export of photoassimilates into the phloem, which then results in an accumulation of substances, including starches, proteins, carbohydrates, and possibly others.

It should be remembered that viruses are too large to move through healthy cell membranes—only ions are able to pass through them. This keeps their movement restricted through vessels such as the phloem or through the symplastic pathway, also known as the plasmodesmata. This network of cylindrical pathways connects cells together and allows larger products such as proteins, amino acids, vitamins, and carbohydrates to pass from cell to cell. Some viruses can inflame these passages in order to pass through. If viruses are able to pass through this system, they will be able to gain access and infect the entire plant rather quickly.

Although most research has detailed the effects of bacterial and fungal infections, research that explains the effects of viral infection is lacking. However, according to Marschner, once a virus has gained entry, multiplied and infected an entire organism, the virus's multiplication is restricted only to the living cells, and their nutritional requirements are limited to amino acids and nucleotides. Generally, nutritional requirements of the host plant tend to also benefit the virus, such as nitrogen, phosphorus, and potassium. A strong correlation between the mineral nutritional status of a plant and the success of a virus is not always evident. However, some studies have shown that supplemental mineral nutrition in deficient plants can alleviate some of the symptoms of the disease and eventually provide the plant with the tools necessary to eradicate the virus.

The main intent of a virus is not to kill the plant. Instead, it tends to weaken the plant by causing discoloration due to chlorosis in leaves and flowers, such as yellow rings or lines in the tissues. Plants that exhibit stunted growth in stems, leaves, flowers, and fruits may be infected with a virus. Some viruses can cause catastrophic damage, such as premature fruit ripening and overall crop quality to decline. Viral diseases are oftentimes very difficult to diagnose. One virus can display many different symptoms that can easily be misinterpreted as a mineral deficiency. A sample of plant tissue can be analyzed in a laboratory to determine if there is a viral infection.

Once again, this reveals how the mineral nutrition of plants influences the severity of viral infection. Minerals affect the virus as well as the vectors that spread the virus.

For example, once a virus is injected into a plant, the impact of the viral infection can be lessened with high amounts of zinc. This element depresses the watercress infection of the fungus Spongospora subterranea, which is responsible for crook rot disease. Zinc's ability to impact viral infections stems from its effectiveness against fungal infections, since many fungi are vectors of viruses.

■ ■ ■

As with all living organisms, a balanced nutrient supply is critical to the organism's development, growth, infectious resistance, and tolerance. According to Marschner, studies have shown an inverse relationship between the nutritional health of the plant and growth, on one hand, and the severity of bacterial infection on the other. It is easy to conclude that plants with an optimal level of mineral nutrition tend to have the highest levels of resistance and tolerance to infectious organisms, and that vulnerability tends to increase as this optimal nutrition level decreases. When plants are already suffering from mineral deficiencies, tolerance to pests and invading microbes also tend to decline, unless they are resupplied with appropriate mineral levels.

Even during periods of storage following the harvest, plant tissues and fruits are still susceptible to fungal attacks. Again, due to calcium's low mobility, fungal and bacterial invasions become much more likely to gain entry through the tissues, especially once the fruit is away from the protection of the tree. Premature fruit rotting can result. Growers will continue to treat their harvested fruit with foliar sprays of calcium and other minerals to prevent post-harvest disorders.

Nutrient deficiency is more than just a measurable low level of a mineral. When the term "deficiency" is used in conjunction with mineral levels, this refers to the condition where plants receive nutrients in such low amounts that their growth is stunted and impairment of its development and metabolism is a result. In other words, plants experiencing deficiencies of minerals are unable to maintain their health. The normal metabolism of plant development can slow down, which slows the growth of the plant and creates poor crop harvest. When a nutrient is found in excess, toxicities can result and even decrease the growth and development of a plant. The best way to identify whether a deficiency or toxicity is causing impairment of growth and development is to understand the mineral's function in plant metabolism and its mobility inside the plant.

Only in the past 100 years have mineral deficiencies besides the macronutrients nitrogen, phosphorus, and potassium, been discovered. Most minerals have been researched enough since then to discover what diseases will result when sufficient levels of each mineral are lacking. Not all deficiency symptoms are easily recognizable. Some symptoms can be subtle enough to create stunted growth over long periods of time or even reductions in crop yields. Reductions in growth can occur without showing visual symptoms first, or can occur long before the symptoms appear.

Epstein has documented direct evidence that supports the paramount role of calcium in the structural integrity of membranes using electron microscopes. Researchers have studied barley and corn that were calcium deficient. According to Epstein, the cells always resulted in "structureless areas, fragmented membranes, and various vesicles and amorphous inclusions." Even when magnesium levels were low these symptoms did not occur; only calcium deficiencies caused this much havoc on the cells of the plants. Other areas of the plant that resulted in disintegration were membranous organelles and chloroplasts.

Studies have documented how too much potassium in a plant can hinder calcium absorption, Subsequent experiments have observed how this increase in potassium may not automatically mean the plant is now exposed to high levels of infections. Instead, if calcium levels can remain high, the plant's defense mechanisms remain intact, but when calcium levels drop, the plant's ability to ward off bacterial and fungal invasions declines.

Macrominerals are not the only minerals that help plants fight off infections. Many observations also document the effects of microminerals on resistance to infectious diseases. Two of the plant's defense mechanisms include phenolics and lignin. Microminerals such as boron, manganese, and copper all have specific responsibilities in phenol metabolism and lignin biosynthesis. Microminerals have also shown an ability to resist diseases indirectly. When plants are deficient in microminerals, researchers such as Marschner have observed that plants can become a more suitable feeding substrate. Zinc deficiencies, for example, result in sugars which can leak onto the surface of some plant species, which increases the impact of infections from parasites such as Oidium. When plants such as wheat lack sufficient boron concentrations, powdery mildew penetrates easier and spreads more rapidly than in wheat with sufficient boron levels.

Some crop management organizations use copper as a fungicide, due to its ability to resist leaf infections, such as powdery mildew in wheat, and control stem pathogens. When used as a foliar application, as much as 10-100 times the normal copper concentrations can be used, not only to reduce infections but also to correct soil deficiencies. Marschner has observed that foliar application of copper is more successful than when applied as a soil fertilizer, since copper can bind strongly to the soil matrix. Researchers have concluded that crop yields increase substantially when fertilizers containing microminerals are applied, marking dramatic improvements in the plant's nutritional status, quality of harvest, and suppression of parasitic diseases.

Plants have a natural and instinctive ability to resist the proliferation of diseases, and calcium and phosphorus are two of the most important mineral elements that contribute to this success. Although billions of dollars are spent every year in crop management practices using chemicals and pesticides, this only addresses the symptoms of pest infestation, rather than the underlying causes of the symptoms. These two elements, when deficient, tend to predispose the plant to infectious attack since the plant's cellular membranes are then susceptible to a weakened state.

Phosphorus is caught in a dilemma that both benefits and hampers the plant's ability to fight infections. One on hand phosphorous is necessary for the root system to maintain strong rates of growth, but on the other hand if it is found in too high concentrations, the susceptibility of plants to viral invasion increases. However, sufficient phosphorus does strengthen the roots and allow for healthy root tissues to expand and multiply. In soils where fungi and multi-cellular parasites called nematodes are numerous, the root's ability to function declines, and the roots' own ability to absorb more phosphorus will also decline.

Some disease symptoms are more visible than others, but it is becoming apparent that minerals play key roles in plants, such as building cellular structures, enzymatic processes, respiration, vascular processes, and protection against infections. A lack of one can cause malabsorption of another. Minerals are absolutely vital to a plant's health and critical to the enduring production of normal fruit and flowers. Without an adequate supply of minerals, the plant weakens and becomes susceptible to infectious attack.

Chapter 8

Elements in an Apple

A discussion about minerals would be incomplete if it only talked about what minerals were found in plants without emphasizing what form these minerals were found in. Minerals come in all sorts of forms. We have seen in earlier chapters how minerals in the Earth are broken down into smaller and smaller particle sizes in order for microorganisms in the soil and the dissolving power of water to provide the final breakdown process. It is this final breakdown process that dissolves the mineral particles into their smallest form—the atom, which is the smallest particle of an element that still retains the element's identity. In Chapter 2 I explained that when one of these atoms gains or loses one or more of its electrons that orbit its nucleus, it becomes charged—either positively or negatively. At that moment, the atom is no longer considered an atom; it is then called an ion.

During periods of geologic activity, some minerals can become mixed with others to form compounds. As previously discussed, most rocks we see in deserts and mountainsides are usually a composite of two or more minerals. Calcium carbonate forms when atoms of calcium become bound with atoms of carbon, creating such features as limestone in the ocean and even regular chalk. This compound is also known as "calcite," and is sometimes used in toothpaste since it is mildly abrasive. It is one of Earth's most common mineral compounds, comprising almost 4% of Earth's crust. When calcium carbonate is present in large amounts, and given millions of years to grow, calcite crystals will form. Mining operations throughout Mexico have located vast caverns more than 300 feet long, 50 feet wide, and 20 feet in height, lined with calcite crystals.

Another example of a compound is when calcium bonds with sulfur, forming calcium sulfate. This compound can also be called hydrated calcium sulfate when large amounts of water were once present. Hydrated calcium sulfate is also known as "gypsum," which is in reference to the fact that when crystals form within calcium rich beds of sand, the sand is trapped within the structure of the gypsum crystals as they grow. Gypsum is a soft compound that is typically used as an industrial material and included as a primary ingredient in "plaster of Paris." When allowed thousands of years to form, crystals of gypsum can grow to 10 feet in length.

Although there are over 100 pure elements found in the Periodic Table of Elements, there may well be thousands of different mixtures of compounds found anywhere on Earth when these elements bond together. Copper atoms can mix with carbon and form "copper carbonate." Magnesium atoms can bind with chlorine atoms to form "magnesium chloride." Potassium atoms can bind with iodine and form "potassium iodide." And sodium, aluminum, and silicon atoms can bond to create "sodium aluminum silicate." Other such compounds are found in various locations around the world, such as copper aluminum phosphate in Arizona and beryllium aluminum silicate in Brazil.

As you can see, just about any two or more elements can mix together and create some kind of compound. This is what we find in rocks throughout Earth's crust, mantle, and core. Museums have large displays of various mixtures of elements such as calcium chloride and large chunks of copper aluminum phosphate that have been discovered in mining operations; some of their largest samples on display weigh hundreds and thousands of pounds. Other examples of minerals and their use as industrial compounds can be seen in Appendix B.

It is rare to find a large crystal or rock anywhere that is just 100% pure element and not bound together with another element. Even when heavy metals such as gold, silver, iron, copper, zinc, beryllium, and molybdenum are mined, miners usually find them bound together with another element. These compounds are melted down, or refined, to separate the two elements before their values can be extracted.

■ ■ ■

What does this discussion about compounds have to do with minerals found in plants? Everything. We have learned that in order for plants to absorb minerals found in soils, the minerals cannot exist in any type of compound. In fact, plants cannot even absorb the mineral if it is comprised of several of its own atoms bound together, in the form of a molecule. A molecule is when two or more of the same atoms are tightly bound together. Plants can only absorb minerals that have been broken down to their smallest size—the ion. In some rare circumstances, ions may form ionic compounds, but with regard to plant absorption, ions must remain independent and cannot be bound with other elements, carbon, amino acids, vitamins, or any other type of compound if they are going to be absorbed into a plant.

What should be understood at this point is that there are some natural geologic processes that have created huge deposits of mineral compounds that have bonded together into large chunks, while other natural processes are busy breaking down these compounds to prepare them for absorption into living organisms such as plants.

What many people do not realize is that just about any of the naturally-occurring elements listed on the Periodic Table of Elements can probably be found deposited in various agricultural soils somewhere around the world. Although one or two minerals may dominate the soil's mineral concentration, such as calcium or potassium, other soils may be deficient in certain minerals, while other soils may contain optimal combinations. This means that eventually these elements, some rare and some more common, could end up absorbed into plants and contributing to its overall mineral nutrition.

For example, aluminum is the third most abundant mineral (8%) in Earth's crust, following hydrogen (47% by weight) and silicon (28% by weight). There is not a square inch of soil that doesn't contain a small trace of aluminum. If the soils are rich in aluminum, then the plants will be able to use whatever benefit aluminum ions are able to provide. In fact, plants can only absorb the elements that the roots can find in the soils.

The nutritional needs of plants do vary somewhat. Some plants require larger quantities of various elements than others, insomuch that roots will continue to drill and mine deeper and deeper for those elements. But generally since plants are not always selective about which minerals to absorb or which to avoid, we can conclude that if an element is found in soils it will likely be found in the plant's tissues.

I have had the chance to speak to many people, including MD's and nutritionists from well-known universities, and I have asked them, "Would you ever eat something if you knew it had arsenic, lead, mercury, aluminum, titanium, barium, or nickel in it?" The answer always seems to be an emphatic "No way!" It is thought that minerals such as these are harmful and anything that contains these elements should be avoided. This goes to show how little we really understand about minerals, how our bodies work, and mineral nutrition.

A chemical analysis was performed on a random sampling of various fruits and vegetables grown under normal soil conditions. According to the ALT Agronomy Handbook, the following foods were analyzed and contained those trace minerals many people mistakenly think are harmful:

- Almonds—aluminum, barium, nickel, rubidium, silicon, strontium, sulfur, and titanium
- Apples—aluminum, arsenic, barium, lead, nickel, silicon, and titanium
- Broccoli—aluminum, nickel, silicon, strontium, sulfur, and titanium
- Carrots—aluminum, nickel, silicon, strontium, sulfur, and titanium
- Grapes—aluminum, barium, lithium, nickel, rubidium, silicon, strontium, and titanium
- Tomatoes—aluminum, barium, bromine, lithium, nickel, silicon, strontium, and titanium

If you are going to eat a lot of fruits and vegetables, you are going to be consuming a lot of aluminum, arsenic, barium, nickel, titanium, lithium, mercury, and lead. The important thing to remember is that many different elements can be found in any plant tissue at any given time. These elements are found as ions in the fruits, flowers, and plant tissues, and provide their various benefits to the plant that absorbed them. However, many people mistakenly think that minerals found in organic matter, such as plant tissues, are different than when the exact same minerals are also found in synthetic manmade materials.

For example, open your wallet and take out a penny. This penny is made of copper, right? Now set that penny next to a piece of broccoli. The broccoli will have many different minerals contained within it, including copper. Both the penny and the piece of broccoli contain copper. But what is the difference? Is the copper in the piece of broccoli any different than the copper in the penny?

If you swallowed the penny, you would likely get sick. But if you ate the piece of broccoli, your body would digest the broccoli and absorb the copper into the bloodstream and eventually into the cells. Why wouldn't your body react in the same way as the penny? What is the difference between these two sources of copper? After the discussion on ions and compounds, you should already be able to picture in your mind the difference between the two sources of copper, and instinctively know which form will be used and absorbed by the body and which one could cause trouble. Both contain the same copper, yes, but the piece of broccoli contains water soluble copper ions, while the penny is one large compound. The human body only has use for water soluble ions—the same as those found in plants!

Now, if you were to take the penny and bury it deep in soil, within a few years the dissolving power of water and the activity of the microorganisms in the soil would dissolve the penny until the individual copper ions were liberated and released into the soil. Even an inorganic, manmade copper compound such as a penny contains the same inorganic copper as a piece of broccoli, but until the ions are liberated from the compound, the copper is of no use to plant or human nutrition.

Similarly, people who lack iron would not gain anything by eating a nail, just like someone who is lacking calcium would not benefit from eating limestone or chalk. For the same reason, someone who swallows a nugget of "copper sulfate," for example, is unlikely to receive much benefit from copper or sulfate. Rather, copper sulfate is an insoluble compound that is a mixture of copper with sulfuric acid, and is used as a drain cleaner and to induce vomiting, and it can contaminate water supplies (see Appendix B). Consuming minerals in the form of water soluble ions is the only way living organisms can maximize their possible benefit from mineral nutrition. No matter how hungry you are, you could never gain any mineral nutrition by eating a penny, a nail, chalk, soil, or a drain cleaner.

■ ■ ■

In a study conducted by Utah State University in Logan, Utah, I submitted an organically grown and randomly selected apple to be analyzed for its mineral content to Dr. Jeff Hall of the Department of Veterinary Medicine. The apple was first homogenized to a uniform analytical sample, and then digested in trace mineral grade nitric acid. Using an ICP-MS Mineral Analysis, the apple was analyzed and it was determined that the following minerals were present in the apple (results in parts per million):

- Potassium (1,283.43)
- Phosphorus (131.70)
- Calcium (64.51)
- Magnesium (60.97)
- Sodium (37.85)
- Silicon (12.61)
- Copper (7.72)
- Boron (3.70)
- Zinc (3.29)
- Iron (2.78)
- Aluminum (0.85)
- Nickel (0.69)
- Manganese (0.48)
- Tin (0.34)
- Barium (0.29)
- Chromium (0.21)

- Strontium (0.22)
- Lead (0.12)
- Molybdenum (0.04)
- Selenium (0.01)
- Arsenic (0.01)
- Lithium (0.01)

And the following minerals were either not present or found in quantities too small to be detected

- Silver (<0.01)
- Beryllium (<0.01)
- Cadmium (<0.01)
- Cobalt (<0.01)
- Antimony (<0.01)
- Thallium (<0.01)
- Vanadium (<0.01)

That is quite an array of elements! You will notice that the macronutrients, such as potassium, calcium, and phosphorus, are present in large quantities, while the micronutrients are found in much smaller concentrations. The numbers next to the element's name represent "parts per million." For example, it was discovered that for every million particles in this apple, which include carbohydrates, amino acids, proteins, and other substances, there are 3.29 zinc ions. The number of parts per million can be viewed the same way as milligrams, which most nutritional textbooks recognize as the standard in analytical measurement. Therefore, generally speaking it can be said that this organically grown apple contained 1,283.43 milligrams of potassium.

The results of this mineral analysis show how it is possible that many different elements can be found in plant tissues at any given time, including those elements that are mistakenly feared, such as mercury, lead, arsenic, lithium, aluminum, nickel, and tin. We must remember that when an element is found in plants and fruits such as apples, their consumption does not pose any risk or have potential to become problematic. The concern about minerals is not necessarily which mineral is consumed, but rather in what form the minerals are found. If these very same elements were consumed in a compound, only then would the minerals pose a hazardous risk.

■ ■ ■

Ions from each element will all have their own level of water solubility. Solubility allows them to be transported and suspended in water, which allows them to maintain their ionic individuality and keep them from bonding together again to form molecules or compounds. For example, if an eight-ounce solution of water containing silver ions evaporated, the silver ions would bond together again and form silver molecules, making the silver no longer water-soluble and they would no longer be ions. If all the water in the solution evaporated, the silver ions would all bond together forming a tiny crystal of silver, probably worth less than one cent.

Water solubility is an extremely important concept that allows ions to float freely in water and exist without bonding and forming molecules or compounds. Due to the high water content in plant tissues, fruits, and vegetables, water solubility allows the ions to remain in their ionic state. However, the high mobility of mineral ions also makes them fragile and more prone to leaching. When ions exist freely in the soils, they are easily leached by rain, wind, and other weather conditions, and even when these water-soluble ions exist inside the leaves of plants, heavy rainfall can leach them out of the plant's tissues.

Dr. Emanuel Epstein explains that the fact that a certain element found in a plant does not necessarily imply that it has any real significance in the health of the plant. It is probable that just about any of the naturally-occurring elements found in the Periodic Table of Elements could be found in almost any soil sample taken at random across the Earth, all in varying quantities. Any plant has the potential to contain extremely trace amounts of almost any combination of most of the elements. This includes the elements needed in large quantities as well as those that are not as necessary, but are still absorbed because the plant does not make any absolute selection between elements considered essential and other elements.

Interestingly, the mineral elements considered “essential” or “beneficial” to plants closely resembles the list of minerals that are also essential or beneficial for humans. The remainder of this book will discuss the role these very same mineral ions play in human health.

Chapter 9

The Macrominerals in People

The lists of which minerals are considered macrominerals (comprising over 100 mg/day, or at least 0.01% of body weight) and microminerals (comprising less than 1 mcg/day) for humans closely resembles those for plants. Most researchers consider an element to be "essential" for humans if it meets the following criteria: 1) a lack of the mineral results in specific deficiency symptoms that respond when the mineral is supplemented, 2) adding it to the diet impacts the health, 3) it significantly contributes to tissue, fluid, or regulatory processes, and 4) it is a required part of some other essential mineral. Macrominerals considered essential are calcium, chloride, magnesium, phosphorus, potassium, sodium, and sulfur. Microminerals are also considered essential, but they are needed in fewer quantities. They are chromium, cobalt, copper, fluorine, iodine, iron, manganese, molybdenum, selenium, and zinc.

Researchers don't yet know all the minerals that we need to maintain a healthy existence, but some theorize that as many as 60 of the known 118 elements could provide dramatic health benefits. These other minerals may not necessarily be absolutely essential, but they may be able to provide various beneficial results. Many of them are considered "beneficial," such as boron, gold, lead, lithium, nickel, silicon, silver, tin, and vanadium, and will be discussed in later chapters.

However, another list of minerals should include "Honorable Mention," since there are still other minerals that also provide benefits only recently discovered and that are undergoing further research. This list includes, but is not limited to, arsenic, bromine, cadmium, and lead. Furthermore, the low quantities of these elements required are no measure of their contribution to human health. It should also be understood that the aforementioned lists of elements provide some benefit only if they are in their water soluble ionic state. See Appendix C for a side-by-side comparison of essential elements for plants and essential elements for humans.

Calcium

"Calcium" comes from the Latin word for lime, calx, and is one of Earth's most widespread minerals. Calcium is the fifth most abundant element on the planet and comprises 4.2% of Earth's crust. Because calcium binds so well with other elements, it is almost never found freely, other than the calcium ions found in plants. Rather, calcium is a metal that is usually bound to other elements to form compounds, such as calcium carbonate, calcium sulfate, or calcium lactate. Calcium carbonate is formed through intense heat to create quicklime, which is then added to water to eventually form slaked lime, a material widely used in chemical processes. It is also used to produce cleansers, white paint, stomach antacids, chalk, and toothpaste. Gypsum is a form of calcium sulfate and is used to manufacture plaster of Paris and dry wall.

Industrial uses of metallic calcium include the refining of other minerals, such as zirconium, thorium, and uranium, and helping to remove impurities such as sulfur, carbon, and oxygen, from other alloys. Calcium's strong binding ability with other alloys allows it to bind commonly with aluminum, beryllium, copper, lead, and magnesium in industrial processes. Calcium is even used in vacuum tubes to extract and remove trace gases.

Studies have shown high levels of calcium in various rocks, such as 41,500 ppm in igneous rocks, 39,000 ppm in sandstone, and 302,000 ppm in limestone. Calcium can also be found 400 ppm in ocean water, 15 ppm in fresh water, and since calcium is an extremely alkaline mineral it is not found in high quantities in acidic environments. Acidic soils have only 7,000 ppm, but alkaline soils can contain as much as 500,000 ppm calcium carbonate.

In 1808, Sir Humphrey Davy first used lime and mercuric acid to isolate calcium. In order for calcium to become useful for absorption into cells, it must first be broken down just like any other element into its water soluble ionic state. After calcium compounds such as those mentioned have been dissolved through the actions of chemical processes, weathering, and microorganisms in the soil, the liberated ions that will be found in plants are positively charged (Ca^{++}) cations. This is the only form of calcium that can be fully utilized by the body.

Calcium ions are used throughout the body for many different functions. Inside the body it can be found in three different forms: 1) as free ions (about 50% of the calcium in the fluids), 2) bound to proteins (about 40% of the calcium in the fluids), and 3) complexed with other ions (about 10% of the calcium in fluids). The widespread benefits of calcium make it one of the most important and useful elements in the human body.

Ninety-nine percent of the body's calcium can be found in the teeth, bone tissues, and bone marrow. The remaining 1% is located in blood and in bodily fluids. The calcium found in fluids outside the cells is tightly controlled and must be in very precise amounts to allow for normal physiological processes to occur optimally. Calcium's presence in the blood and fluids helps maintain the acid-alkaline balance and activates some enzymes. Males have an average of 1,200 grams and females usually have 1,000 grams of calcium, which comprise between 1-2% of total body weight, as well as 39% of our total mineral reserves. Tissue samples of animal bones have shown calcium concentrations to be 260,000 ppm, while softer tissues have 200 to 500 ppm and red blood cells around 5 ppm.

Bones are the storage sites for calcium reserves. With 99% of calcium being found in bones and teeth, it is evident that calcium plays a significant role in bone structure and teeth development. An interesting feature of bone tissue is that it is constantly undergoing a remodeling process by being dissolved and replaced. Osteoclasts are bone cells that begin this process by dissolving or resorbing bone tissue. This is followed by the osteoblasts, which are bone cells that replace the old tissue by creating new tissue. During periods of growth, such as infancy or adolescence, bone growth is greater than bone resorption.

In bone tissues and in the dentin of teeth, calcium is found as a hydroxyapatite salt, which is made up of phosphate, carbon, and calcium combined to form a crystal structure that is bound to a protein framework. In other areas of the body, the role of calcium is so profound that if calcium ions are not being consumed, the body is forced to begin taking calcium from its own bone tissues, effectively stealing from its reserves. When this occurs, the bones will begin to deteriorate and skeletal growth deformities can result.

Calcium is closely associated with hormonal activity. In fact, the level of calcium in the blood and bones is actually monitored and regulated by hormones. This is important because our internal and external environments are always changing, and in order for the body to meet this challenge it is important that our organs and tissues be able to communicate with each other. This type of internal communication is the responsibility of hormones and the circulatory system. Certain tissues and glands secrete chemical messages (hormones) into the blood to influence metabolic activities, give instructions about responding to certain conditions, and communicate with other organs.

The largest of these types of glands is the thyroid gland, which is located at the base of the neck. It secretes three hormones, two of which are made largely from iodine, and the third hormone is called calcitonin, which is made from amino acids. When the body senses that calcium levels in the blood are too high, the calcitonin hormone is secreted into blood which signals the osteoblast cells to start absorbing the excess calcium back into the bone.

However, the body also needs to have a way to respond when calcium levels are too low. The thyroid is surrounded by four very small parathyroid glands ("para" means "near"). With the help of magnesium, these four parathyroid glands secrete a hormone called parathormone, which regulates the amount of calcium, phosphate, and magnesium that are found in the blood. When this hormone is secreted, it initiates the conversion of vitamin D to another form known as calcitriol (not to be confused with calcitonin) in the kidneys to increase the absorption of calcium in the small intestines and into the blood. Together, parathormone and calcitriol sense when calcium levels in the blood are too low, and they stimulate the osteoclast cells in bone tissue to start releasing calcium from the bone reserves back into the blood. However, an adequate magnesium level largely determines the responsiveness of the osteoclasts.

Calcitriol and parathormone also work together to protect the current level of calcium by increasing its absorption into kidneys, which decreases the amount that is lost through the urine. Eventually, when the calcium in the blood reaches its optimal level, these glands stop producing the parathormone and the kidneys are free to excrete excess calcium through the urine as necessary. Through these efforts, calcitonin and parathormone are constantly trying to balance the calcium levels in the blood at an optimum level.

This system of checks and balances provides a tight control and regulation of the calcium in the blood, even at the expense of the bones. When any of these glands are unable to produce hormones, or if there is a magnesium deficiency causing these glands to malfunction, or if they are injured or accidentally removed during surgery, an imbalance of calcium can result, causing either too much calcium to be removed from the bones or too little calcium to be found in the blood. Either of these conditions will cause problems. It is important that these glands work properly because calcium has other important roles than just bone density, growth, and development.

As early as the 1960s researchers suggested that osteoporosis could be the result of improper hormonal activity. Dr. Frederic Barker of the National Heart and Lung Institute in Bethesda, Maryland stated that when blood levels of calcium are low, the parathyroid hormone is over-activated to dissolve bone in order to get blood levels of calcium normalized. If the calcium levels in blood are too low, this could suggest a malfunctioning parathyroid gland.

Calcium's role in hormonal activity also includes the secretion of insulin. Pancreatic cells must have adequate calcium in their outer cellular fluids in order to properly produce and secrete insulin. During periods of high glucose levels, insulin is supposed to be secreted to lower these levels. When calcium is lacking, insulin production is impaired from reaching its full optimal level.

A university study that was conducted in Greece showed was conducted using people who suffered from Type II diabetes and hypertension. For eight weeks half of them were given a calcium supplement and the other half were given a placebo. The study found that those who received the calcium supplement experienced higher insulin sensitivity, while the group who took the placebo did not experience any change. The study concluded that oral supplementation of calcium improves insulin sensitivity in patients who suffer from Type II diabetes and hypertension.

Calcium also plays a critical role in the central nervous system. Nerve cells, called neurons, do not look like other types of cells because their function is so different. A neuron has a central body and a long tentacle that extends outward called an axon, which can be anywhere from a few micrometers to several meters in length. Axons longer than a few micrometers are usually wrapped in a fatty layer of insulation called the "myelin sheath," which insulates the axon from the outer fluids. A disease called Multiple Sclerosis occurs when the myelin sheath deteriorates and exposes the axon to the outer fluids, which slows down or completely stops the electrical impulses traveling down the axon.

The inside of neurons contains ions from many different elements, although potassium is usually the most concentrated. Outside the neuron, sodium is highly concentrated. The cell membrane of neurons has ion channels for most elements, but again, these membranes are mostly comprised of sodium, potassium, calcium, and chloride ion channels. Fortunately, the inside of neurons contains many organic products, such as amino acids, that are negatively charged because the important ions such as sodium, potassium, and calcium are positively charged (except for chloride, which is negatively charged and is highly concentrated on the outside of the neuron). This strong negative charge helps keep the positively charged ions inside the neuron.

Neurons are always undergoing electrical changes and transmitting electrical impulses through the axon. This is how neurons are able to signal with each other, or transfer information, from one neuron to another. According to Irwin B. Levitan and Leonard K. Kaczmarek, authors of The Neuron, signaling is an important way for a person to sense information about its environment, import the information into the brain where it can be processed, and ultimately generate a behavioral response.

These electrical charges travel down the axon where they eventually reach the end. The tips of the axons do not actually touch each other; there is a small space that separates each axon from one another called a synapse. Electron microscopes have shown this gap to vary between 200 and 300 angstroms across, an area somewhat larger than the space between other cells in the body. In order for the electrical charge to travel across a synapse and reach the next neuron, a process occurs that will carry the charge across. This flow of ions through the neuron is responsible for the transfer of all electrical impulses.

According to The Neuron, it has been known since the 1800s that calcium is crucial to the transfer of electrical charges between neurons. When an electrical charge reaches the end of an axon and needs to be transmitted across the synapse, calcium in the outer fluid quickly travels through the ion channels into the axon. The calcium stimulates the secretion of a chemical fluid called a neurotransmitter that will be secreted from the axon and will carry the electrical charge across the synapse and into the neighboring neuron. At most synapses, if calcium ions are lacking in the external fluids, the axons are unable to release neurotransmitters and the transfer of electrical impulses is stopped. However, if the level of calcium in the outer fluid is highly concentrated, the amount of neurotransmitter that is released is greatly enhanced. Using electrical measurements, it is understood that the release of neurotransmitters depends largely upon the presence of high concentrations of calcium, release is more sensitive to calcium than any other ion, and release is rapid once calcium enters the neuron.

For everyday thought, reasoning, and other mental activities, humans use, on average, over 60 different neurotransmitters that all provide their own unique function. Interestingly, it is possible for one neuron to produce more than one neurotransmitter, and each neuron can have as many as 10,000 synapses, altogether producing a wide range of messages that can be sent and received.

Other ions present in the outer fluids can either impede the work of calcium or stop it altogether. These ion channels are so sensitive that if other elements such as cadmium, nickel, cobalt, manganese, or lanthanum are present, they can act as a channel blocker for the more important calcium ions, thus preventing the release of neurotransmitters. Other elements such as strontium or barium can substitute for calcium and enter the neuron through the calcium ion channels, but the release of the neurotransmitter will be much slower. However, if calcium is found in high concentrations in the outer fluids, neither of these two scenarios are likely.

Neurotransmitters keep brain signals properly communicating and ensure proper transmission of nerve impulses. These nerve impulses are important to muscle contraction and also help to regulate heartbeat and nerve stimulation, which helps with muscle growth and reflexes. Some well-known neurotransmitters affected by calcium include serotonin, acetylcholine, dopamine, and norepinephrine. Calcium ions are also used by the body to transport energy produced during protein synthesis (ATP) to allow for the transmission of electrical impulses from nerves to muscles. A severe lack of minerals such as calcium, potassium, cobalt, copper, manganese, and sodium can result in many different nervous system and behavioral disorders, such as cramps and convulsions, and even a deterioration of the myelin sheath, resulting in conditions such as Multiple Sclerosis.

The release of neurotransmitters is ultimately dependent on calcium's presence inside the neuron and in the outer fluids. However, as essential as calcium is in contributing to the release of neurotransmitters, its role is even more important for the interior of neurons. After calcium ions travel through the ion channels and enter the neuron, they interact with proteins to activate enzymes and they help regulate the ion channels of other minerals.

Calcium's role in the nervous system also influences muscles. According to the Linus Pauling Institute at Oregon State University, when a muscle fiber receives a nerve impulse stimulating it to contract, calcium ion channels open up to allow a few ions into the muscle cell, which then become bound to activator proteins that trigger the flood of calcium ions to be released from storage compartments inside the cell. Calcium can bind with a protein called troponin-c, triggering a series of steps that results in muscle contraction, or it can bind with the protein calmodulin to activate enzymes that break down muscle glycogen (sugar), which provides energy for the muscle contraction.

Most people don't realize that in order for calcium to perform many of its roles in the body, certain other substances such as vitamins A, C, and D, and the minerals phosphate, iodine, boron, copper, and magnesium, as well as the hormone calcitriol which is made from vitamin D, must be present. Lack of any one of these nutrients can lead to improper utilization of calcium. In soils, plants, and in people, calcium ions are not very mobile. Fortunately, elements such as magnesium help regulate the movement of calcium throughout the body. Magnesium is widely known as a calcium-catalyst because it assists calcium with its movement inside the cells.

Since magnesium is critical for the proper utilization of calcium in the bones, supplementing with magnesium can help maintain bone tissue and structure. Women who have taken water-soluble magnesium and calcium have reported relief from premenstrual cramps. Over time, if magnesium is missing in the diet, or if calcium compounds are consumed, either one of these conditions can result in unusable calcium. This can cause calcium to be leached from the bones and be deposited in various soft tissues throughout the body, where up to 30% of the energy created in the cell is being used to pump the calcium out of the bone tissue. Using this much energy for this purpose could explain why some women exhaust so easily. It is suggested that Premenstrual Syndrome (PMS) is this calcification of female body parts, which is provoked by insufficient magnesium or regular consumption of insoluble calcium compounds. Furthermore, it should also be mentioned that when magnesium levels in the body are adequate, the body uses all the calcium ions it needs and discharges any excess without any toxicity. Clearly this is one example of how a deficiency of one mineral can result in an excess or shortage of another.

In 1966, Dr. Lewis Barnett studied magnesium's relationship with calcium by examining the drinking water of two Texas cities, Dallas and Hereford. According to his observations, femur and neck fractures were noticeably higher in Dallas than in Hereford, and he sought to find out what could be the cause. His investigation showed that the average age of a fracture in Hereford was 82 and experienced healing within 8 weeks. However, in Dallas the average age was 63 and it took them an average of six months to heal. Water samples from both cities showed that Hereford's magnesium content was double (8 ppm) that of Dallas. Also, bone samples of subjects in Dallas showed magnesium's concentration in the bone was only 0.5%, while Hereford's bone samples showed a remarkable 1.76% magnesium content. This was one of the first studies that clearly showed the relationship between magnesium and calcium. He concluded that magnesium prevents the pituitary gland from over-functioning.

Some municipal water systems add calcium and magnesium to its water, creating what is commonly known as hard water. Although the intent is to provide extra minerals to the users of the water, there are a few instances where the results can be negative. These minerals can react with soap residues to form soap scum, commonly found as the buildup in baths and shower stalls. Also, insoluble compounds may form if the water is ever heated, which would deposit and begin to build up inside the plumbing system or on the bath or shower walls. When water that contains calcium and carbonate ions is heated, carbon dioxide evaporates, leaving behind a highly alkaline and insoluble compound known as calcium carbonate, which lines the inner surfaces of pipes, causing a buildup known as "scale." This buildup decreases the flow of water and heating efficiency. In order to remove these insoluble compounds, water is "limed," which is an acidic treatment used to decrease the pH in an effort to "soften" the water.

Researchers in England studied the role of calcium on spinal development and health just by studying users of hard water versus soft water. In their observations, infants experiencing deformed brains and spinal cords tended to use soft water, while hard water households rarely experienced symptoms of spina bifida or other nervous system disorders. Calcium and magnesium are major ingredients in hard water.

When an excess of insoluble calcium is consumed, certain symptoms considered normal could result. According to Dr. D. H. Copp, a retired professor at the University of British Columbia, the thyroid controls and regulates the calcium levels. Calcium deficiencies can possibly be a direct result of improper calcium management from a malfunctioning thyroid or excess insoluble calcium. Kidney stones, gallstones, and even cardiac problems are all characteristics of accumulations of insoluble calcium, or calcium deficiency resulting in the buildup of saturated fats.

Water-soluble calcium serves many functions in the body, including the removal of insoluble calcium compounds that have accumulated in bone, teeth, and soft tissues, as well as compounds that have been deposited in other places, forming kidney stones or arthritis. Although some have theorized that excess calcium compounds result in kidney stones, proper calcium ions are known to inhibit these formations and other conditions such as gallstones, arthritis, and high cholesterol. Water-soluble calcium can also reverse conditions characterized by a calcium deficiency such as osteoporosis and cardiovascular irregularities.

Calcium ions perform other functions in the blood, such as activating the fibrous protein fibrin and stimulating the production of red blood cells responsible for blood clotting. If the calcium found in blood is water-soluble, it softens and relaxes blood vessels, helping to normalize blood pressure. However, insoluble calcium compounds float around in the blood where it settles, hardens, and gums up the tissues of blood vessels, in much the same way as it does to household plumbing. Water-soluble calcium is so effective at regulating blood pressure that someone could have high sodium intake but not have high blood pressure if they are consuming the right form of calcium.

Some studies have shown an extreme lack of calcium in patients with untreated hypertension. A four-year investigation involving over 58,000 nurses showed salt sensitivity was much more likely to occur in those who consumed low levels of calcium. The body uses over one-half of the calcium ions that exist in the blood for this and other arterial purposes.

Cells are bound together to form bones, organs, and our skin, to create the architecture of our tissues through cell adhesion. Cell adhesion occurs when various forms of proteins are uniformly distributed and held together along the outer plasma membranes that come into contact with other similar cells. This region is stabilized and specialized to allow or prevent ions and molecules from passing from one cell to another through gap junctions—a tight system of channels that connect and hold similar cells together. There are three different forms of these cell adhesion proteins: the cadherins, selectins, and immunglobulin superfamily. The first two, cadherins and selectins, depend upon calcium ions. The cadherins are a group of calcium dependent molecules needed for tissue differentiation and structure, and the majority can be found in the brain. Thus, cell adhesion is literally the glue that holds us together, and is inoperable unless calcium ions are present.

Deep inside the tissues, calcium, along with zinc, aids the transport of substances into and out of the cell membranes. It permits other mineral ions, vitamins, and other necessary substances to enter the cell, while allowing the excretion of toxins to exit the cell. When proper water-soluble calcium ions are deficient, cellular breakage can occur, allowing improper substances to enter the cells and mineral ions to exit. Calcium's ability to regulate the entry and exit of products from the cell also provides protection against infectious organisms, such as bacteria, molds, parasites, and viruses.

Calcium performs other critical functions inside the cells. Its presence helps the cell communicate with others cells, a process known as cell signaling. Calcium also helps to raise the body's pH level to a safe, neutral range. This is important because infectious pathogens are unable to live in an environment of high pH. Some have reported putting water-soluble calcium ions in water vaporizers and watching children's coughs disappear within 30 minutes. Pure calcium ions prepared in clean water can also be used as a non-toxic optical eyewash to clear out bacteria or other contaminants, even being mixed with zinc and silver, without causing any type of irritation.

Calcium's responsibility to govern what enters and exits a cell also allows it to protect against atmospheric pollutants and industrial contaminants. There are two ways that calcium can protect against lead toxicity. An increase in dietary calcium reduces the absorption of lead in the intestines where it would have become deposited in bones, and can remain there for more than 20 years. Also, during periods of bone growth, calcium provides some protection against lead that has become remobilized back into the bloodstream.

Certain acids can inhibit the absorption and utilization of calcium. Phytic acid, found in wheat and bread products, can interfere with calcium absorption because it can induce the formation of insoluble calcium phytate (known as precipitation) on the walls of the gastrointestinal tract. Cereals and other bread products, coupled with this lack of soluble calcium and a lack of vitamin D, can result in a condition known as rickets. Also, pharmaceutical drugs such as penicillin, neomycin, and Chloromycetin tend to increase the body's requirement for calcium, while steroids such as prednisone and dexamethasone can decrease the body's rate of calcium absorption.

In studies using animals, increased sodium intake resulted in excess loss of calcium through the urine. It is theorized that this results from competition between calcium and sodium for absorption into the kidney, or the sodium has a negative effect on the parathyroid. Some animal studies observed increased bone loss during periods of high salt consumption. Other experiments have shown high protein consumption corresponding with increased urinary loss of calcium. As a result, the recommended daily intake of calcium is greater than that found in other countries due to our tendency to eat high amounts of protein. Some have reported that for every gram of protein consumed over and above the RDA limit, a loss of 1.75 mg of calcium per day results.

Phosphorus-rich foods such as carbonated soft drinks and high-protein foods can decrease the amount of calcium being absorbed, thus increasing the amount of calcium being lost through the feces. Caffeine increases the loss of calcium through the urine. High-protein diets and low calcium-rich foods can decrease the amount of parathormone secretion. Some nutritional researchers are concerned about the amount of calcium being lost due to heavy consumption of soft drinks.

High fat diets can influence the utilization and effectiveness of calcium. Excess consumption of saturated fat (bad fat) can raise LDL-cholesterol, increase susceptibility of colorectal cancer, and increase the likelihood of forming gallstones. However, calcium ions can bind with saturated fats, which prevents their absorption into the intestine and blood. Thus, adequate calcium can lower risks associated with high LDL-cholesterol levels and similar cardiovascular conditions. However, the calcium ions that bind with saturated fats will then be utilized and unable to perform various other functions.

Calcium and vitamin D both help to produce stomach acidity. Water-soluble calcium ions taken as a supplement are absorbed in the upper stomach by immediately passing through the tissues' ion channels through simple diffusion, skipping the usual digestion process if they would have been supplied through plants. They are immediately routed directly into the body's fluids where they go to work neutralizing the pH of the body.

Laboratory studies using animals have shown calcium to play a preventative role against various intestinal cancers. People supplementing with 1,200-2,000 mg/day calcium have shown a marked decrease in precancerous polyps. Although this decrease was not significant, it does show the potential of the human body once it has minerals in place, and studies such as these would very likely experience dramatic results when using pure calcium ions rather than compounds in their research.

Some people develop a condition known as hypercalcemia, which is a toxic accumulation of insoluble calcium compounds, characterized by a loss of appetite, vomiting, nausea, frequent urination, abdominal pain, and constipation. Extreme cases can include mental disorders such as confusion and delirium, along with coma and even death. This condition never develops from plant food sources containing water-soluble calcium ions. Instead, it develops only in cases where calcium compounds in a supplement were heavily consumed, especially when being combined with antacids. Hypercalcemia was more common when peptic ulcers were being treated with milk, calcium carbonate, and sodium bicarbonate.

Such conditions make the kidneys and urinary tracts work overtime. They are busy trying to excrete as much of this unusable calcium as they can that did not end up deposited in tissues. Kidney stones, arthritis, and cardiovascular problems arise during periods of high kidney and urinary excretion of insoluble calcium.

Most of the research with calcium has involved calcium compounds rather than true, non-toxic, water-soluble calcium ions in the same form as those found in plants. As early as 1968, researchers such as Dr. Carla J. Pfeiffer, who was at that time director of the Institute of Gastroenterology, suggested a problem in relying on the current governmental recommended daily allowances of certain minerals, including calcium. The problem occurs when a person follows the guidelines but still doesn't get enough calcium, because it may have been bound to another element, excreted through the digestive system too fast and not absorbed, or was removed from the blood by the kidneys. What should be realized at this point is that these studies and the Recommended Daily Allowances were studied using insoluble calcium compounds, such as calcium carbonate, in their research. Ionic calcium, such as that found in plants (Ca^{++}), is water-soluble and will not result in the dire circumstances that Dr. Pfeiffer mentioned, or in the health conditions described.

Another research study centers on the over-consumption of calcium compounds as being a catalyst for prostate cancer. After studying over 50,000 male health professionals from around the United States for eight years, those who consumed over 2,000 mg/day of calcium compounds had three times the risk of developing advanced cancer in their prostate glands when compared to those who took 500 mg/day. Similar findings were reported in Sweden, although another study using calcium did show a decrease in prostate cancer risk when calcium consumption was high. Even more evidence from studies has shown increased rates of prostate cancer among men who consume large amounts of dairy products, which also contain calcium compounds. These complex interactions could probably be better understood if the form of the calcium being consumed was investigated. Such symptoms do not occur when the calcium being consumed is derived from plants in its water-soluble ionic state.

Calcium is needed in every organ in the body, including the thyroid, pancreas, heart, and brain. It is called the "knitter" because of its incredible healing properties, and is valuable for muscular strength, energy, endurance, power, and tone. It helps transmit electrical impulses in the nervous system, regulate heartbeat, normalize blood pressure, regulate metabolism, normalize the body's pH, and blood clotting. Many elements, vitamins, and hormones help increase the absorption of calcium, while sodium ions help to keep calcium in a soluble form. Calcium can also help with iron and vitamin B12 absorption.

Symptoms of long-term calcium deficiency, other than what has already been mentioned, can include insomnia, irregular heart patterns, muscle spasms, arthritis, acidosis, asthma, attention deficit disorder, constipation, cavities, cataracts, enlarged heart, Bell's palsy, and high cholesterol.

Sources of water-soluble calcium ions include nuts and seeds such as almonds, walnuts, and pecans. Other vegetative sources include green leafy vegetables. Fruits also contain calcium in quantities large enough to help the fruit develop and ripen, but due to calcium's low mobility, they will contain less calcium when compared to green leafy vegetables or nuts and seeds.

Chlorine

"Chlorine" comes from the Greek word for greenish yellow, chloros. It is a poisonous gas that can burn the skin and irritate mucous membranes, and is so reactive that it continuously tries to bind with other elements to create compounds. It is the 17th atomic number on the Periodic Table of Elements, which means that each atom of chlorine contains 17 protons inside the nucleus and has 17 electrons orbiting it. Remember, at this point regular chlorine atoms are not positively or negatively charged—they are neutral. However, when a chlorine atom gains an extra electron, making the total 18, it becomes negatively charged, which changes the entire chemical structure of the element. It then becomes an ion, and is no longer known as chlorine, but is referred to in its ionic form as chloride (Cl-), which is what is found in plants. Chloride should never be confused with chlorine—they are extremely different.

Chlorine was first isolated by the German scientist Carl Wilhelm Scheele in 1774. It easily binds with other elements, which means chloride is rarely found in nature, other than in plants and soils. For example, when an atom of sodium binds with an atom of chlorine, one of the 11 electrons from the sodium atom will leave and join the 17 electrons in the atom of chlorine. The sodium atom will now have 10 electrons, making it positively charged since it has lost one of its electrons, and the chlorine atom will now have 18 electrons, making it negatively charged since it has gained a new electron. The chemical compound that results when this occurs is sodium chloride (commonly known as table salt).

Chloride is an essential mineral and benefits the human body, and it is uncommon to have a chloride deficiency since it is found in so many foods. When consumed through food, chloride is usually absorbed in the gastrointestinal tract and aids in both digestion and metabolism. The body absorbs chloride into the gastric lumen, which is then exchanged for a positively charged ion in order to maintain a neutrally charged environment in the stomach membrane.

Chloride is a component of gastric juices, where it acts as a cofactor in the enzyme amylase that breaks down starches. It also binds with hydrogen in the stomach to make hydrochloric acid, which is the fluid that breaks down protein before they become part of enzymatic processes. Hydrochloric acid also helps produce the intrinsic factor, which is the protein that aids in vitamin B12 absorption (see cobalt). Once the chloride is used in the production of hydrochloric acid, some chloride passes through the tissues and is absorbed into the bloodstream where it reaches most of the body's fluids.

There are not too many other elements in the blood that are negatively charged, so chloride represents about 70% of all negatively charged ions. Although potassium's concentration inside the cell is thirty times greater than outside and is one of the most common elements inside cells, the concentration of chloride is ten times larger outside the cell walls than inside cells. In this role, chloride helps to regulate water, fluid balance, and pressure in the body, and it helps to control the flow of ions and waste products into and out of cells. When the negatively charged chloride moves into the nerve cells, it helps to stimulate the nerve's electrical potential.

Chloride is water-soluble, which allows chloride to work with other ions, such as potassium and sodium, to assist in the electrical conduction of impulses. When these three minerals first dissolve and become ions, chlorine has gained an electron and becomes negatively charged, while potassium and sodium have both lost an electron, making them positively charged. One of the most interesting aspects of chemical elements in nature is that many times a positively charged ion will be accompanied by a negatively charged ion; therefore, in the body sodium and potassium are frequently accompanied by chloride to provide some electrical balance of charges in the blood. Chloride is absorbed both passively and actively, and is constantly being exchanged with bicarbonate between red blood cells and the blood plasma. This regulates both the pH balance and the transport of carbon dioxide, which is a waste product of respiration.

The body's highest concentration of chloride can be found in the digestive organs and in the cerebrospinal fluid. However, chloride can also be found in bodily fluids such as blood plasma and optical fluids. It makes up as high as 3% of the total mineral content of the body and it can represent 0.15% of body weight. Events that are known to expel sodium, such as sweating, vomiting, and diarrhea, can also excrete chloride. Chloride has even been observed stimulating the liver, regulating the spread of hormones throughout the body, and keeping collagen firm and strong, thus keeping skin, tendons, and joints in good condition.

Chlorine (not chloride) is used as a cleansing agent in swimming pools and municipal water systems. According to Dr. Gary Price Todd, MD, chlorine acts as an oxidant and destroys vitamin E. Studies conducted during the 1950s proved that chlorine's presence in drinking water resulted in hardening of the arteries, or atherosclerosis, in chickens. The cooking and canning processes, which use chlorine, as well as bleaching of flour, also result in the loss of vitamin E.

Although rare, chloride deficiencies can result in severe conditions. The acid/alkaline balance of the body is always in constant flux. During chloride deficiencies, the body's pH level can become disrupted, resulting in a condition known as alkalosis, which is where the blood pH level becomes extremely alkaline for a prolonged period of time. This condition can also occur when sodium levels are too low, such as after a prolonged sweating, diarrhea, or even vomiting. Low levels of chloride can result in poor muscular contraction, muscle weakness, heartburn, improper elimination, impaired digestion, loss of appetite, dehydration, fatigue, and even hair and teeth loss. Infants who were inadvertently fed chloride-deficient formulas experienced lack of stamina, anorexia, and overall weakness during their first 12 months.

Healthy sources of chloride include kiwi fruit, coconuts, olives, seaweed, tomatoes, avocadoes, celery, lettuce, and any other fruit or vegetable that usually has a "salty" taste.

Magnesium

Named after Magnesia, an area in Thessaly, Greece, magnesium is the 8th most plentiful element in the universe, and is the 7th most abundant element in Earth's crust. Although it is almost always bound to other elements, magnesium ions can still be found readily available in soils for plant absorption. In 1808, Sir Humphrey Davy first isolated and identified magnesium.

Magnesium alloys are usually comprised of magnesium and aluminum in the manufacture of aircraft parts, missiles, and rockets. Epsom salt, also known as hydrated magnesium sulfate, was discovered in 1618 by a farmer whose cows refused to drink the water from a certain well. After tasting its bitterness, the farmer noticed that it helped to heal scratches and rashes on his skin. Even today, Epsom salt is still used for similar applications. Magnesium carbonate is a compound that is used in dyes and paints and prevents caking in table salt.

Magnesium is one of the most essential of all minerals. It is second only to potassium in total content of all positively charged ions (cations) inside cells. A normal adult body contains between 20 and 30 total grams of magnesium, comprising approximately 0.05% of their total body weight. Most estimates show that 60% of the total magnesium content is found in the bones, 27% is contained in liver and muscle tissues, 6-7% can be found performing functions in other various tissues, and the remaining is usually found outside the cells.

Some cellular processes such as energy production require magnesium in order to function. It is required for all of the body's major biochemical processes, including, but not limited to, the production of cellular energy (ATP), the metabolism of glucose (blood sugar), and even the synthesis of various types of proteins and nucleic acids. ATP is a molecule that provides energy for most of the body's metabolic processes. One of the roles of mitochondria inside the cell is to synthesize protein by using ATP produced from magnesium. When magnesium and calcium are found in the fluids outside the cell walls, they aid the body in transporting other cells from one place to another, which is an important part of healing.

Essential molecules inside cells need magnesium in order to function properly. Magnesium-containing ATP is involved in the production of cyclic adenosine monophosphate, a molecule involved in cell signaling as well as many other cellular processes, such as the secretion of the parathyroid hormone (PTH). Also, magnesium's role in DNA and other types of substances and metabolic processes is profound. Nucleic acids are substances found in all cells that carry the genetic code called DNA, which is found in the nucleus of the cells. Nucleic acids such as DNA, RNA, and proteins, as well as glutathione, a powerful antioxidant, need magnesium during some of the stages of their synthesis.

There are more than 300 enzymes that need various magnesium-ATP complexes as a cofactor. Also, the energy known as ATP cannot be produced unless magnesium is inside the cells. ATP is found in all cells, and this energy is used for several different biochemical processes including the metabolism of other minerals and muscle contraction. This energy is then used to transport other minerals and substances into the cells through ion channels and protein transport systems. The electrical potential of cellular membranes is also governed by magnesium's presence, while the structural integrity of membranes and chromosomes is greatly increased when magnesium is present.

There is evidence that magnesium is required for both the electrical transmission of nerve impulses and muscle contractions. The health of the nervous system requires magnesium's presence outside the cells (extra-cellularly), especially in the nerve endings where electrical impulses get transferred from one nerve ending to another. All movements of the body are initiated by the electrical impulses transferred through the nervous system, which triggers movement in the muscles. The primary regulator of this electrical activity in the human body is magnesium. Energy produced during protein synthesis is transferred to provide for the excitability of nerves, which then results in the contractions of the muscles. Some observations have shown relieved tensions and an overall feeling of relaxation after taking magnesium supplements.

Long-term deficiencies of magnesium in the nervous system include behavioral disorders such as depression, loss of appetite, anorexia, confusion, apathy, and irritability, as well as other nervous system problems such as menstrual migraines, neuromuscular problems, tremors, headaches, muscle weakness, loss of balance, and poor coordination. An experiment performed by the Southampton General Hospital in England observed patients suffering from chronic fatigue syndrome (CFS) experienced heightened mental states and elevated energy levels after supplementing with magnesium.

Using laboratory rats, investigations into the role of magnesium on behavior has shown this element to have a complex relationship with aggressive behaviors. According to Dr. Melvyn Werbach, a deficiency of magnesium increases aggressive behaviors, but also increases defensive aggressive behavior. Decreased levels of magnesium usually resulted in increased attacks on intruders, while adequate magnesium levels decreased such attacks.

In the December 2, 2004 issue of Neuron, researchers at the Massachusetts Institute of Technology examined how magnesium affects learning and memory. They discovered that this mineral helps regulate an important brain receptor and that its presence in the cerebrospinal fluid "is essential for maintaining the plasticity of synapses."

Plasticity refers to the ability to change, which is critical to brain activity. In their study the researchers realized how important magnesium is to someone's ability to learn and remember. Their findings suggest that magnesium deficiency can decrease someone's ability to learn and memorize. It is estimated that the average American adult consumes less than half the recommended requirement of magnesium.

Dr. Werbach also explains how other studies have shown how magnesium deficiencies result in increased secretion of catecholamine and increased sensitivity to stress, all of which encourage aggressive behavior. When secretion of catecholamines increases, intracellular magnesium is lost, followed by increased urinary excretion of magnesium. Some have suggested that the Type A behavior, characterized by chronic stress and aggressive behavior, could be caused by magnesium deficiencies.

Another investigation into magnesium's effects on psychological conditions was performed by the French scientist M.L. Robinet, who observed soil samples taken from various parts of the country. Strangely, in areas where magnesium levels were low, the rate of suicide was consistently higher. He also acknowledged that people who had healthy magnesium levels tended to have a more stable equilibrium. In the Journal of Orthomolecular Medicine (1995), Dr. Melvyn Werbach explains that suicide attempts, which are violently aggressive acts against the self, can be attributed to low magnesium levels in the cerebrospinal fluid.

A retired orthopedic surgeon, Dr. Lewis Barnett, observed magnesium's role in the function of the pituitary gland. When magnesium is lacking, this gland is unable to perform its thermal static control over the adrenals, which then results in an overproduction of adrenaline. He noted huge surges of adrenaline would often be followed shortly thereafter by suicide attempts. Dr. Barnett's findings also showed that those who over-consume protein were much more likely to suffer from magnesium deficiencies, and more prone to these types of conditions.

With regards to regulating nerve impulses and muscle contraction, magnesium plays a very important role in the cardiovascular system. Recent data shows how magnesium affects heart disease and irregular heartbeat. Some pharmacological evidence points to magnesium ions being supplemented and helping in the treatment of cardiac arrhythmia, possibly due to its role as a blocker of insoluble calcium. Some epidemiological observations using people and animal subjects have shown protection from atherogenesis and an improved blood lipid profile when their diets were supplemented with magnesium.

Many studies have found a relationship between cardiovascular mortality and the level of calcium and magnesium in drinking water, otherwise known as hard water. As early as 1966, an orthopedic surgeon named Dr. Lewis Barnett studied magnesium's relationship with calcium by examining the drinking water of two Texas cities, Dallas and Hereford. According to his observations, femur and neck fractures were noticeably higher in Dallas than in Hereford, and he sought to find out what could be the cause. His investigation showed that the average age of someone with a fracture in Hereford was 82 and they experienced healing within 8 weeks. However, in Dallas the average age was 63 and it took them around six months to heal. Water samples from both cities showed that Hereford's magnesium content was double (8 ppm) that of Dallas. Also, bone samples of subjects in Dallas showed magnesium's concentration in the bone was only 0.5%, while Hereford's bone samples showed a remarkable 1.76% magnesium content. This was one of the first studies that clearly showed the relationship between magnesium and calcium. He concluded that magnesium prevents the pituitary gland from over-functioning.

Another study was conducted in Sweden that collected data on 27 municipalities and the level of hardness in their drinking water. An inverse relationship was found between hardness and cardiovascular death. The study concluded that the data supports results from previous studies that suggest that a high magnesium level in drinking water reduces the risk of death from ischemic heart disease, especially among men.

Some municipal water systems add calcium and magnesium to its water, creating what is commonly known as hard water. Although some municipal water systems add calcium and magnesium to their water to provide extra minerals to the users of the water, there are a few instances where the results can be negative. These minerals can react with soap residues to form soap scum, commonly found as the buildup in baths and shower stalls. Also, insoluble compounds may form if the water is ever heated, which would deposit and begin to build up inside the plumbing system or on the bath or shower walls. When water that contains calcium and carbonate ions is heated, carbon dioxide evaporates, leaving behind a highly alkaline and insoluble compound known as calcium carbonate, which lines the inner surfaces of pipes, causing a buildup known as "scale." This buildup decreases the flow of water and heating efficiency. In order to remove these insoluble compounds, water is "limed," which is an acidic treatment used to decrease the pH in an effort to "soften" the water.

Researchers in England studied the role of calcium on spinal development and health just by studying users of hard water versus soft water. In their observations, infants experiencing deformed brains and spinal cords tended to use soft water, while hard water households rarely experienced symptoms of spina bifida or other nervous system disorders. Calcium and magnesium are major ingredients in hard water.

Adequate magnesium levels have also been recognized to control blood pressure. As the editor of the British Journal of Clinical Practice, Dr. Eric Trimmer observed that when magnesium levels decrease, this marks a corresponding increase in blood pressure. He further observed that when large doses of magnesium were infused into patients who suffered from hypertension, blood pressure decreased rather quickly. Some have observed magnesium affecting cholesterol levels since it influences how choline prevents the buildup of cholesterol. Also, experiments performed by the University of Naples in Italy watched older people improve insulin resistance after supplementing with magnesium.

Other experiments using rats have shown magnesium's role in decreasing the susceptibility to peroxidation of tissues and lipoproteins, and some emergency rooms use magnesium to alleviate and control damage in heart attack victims. Some cardiology journals have compared those who entered and eventually exited emergency rooms from heart attacks is determined largely on the magnesium supply in their blood. Different experiments have injected magnesium into heart attack patients as soon as they arrive in the hospital—doubling their chances of staying alive.

One study involved a randomized, placebo-controlled study using over 2,000 patients and found a decline in mortality by more than 10% in patients who were provided with supplemental magnesium shortly after suffering a heart attack. Within five years after the heart attack, patients who continued to take magnesium supplements were 21% less likely to suffer from other forms of cardiovascular disease. Other studies suggest that there are higher death rates from ischemic heart disease in areas of the country that use soft water. Soft water does not contain calcium or magnesium—hard water does.

For many years, magnesium and calcium were provided to pregnant women to relieve suffering from a condition known as preeclampsia, which is characterized by high blood pressure, swelling, and urinal discharge of protein, usually occurring after the 20th week of pregnancy. If this condition becomes severe, seizures can occur, causing a condition known then as eclampsia, largely the result of spasms in blood vessels that restrict blood flow to the brain.

A Journal of the American Medical Association article reported a group of researchers who studied 1,033 hospital patients and found that 54 percent of those suffering from heart problems were lacking magnesium, who eventually died of magnesium-related problems. If studies such as these are accurate, more importantly it suggests that people's diets are inadequate.

Cells that line the inside of arteries that are in constant contact with the flowing blood are known as endothelial cells. These cells are responsible for continuous blood flow and the formation of blood clots. However, the arteries can develop an arterial plaque which lines the inside of the blood vessels and impairs the functioning of these endothelial cells, which is a condition known as atherosclerosis. This increases the risk of restricted blood flow, which can result in heart attacks or strokes. Supplementing with magnesium has shown some improvement in endothelial cell performance. For example, one observation using a randomized, double blind, placebo-controlled study showed that those who suffer from these cardiovascular conditions experienced a 12% improvement in blood flow, and an improved ability to exercise, following magnesium supplementation.

Low levels of magnesium can result in irregular heartbeat, resulting in a potential heart attack. An interesting study was conducted by researchers Ilseri and co-workers using magnesium on patients who suffered from ventricular dysrhytymias. Blood samples showed that sufficient magnesium was present in the blood. However, magnesium was deficient inside the cells, suggesting that either the form of magnesium that was in the blood was an insoluble compound and not capable of passing through the ion channels to reach the inside of the cells, or there was not enough magnesium to prevent the cardiovascular problems in the first place. Only water-soluble magnesium ions are going to provide appropriate benefits. Researchers Kohen and Kitzes also documented such findings.

It is inside the cell where magnesium will really provide the benefits people need. Some research suggests that when magnesium levels are low, the ribosomes containing nucleic acids and DNA will weaken, and functions involving the mitochondria become impaired. Samples of blood can show misleading magnesium levels as it may not reflect the magnesium concentrations inside cellular membranes. Some researchers have explored a new testing procedure called the Essential Metabolic Analyst to perform such examinations. Researchers Pike and Brown state, "Whatever the nutritional potential of an element or food, that contribution is nonexistent if it isn't absorbed." They further explain, "Nutrients that never pass through the intestinal muscosala cell to enter the circulation, for all nutritional intent and purposes, have never been eaten or utilized."

Investigations using magnesium to help diabetics have recognized that 25-38% of insulin dependent and non-insulin dependent diabetics are lacking proper levels of magnesium. This deficiency of magnesium could be the result of excess urinary excretion of glucose. Preliminary studies have shown that magnesium may be beneficial in controlling glucose levels and improving glucose tolerance.

Magnesium ions are required for the optimal absorption of other minerals, such as phosphorus, potassium, sodium, and calcium, by helping to transport them across the ion channels and into the cells. In fact, the pump that pumps potassium into the cell is a magnesium-dependent enzyme that needs magnesium in order to function. Therefore, a magnesium deficiency can result in conditions usually attributed to intercellular deficiencies of other minerals. By providing for the ion transport of potassium, calcium, and other minerals, it can be said that magnesium is critical to muscle contraction, nerve impulses, and even maintaining a regular heartbeat, since both calcium and potassium are responsible for such roles.

Many people don't realize that calcium requires magnesium to be present in order for it to be effective in many of its capacities. Calcium stimulates contraction in muscles, while magnesium is a relaxant and governs calcium's absorption into cells, where one of calcium's responsibilities is to keep the heart beating. However, without sufficient magnesium, this role of calcium is jeopardized.

In experimental studies of rats, magnesium was shown to prevent toxic accumulations of calcium, which would result in the formation of kidney stones. If magnesium is lacking, deposits of calcium, especially insoluble forms of calcium, can form in and around tissues of the heart, kidneys, and arteries. This results in a gradual deterioration of the tissues and provides conditions where these forms of calcium can bond with other elements to create large molecules, or compounds, of calcium. Such toxic compounds can include large formations of insoluble calcium-oxalate (kidney stones). Thus, magnesium provides for proper utilization of calcium, decreasing the likelihood of such ailments.

Most people credit calcium to having strong bones and healthy teeth. While calcium is indeed important in that regard, once again it is unable to perform these roles unless magnesium is present. Magnesium is responsible for enhancing the absorption of other minerals into the bone. When magnesium levels are low, teeth are only able to produce soft enamel. Calcium builds the tooth structures and root system, while magnesium creates the hard dental enamel layer on the top of the tooth that protects against acids that result in cavities.

There is an even stronger connection between calcium and magnesium. Since these minerals work together with boron, fluorine, and vitamin D to maintain strong bones and teeth, adequate magnesium levels have been reported to help people feel younger. Magnesium deficiencies can cause calcium to migrate from the bones to the softer tissues where it collects in various places around the body, as mentioned earlier. If magnesium levels decrease, some estimate that up to 30 percent of the energy created in cellular processes will be used to remove what is then considered excess calcium out of the bones, thus decreasing a person's overall energy level.

Doctors at the Royal Sussex Country Hospital in Brighton, England conducted research using magnesium and were surprised to learn that low magnesium levels resulted in symptoms that resembled premenstrual syndrome (PMS). Their investigations were inspired from earlier studies performed in the United States by Dr. G. E. Abraham, who originally suggested that most of the characteristics of PMS could be caused by a lack of magnesium. Magnesium deficiencies have been known to result in various forms of cramps, headaches, appetite changes, and mood swings. Some women who increase their magnesium intake have reported no longer suffering from PMS. This discomfort can be caused either by lack of magnesium or consuming insoluble forms of calcium, such as calcium carbonate (limestone).

Most attention to osteoporosis in postmenopausal women involves the use of hormone-replacement therapy (estrogen) and supplementation of calcium and vitamin D. What isn't mentioned is magnesium. First, it should be realized that the thyroid, which gets its functioning from minerals such as iodine, regulates hormone levels. Second, many studies show deficiencies of magnesium in osteoporotic women. Osteoporotic bone mass typically has 12 percent lower levels of magnesium than healthy bone mass.

A study conducted in Israel experimented with osteoporosis by supplementing 250-750 mg/day of magnesium. The results showed that either bone density increased by 8 percent during a 24 month period or bone loss was stopped in 87 percent of the cases. Some of the subjects reported both an increase in bone density and a decrease in bone loss. Women who went untreated lost an average of 1 percent per year.

Another study in the former Czechoslovakia involved a study using postmenopausal women suffering from osteoporosis. Their results were similar—within two years almost 65 percent of the subjects became both totally free of pain and did not experience any further deformity in their vertebrae after taking 1500-3000 mg/day of magnesium supplements. The remaining 35% of the subjects experienced either a slight increase in bone density or a decrease in bone loss.

Magnesium comprises around 1% of bone tissue where it helps with bone mineral metabolism. When magnesium levels decline, there results a loss of bone density as the bone crystals become larger, making the bone more susceptible to breakage. And as magnesium levels decline, the amount of calcium also tends to decline, which ultimately results in resistance to parathyroid hormone and vitamin D. One study observed increased bone density in the hips of both men and women who supplemented with magnesium. Another study showed that postmenopausal women who were taking estrogen replacement therapy benefited from improved bone density after taking a multivitamin and magnesium and calcium supplements.

Women who supplement with magnesium also report having increased energy levels, less depression, and enjoy a sex life they haven't enjoyed since they were younger. Because all types of tissues rely on both magnesium and calcium, some women have observed a slight decrease in wrinkled skin when proper calcium and magnesium ions prepared in a solution were taken both orally and topically.

People who regularly suffer from migraine headaches have been known to lack sufficient magnesium inside their red and white blood cells. Many migraine sufferers report a reduction in headaches after supplementing with water-soluble magnesium. One study showed that those who took extra magnesium experienced a modest decline in the severity and frequency of headaches.

Certain conditions can cause minerals such as magnesium to be discharged from the body, causing mineral deficiency symptoms. Examples include surgical removal of intestinal tracts, inflammation of intestines from radiation, diuretics, gastrointestinal problems, alcoholism, and diarrhea, which have all been known to reduce magnesium levels.

Experimental studies of magnesium deficiencies can often show symptoms that are usually characteristic of other mineral deficiencies, such as sodium, potassium, and calcium. When magnesium levels decline, researchers have watched calcium levels also begin to decline, even when extra parathyroid hormones were being excreted in an effort to keep the calcium in the body. Intracellular potassium levels also began to decline when magnesium was deficient. Other conditions that resulted with low magnesium levels were muscle spasms (including tremors), nausea, vomiting, and even slight personality changes.

When the body has sufficient magnesium, it will utilize the calcium it has and discharges any excess calcium without storing it in tissues. This is one example of how a deficiency or an excess of one mineral can result in the underutilization of other minerals. Some vitamins, such as vitamin B6, require magnesium to act as a cofactor for their synthesis, while vitamin E also needs magnesium for its roles in the body.

Magnesium is required in order for plants to grow. Therefore, most plant tissues will contain magnesium. Well-known plant sources include artichokes, broccoli, avocadoes, chard, spinach, okra, and most green vegetables. Nuts and seeds, such as peanuts and hazelnuts, as well as many well-known herbs like dandelion, fennel seed, yarrow, sage, peppermint, and yellow dock, are also known to contain magnesium.

Chapter 10

The Macrominerals in People (continued)

Phosphorus

Phosphorus comes from the Greek word phosphoros, which means "light bearer" and was the ancient name for the planet Venus. In 1669, the German physician Hennig Brand first isolated phosphorus by boiling and then filtering 60 buckets of urine. This process produced a white material that glowed in the dark and burned brilliantly. Since that time, phosphorescence has been used to describe substances that glow in the dark without burning. Fortunately, today phosphorus is obtained from phosphate rocks. Some phosphorus compounds are used to as a cleaning agent, water softener, and to make china and baking powder. Phosphoric acid is a phosphorus compound that is found in carbonated soft drinks and is used to create fertilizers.

According to Dr. Matthew A. Pasek at the University of Arizona's Lunar and Planetary Laboratory, phosphorus is an important element for all living organisms, and ranks fifth in importance right after carbon, hydrogen, oxygen, and nitrogen. In fact, Dr. Pasek has stated, "there's approximately one phosphorus atom for every 2.8 million hydrogen atoms in the cosmos, every 49 million hydrogen atoms in the oceans, and every 203 hydrogen atoms in bacteria. Similarly, there's a single phosphorus atom for every 1,400 oxygen atoms in the cosmos, every 25 million oxygen atoms in the oceans, and 72 oxygen atoms in bacteria. The numbers for carbon atoms and nitrogen atoms, respectively, per single phosphorus atom are 680 and 230 in the cosmos, 974 and 633 in the oceans, and 116 and 15 in bacteria." These comparisons make phosphorus sound extremely rare when compared to these other important elements. However, the question remains about how phosphorus became so abundant on planet Earth in the first place.

When Earth was first forming, and long before life began, researchers at the University of Arizona theorize that phosphorus was delivered by violent impacts with meteorites that were rich in iron-nickel metals that often contained phosphorus. Dr. Pasek explains that meteorites tend to have various compound minerals that contain phosphorus, with the most important compound being schreibersite, which is extremely rare on Earth.

When this mineral comes into contact with water, various forms of phosphorus compounds will develop, including a form of phosphate that is two phosphorus atoms bound to seven oxygen atoms. This compound is used in photosynthesis and closely resembles ATP, the cellular energy that provides growth and movement. Since phosphorus is required to provide structure to DNA and RNA, it is thought that these iron meteorites that also contained phosphorus landed near fresh water, which eventually formed various phosphate bonds with carbon-containing compounds, and went on to participate in many other types of biological processes.

Meteorites such as these are the building blocks of planets. Ones that contain heavy amounts of iron help to form the metallic core of a planet, while other meteorites that contain silicates deliver elements that form the mantle. According to Dante Lauretta, a University of Arizona professor of planetary sciences, life can originate in solar systems only if there is an asteroid belt that contains these types of meteorites. Then, there must be a large celestial body with a strong enough gravitational pull that causes them to break loose from the belt so they can begin raining upon newly forming planets. In our galaxy, that gravitational pull comes from Jupiter, which "drives the delivery of planetesimals to our inner solar system, thereby limiting the chances that outer solar system planets and moons will be supplied with the reactive forms of phosphorus used by biomolecules essential to terrestrial life." Therefore, the presence of Jupiter provides a strong enough gravitational power to keep any meteors containing iron and phosphorus local to our galaxy, rather than having them orbiting aimlessly and contributing their life-giving phosphorus to other solar systems.

Phosphate is the ionic version of phosphorus that is found in plants, and is one of the most widespread minerals in the human body. This element is involved in just about every chemical process. It is found in every cell and total body content can amount to as much as two pounds.

Phosphate is known as the metabolic twin of calcium. Eighty-five percent of the body's total phosphate is found in bone tissue, making it a component of strong bones and the overall structure of the body. It needs to be found in correct balance with calcium in order for it to be used appropriately; usually a balance of 2.5 parts calcium to one part phosphorus is sufficient. If the phosphorus-calcium ratio becomes out of balance for a prolonged period of time, it is more likely that calcium will be the element that becomes unavailable or deficient. Vitamin D, magnesium, and boron are all elements that affect the absorption of calcium, and phosphorus is no exception.

Phosphate participates in the formation of the calcium phosphate salt called hydroxyapatite, the crystal that comprises bone tissue. Phosphorus also has certain functions with regard to fats, such as combining with fat to form phospholipids. Phospholipids make up a layer of cellular fats and waxes that help transport nutrients across cell membranes. Phosphorus is also a contributing factor in cell signaling and hormones.

Inside the cell, phosphorus plays a key role in the nucleus. It is central to life because it forms part of the nucleic acids DNA and RNA, which carry the organism's genetic code. When damage occurs to the DNA, the cell becomes susceptible to improper protein synthesis. Phosphorus helps to form RNA, which is not located in the nucleus but rather is in the cytoplasm and surrounding fluids. RNA carries the information stored by DNA out of the nucleus and into the cytoplasm where it is used in protein synthesis. A molecule known as 2,3-diphosphoglycerate contains phosphate and binds to hemoglobin found inside red blood cells, which helps with oxygen delivery to tissues throughout the body.

Phosphorus activates certain enzyme systems, especially those concerned with carbohydrate metabolism. Energy gained from carbohydrate metabolism is released into the muscle and nervous systems. Phosphorus is a component of ATP, making its presence required for various cellular processes and transferring some energy to other metabolic systems.

The process where ATP transfers one of its phosphate ions to glucose (blood sugar) is known as phosphorylation. This creates energy that allows the cell to produce specific reactions, making phosphorus required for the transfer of cellular energy.

This type of energy transfer allows for a state of equilibrium. If the DNA is unable to be transported where it can participate in protein synthesis, or if the proteins are defective, an excess of enzymes may become activated prematurely, which could destroy the cell. Phosphorus helps keep this process active and working smoothly.

Fluids and tissues that contain sufficient phosphorus will be able to more effectively utilize some vitamins, including vitamin B12, and balance the pH level of the body. However, if the pH level of soil or the body drops below 5.0, phosphorus becomes insoluble and binds with other elements, creating a dangerous compound.

Phosphate has also been known to participate in brain functions and overall metabolism. It works with potassium to regulate and control normal heartbeat patterns and combines with calcium to increase bone strength. This important element is found in all fruits and vegetables. Human milk provides plenty of phosphate for nursing infants if the mother has appropriate levels.

Phosphorus is absorbed through the intestinal lining of the small intestines, and any excess phosphate will be discharged from the body through the kidneys. Phosphorus and calcium are both regulated by parathyroid hormones and vitamin D. If calcium levels decline, the parathyroid gland senses this condition and responds by increasing the amount of parathyroid hormone in the blood, which stimulates an increase in the conversion of vitamin D to a more active form in the kidneys, known as calcitriol. This action increases the intestinal absorption of phosphorus and calcium. Increases in vitamin D and parathyroid hormone both increase the amount of calcium and phosphorus that is released from bone tissue back into the blood. In an effort to decrease the amount of calcium that is lost through the urine, the parathyroid gland will release more phosphate to keep calcium levels adequate.

Some foods common in today's society can increase urinary loss of phosphate, such as fructose and other artificial sugars. A phenomenon known as "fructose trapping" occurs when fructose is not converted to fructose-1-phosphate in the liver, which results in large amounts of phosphate being used up because the enzyme that phosphorylates fructose is inhibited.

Deficiency symptoms of phosphorus can include weakness, anorexia, malaise, arthritis, osteoporosis, tooth decay, and rickets. Its working relationship with other elements already mentioned makes a phosphorus deficiency characteristic with deficiencies of other elements.

Phosphorus is a nutrient needed in high amounts in order for plants to grow. Most plants will contain sufficient phosphorus, making deficiencies in humans rare. Common sources of phosphorus usually include nuts and seeds such as pumpkin seeds and sunflower seeds. Garlic, corn, and asparagus are frequently cited as having large amounts of phosphorus.

Potassium

Potassium, a very reactive element, is the 8th most abundant element on Earth, making up 2.1% of Earth's crust. In 1807, Sir Humphrey Davy first isolated potassium. When isolated, it is a soft, waxy metal that can be cut with a knife. However, potassium is usually bound to other elements such as sodium which is used in various nuclear reactors. Other potassium compounds are often found in ancient lakebeds and are used in fertilizers, in the manufacture of soaps and detergents, and to make some forms of glass and pyrotechnics.

Potassium is one of the most important elements for healthy human cells. It is essential to all tissues in the human body, where it is always found as a positively charged ion—a cation—and never as a compound.

This element is so profound that it makes up as much as five percent of the total content of mineral ions in healthy bodies.

Potassium can be found primarily inside cells—usually in cellular fluids—making potassium a major cation inside cell cytoplasm. Researchers have observed that as much as 75 - 98% of the total ions found inside cellular fluids can be potassium, depending on which fluid is being studied. This mineral is the principle base in blood cells, which helps to transport oxygen through the blood, and is considered responsible for at least half the carbon dioxide carrying capacity in the blood. Potassium's dominating presence inside cells and fluids makes it required for a wide variety of electrochemical and catalytic functions for enzyme systems.

Although plants require the presence of potassium to activate 46 of its enzymes, including biochemical process such as photosynthesis and respiration, potassium participates as an activator or as a cofactor in several enzyme systems in humans. These enzyme systems are responsible for the transfer and utilization of energy, carbohydrate synthesis, and protein synthesis. Examples of enzymes include adenosine triphosphatase (ATP), hexokinase, carbonic anhydrase, salivary amylase, fructokinase, and pyruvic kinase. And since potassium is also responsible for the absorption of amino acids into cells, this explains potassium's role in human growth and development.

Potassium's activities inside the cell include not only enzymatic activity, but also assist skeletal and heart muscle contraction, release energy from food, and work with calcium in the transmission of nerve impulses. In addition, potassium also appears to carry out many of the same functions inside the cell that sodium performs outside cells in blood plasma and interstitial fluid, such as maintaining a healthy water balance, commonly known as an osmotic equilibrium.

Potassium, calcium, chloride, and sodium are all responsible for regulating the traffic that goes into and out of cells. Potassium is much more concentrated inside the cell than outside, while sodium is more commonly found outside the cell. Balancing the cation-anion relationship in and out of cells also regulates the pH level and the flow of water. These functions are properly regulated when there is sufficient potassium and calcium inside the cells and sodium and chloride outside the cells.

Research indicates that potassium contributes as much as 50% of the overall osmotic activity of intracellular fluids, while sodium and chloride contribute around 80% of the extracellular osmotic activity. Early research explained how the separation between potassium and sodium was originally thought to be handled by an independent sodium pump. However, new technology has now shown that crystalline structures in the cell actually keep the sodium outside the cell, while retaining potassium inside, and at an optimal ratio. Maintenance of these concentration gradients allows the transport of these materials to occur with proper osmotic pressure.

Similar to plant cells, the presence of potassium and sodium inside and outside the cell membranes creates a phenomenon known as membrane potential, which is an electrical potential that is created from their combined electrical energy and the flow of other ions that are transported across the ion channels, and it is maintained by the sodium and potassium ion channels that pump ions across the membrane. These ion pumps use the energy produced inside the cell known as ATP to excrete sodium ions out of the cell in exchange for potassium ions in an effort to keep the proper balance of ions. All of this electrical energy and the action of pumping and balancing ions accounts for between 20-40% of the resting energy in healthy adults. This high energy usage should explain the importance of this process.

The optimal presence of these elements not only regulates the flow of ions but also regulates the movement of water as it diffuses across the cell membranes. In fact, if an imbalance occurs causing a collection of molecules outside the cell to be greater than inside the cell, the cell poses the risk of losing its electrical stability, which can cause the interior of the cell to lose water (and ions) and eventually dry up. This imbalance of ionic buildup outside the cell can create a build-up of fluid, causing edema to develop. Such an improper regulation of fluid balance occurs when potassium is deficient.

The tight cellular regulation of the sodium/potassium balance makes potassium essential in the functioning of the muscular and nervous systems. Potassium is also referred to as an "electrolyte," which is a term that describes any substance that dissolves into electrically charged ions and has the ability to conduct electricity. Therefore, potassium plays a strong role in the transmission of nerve impulses and muscle contractions.

If sufficient minerals are present, the body will be able to naturally balance potassium, sodium, calcium, and magnesium ions in order to properly control cellular excitability of nerves and muscle contractions. These functions in the nervous system make potassium responsible for reducing or preventing neuromuscular irritability. When combined with sodium, potassium protects or restores membrane potential in nerve synapses. These functions explain why potassium and sodium have been known to relieve pain.

Understanding potassium's role in the nervous system leads us to understanding potassium's roles in the cardiovascular system. An influence on the nervous system allows potassium to help regulate the heartbeat. With responsibility in various nerve functions and muscle contractions, potassium helps to prevent heart palpitations and fluttering heart conditions. With its functions in cellular activity, including regulation of water and ion balance, potassium is helpful in regulating blood pressure, especially since sodium and potassium work together to regulate the transport of nutrients into the cell and excrete waste products out of the cell, which reduces cholesterol build-up. These functions make potassium useful in preventing strokes and other similar conditions, and some studies have shown high-potassium diets are less likely to result in elevated blood pressure (hypertension).

Over 17,000 adults participated in the third National Health and Nutritional Examination Survey to determine the effects of dietary potassium on blood pressure. Those who participated experienced lower blood pressure after supplementing with potassium. An investigation by the Dietary Approaches to Stop Hypertension showed that those who consumed over eight servings per day of fruits and vegetables were able to lower their blood pressure by an average of 2.8/1.1 mm Hg in those who had normal blood pressure, compared to 7.2/2.8 mm Hg in those suffering from hypertension. Interestingly, when the same subjects also supplemented with calcium, their blood pressure was even lower.

Some studies show a correlation between potassium intake and the risk of developing strokes. In one study, over 43,000 men were observed over an 8-year period. It showed that those who were in the top 20% of potassium supplementation were able to reduce their risk of having a stroke by almost 40% when compared to the lower percentile. Later, using the same population in their research, it was discovered that those who supplemented with much as 1,352 daily grams of potassium were only 72% as probable to develop a stroke.

Potassium's role in keeping the cardiovascular system working optimally doesn't stop there. Some heart conditions are a result of an excess of the compound sodium chloride, otherwise known as table salt. Fortunately, potassium ions are an effective diuretic, and while ridding the body of excess water and other fluids, potassium is also able to excrete excess sodium chloride from the body, an effect called natriuresis. Dr. George R. Meneely, Emeritus Professor of Medicine at the Louisiana State University Medical Center, studied potassium's effect on excess sodium chloride. He observed that the hypertensive effects of excess sodium chloride are counteracted with extra dietary potassium.

Although this relationship is still under investigation, researchers J. He and coworkers theorized that the effects of potassium on sodium chloride could be the result of potassium's influence on other minerals, and not necessarily potassium acting alone. Their research showed that low potassium levels consistently resulted in higher sodium chloride levels, while sufficient dietary potassium resulted in a decrease of excess sodium chloride. Either way, potassium's influence on the body seems to include not only regulation of the cardiovascular system, but also the regulation and excretion of excess fluids and materials, including table salt.

Researchers in Israel studied the eating habits of 98 vegetarians who averaged 60 years old and compared them to regular meat eaters. They all ate the same amount of table salt during the study, and all had relatively similar predisposition to high blood pressure. It was discovered that the vegetarians, with a plant-based diet that included potassium, did not develop hypertension, suggesting that lack of potassium, rather than an excess of salt, is contributing to hypertension.

Overall, potassium plays key roles in cardiovascular and muscular functions. It works with sodium to neutralize acids, restore healthy alkaline salts to the bloodstream, and regulate water, fluids, and other materials in and out of cells. These functions make potassium effective in keeping nerves working properly, regulating heartbeat, and keeping blood pressure normal. Potassium also helps the body eliminate wastes, relieve pain such as headaches and migraines, promote faster healing of cuts and bruises, and generally contributes to a sense of well-being.

A deficiency of potassium can result in nerve disorders, slow or irregular heartbeat, bad circulation, heart palpitations, hypertension, chest pain, or muscle damage. Severe and prolonged deficiencies can also result in muscle weakness, hypokalemic cardiac failure, and even paralysis. Too little potassium or too much potassium compounds can interfere with the electrical connectivity of the heart muscle, which can result in a mistaken diagnosis of heart disease from an electrocardiogram.

There may be a relationship between a decline in bone mineral density and potassium deficiencies in pre-, peri-, and postmenopausal women and older men. One study observed that those who consumed high fruits and vegetables, amounting to at least 3,000 milligrams a day of potassium and other minerals, had significantly greater bone mineral density. Common Western diets tend to include acidic foods such as dairy and meat products, and not enough alkaline foods, such as a plant-based diet comprised mainly of fruits and vegetables.

The sodium and potassium ionic balancing act is useful in buffering against acids introduced in the body. However, if these ions are deficient, the body's pH level declines, forcing the body to remobilize alkaline calcium salts from bone tissue in an effort to neutralize the acids being consumed. Increasing the amount of fruits and vegetables into the diet brings the body's pH level to a neutral range, thus preserving the calcium content in the bone tissue where it should be, rather than having to be released into the blood to buffer against acids. One study used 18 postmenopausal women who supplemented with potassium to study this phenomenon. The results were a decline in urinary acid and calcium loss from bones.

When the body is forced to excrete calcium through urine, the risk of kidney stones increases. Those with acidic dietary habits tend to have the most common occurrences of kidney stones. Several things have shown to be effective in reducing this calcium excretion, including an increase in fruits and vegetables or supplementing with potassium. One study that observed 45,000 men for over 4 years showed that those who supplemented with high amounts of dietary potassium were only half as likely to develop kidney stones versus those who regularly consumed low potassium amounts. A similar study that followed over 90,000 women for 12 years showed that those who consumed the highest amounts of potassium were only two-third as likely to develop kidney stones when compared to those with the lowest potassium intake. In both of these studies, the dietary potassium was derived from potassium ions in fruits and vegetables, once again showing not only the need for potassium, but the need for potassium in the right form.

Other ailments known to occur in the presence of low potassium levels include acidosis, nervousness, insomnia, nausea, loss of appetite, and neurological symptoms such as mental apathy and altered mental states (leading to addiction to alcohol and drugs). Other symptoms include chronic fatigue syndrome, a bluish tint to skin, earaches, diabetes, edema, headaches, prolapsed uterus, oppressive breathing, swollen glands, tissue anemia, water retention, and even pain in the eyes.

Prescribed diuretics, prolonged diarrhea, vomiting, alcoholism, or overuse of laxatives can inadvertently remove potassium from the body, causing a potassium deficiency in the blood, a condition known as hypokalemia. Symptoms of this condition can be attributed to changes in cellular metabolism or membrane potential. Muscular weakness, fatigue, convulsions, cramps, and various intestinal disorders that include constipation and bloating can occur. Prolonged and severe hypokalemia can result in various forms of muscular paralysis or irregular heartbeat. Eating foods grown in potassium-rich soils can reverse these disorders.

Potassium deficiencies in plants are rare, especially since fertilizers almost always contain extra potassium. Its high mobility, sufficient quantity in the soil, and status as a macromineral makes potassium likely to be found in all fruits, vegetables, nuts, seeds, and grains. Prunes, grapes, citrus fruits, melons, apples, pears, tomatoes, and all vegetables are all good sources of potassium.

Sodium

"Sodium" comes from the English word soda, and from the medieval Latin word sodanum, which, being interpreted means "headache remedy." Sodium is the 6th most abundant element on Earth, comprising roughly 2.6% of the crust. It is a very reactive element that can ignite upon direct contact with water so it is usually stored in a moisture free environment. Sir Humphrey Davy first isolated sodium in 1807.

Naturally, sodium is normally found in compounds, some of which are used as coolants in nuclear reactors. Sodium vapor can be found in streetlights producing the "caution" yellow light. When combined with chloride, it forms sodium chloride, more commonly known as table salt. It also forms baking soda, caustic soda, and borax.

Even though most people consume far too much sodium, this element has some very important roles in the body. The metabolism of sodium is started by one of the adrenal cortex hormones named aldosterone, which is responsible for controlling the resorption of sodium from the kidneys. This process regulates the amount of sodium that is excreted, helping to prevent sodium deficiency. Unfortunately, when excess sodium is consumed from sodium chloride, an increase in urinary excretion of calcium can result. For every 5.8 grams of salt that is excreted by the kidney, 20-40 milligrams of calcium can also be excreted through the urine.

High amounts of urinary excretion of calcium through the kidneys again pose the risk of kidney stones. An experiment that studied 90,000 women for over 12 years discovered that those who consumed an average of 4.9 grams per day of sodium experienced a 30% higher incidence of kidney stones when compared to the women who took 1.5 grams per day. Although other studies have experimented with men but not found similar results, research studies have shown that decreasing salt intake results in less urinary excretion, which lessens the likelihood of developing kidney stones.

The amount of sodium excreted is largely determined by the amount of water that is lost through sweat, urination, and even defecation. However, during periods of vomiting, diarrhea, or heavy sweating, symptoms of sodium deficiency can result, such as low blood pressure and muscle cramps.

Potassium is the main cation in intracellular fluids, and sodium and potassium work together to regulate the fluid balance inside the cells. Sodium is also influential in cell permeability; together, sodium and potassium help regulate the transport of nutrients into and out of each cell. Their combined actions also normalize the pH balance of the blood, thus keeping other minerals water-soluble and preventing their buildup in tissues.

Approximately 85% of the sodium in the body is located alongside chloride in the fluids that surround the body's cells, such as blood and lymph. Sodium also helps eliminate carbon dioxide from the body, and is an important component in the production of hydrochloric acid in the stomach. It also helps the nervous system by helping to activate the transmission of electrical impulses along the nerve membranes, which helps muscle contraction and nerve stimulation. Symptoms of sodium deficiency include muscle cramps, fatigue, weakness, arthritis, heartburn, intestinal gas, neuralgia, confusion, and short attention span.

Sodium concentrations are typically 10 times higher in blood than in the cells, although much of sodium's contribution to human health is when it works alongside potassium. See "potassium" for more information on sodium.

Plant sources of sodium include most fruits and vegetables. Nuts and seeds also tend to have consistent levels of sodium.

Sulfur

Antoine Lavoisier spent the year 1777 trying to convince other scientists that sulfur was indeed an element. Sulfur would later become recognized as the 10th most abundant element in the universe. Some geologists and paleontologists theorize that sulfur's widespread presence across Earth can be attributed to an asteroid that hit Earth millions of years ago, which contributed to the extinction of the dinosaurs and widespread dispersal of sulfur across the planet. Scientists think that the asteroid was largely comprised of sulfur and vaporized upon impact, sending an estimated 100 billion tons of sulfur dioxide into the atmosphere. The sulfur spread around the world and eventually entered the natural cycles of the environment.

Sulfur is so widespread in nature that it can be found in gypsum, pyrite, cinnabar, stibnite, epsomite, and other inorganic mineral compounds. One-fourth of the sulfur produced today is obtained through petroleum operations or as a residual byproduct when extracting other materials from various ores. The rest of the sulfur we enjoy today is gained through mining operations.

Sulfur compounds are used to make fertilizers, batteries, natural rubbers, insecticides, gunpowder, and as a yellow coloring agent. Hydrogen sulfide is a sulfur compound that smells like rotten eggs. Another compound, sulfur dioxide, is used as a bleaching agent, disinfectant, and a refrigerant. If sulfur dioxide mixes with water, sulfurous acid will result, which is also known as acid rain.

Most people don't realize how widespread sulfur is in the human body—it is the 4th most abundant mineral in humans, comprising around 140 grams, or 0.25%, of total body weight. Fifty-percent of the total sulfur can be found in muscle tissues, while the remaining fifty-percent is spread between the skin, hair, bones, brain, and places that require collagen, such as cartilage, blood vessels, and gums. This mineral is not a metal, but products manufactured from sulfur can be found in every cell of the body and have many useful functions.

Hydrogen, oxygen, carbon, nitrogen, phosphorus, and sulfur are the most common elements that need to be bound to certain biological molecules, such as protein. When sulfur is found in ionic form, such as in the soil or in plants, it is referred to as "sulfate." Sulfate is the form of sulfur that is found in green vegetables, fruits, and grains, and can be destroyed by high heat. Although most minerals in the body are used in their ionic form, sulfur is oftentimes bound with other atoms and used as a building block to create hormones, proteins, amino acids, and even vitamins.

Sulfur helps to activate the B vitamins, all of which participate in the nervous system. Vitamins such as thiamine (B1) and biotin, as well as carbohydrates such as heparin, which is an antiocoagulant found in the liver, are all products created in the body from sulfur.

Amino acids such as cystine, cysteine, and methionine are protein building blocks made from sulfur and are found in hair, skin, and nails, all of which contain keratin, a strong, flexible product that is 6% sulfur. Five of the nutrients needed for good-looking skin cells are sulfur, calcium, zinc, copper, and vitamin C. However, the body is unable to absorb vitamin C unless copper is present, and copper is sometimes inoperable unless zinc is present. Sulfur acts to soften the cell walls of skin, keeping that youthful elasticity and suppleness and preventing wrinkles. This soft firmness also allows harmful toxins to be excreted from these cells.

Glutathione is a product made from cysteine that is used in cellular processes such as protecting membranes against free radical damage. Eventually, cysteine is converted to taurine, which will then aid in the nervous system, and some proteins created from sulfur will eventually be used as enzymes.

Among these various roles as a building block, one of sulfur's biggest responsibilities is to metabolize carbohydrates, an important function, especially for diabetics. Coenzyme A is the enzyme helper made from sulfur and B vitamins, all of which help in the metabolism of carbohydrates and fats. These are important functions when blood glucose levels are abnormal. Hormones are also created from sulfur. Interestingly, sulfur is an important part of the insulin hormone. Therefore, a deficiency of sulfur can lead to inhibited insulin production.

This mineral is used to produce chondroitin sulfate, which is used to create collagen. Collagen is the tough, flexible product found in cartilage, tendons, skin, and the walls of blood vessels. It provides both a strong framework of slippery surfaces for connective tissues and it becomes a lubricant for joints. Sulfur deficiencies can result in inhibited collagen formation, which can lead to a degeneration of cartilage. Ligaments, joints, tendons, and other collagen products could be rendered inoperable during long periods of sulfur deficiency, resulting in conditions such as arthritis or even sickle cell anemia.

Sulfur is also used by the body to eliminate waste products. The liver takes sulfur and binds it with toxins and other products it needs to eliminate or inactivate them in order to flush them from the body. For example, the chemical phenol and the hormone progesterone eventually are rendered as a byproduct. If sulfur becomes bound to these products, phenol becomes phenol sulfate, and progesterone becomes progesterone sulfate, which are then promptly excreted from the body. Some forms of sulfur found in foods may not be beneficial. These activities require an enzyme known as sulfite oxidase, which requires the mineral molybdenum for activation. This enzyme tries to break down harmful forms of sulfur that are known as sulfites, which can be found in food preservatives.

Sulfites are not water-soluble and can irritate the cells, causing allergies or triggering asthmatic attacks. The enzyme sulfite oxidase can break down sulfites into sulfate, as along as the mineral molybdenum is present. One study of asthmatic children revealed 85% of the subjects experienced high sulfite sensitivity, which was attributed to an inability to convert sulfites into sulfate. Taking the right kind of sulfur (sulfate) initiates these cleansing activities, purging the body of these types of toxins. Sulfur can also coat and cleanse the intestinal tract, purging allergic toxins that may reside there. When these children were treated with water-soluble molybdenum and sulfur, they experienced urinary excretion of sulfites and decreased allergic reactions.

Many people report less joint pain after supplementing with sulfur. This most likely occurs because the tissues become softened, allowing fluids to pass easily through the tissues, which can equalize pressure and relieve pain. Nerve endings in the skin signaling pain can be attributed to a loss of flexibility in tissues and atmospheric barometric pressure. Some people suffering from arthritis know when a storm is coming because they can sense when outside air pressure drops. This results in inflamed joints and even pain because their cell walls become hardened and lack the flexibility and permeability they should be getting from sulfur. Sulfur can also provide repair to the myelin sheath that surrounds nerve endings.

Sulfur can also benefit the eyes. The protein membrane in the eyeball contains nerves and fluids. Only certain fluids and nutrients are allowed to flow through the optical membrane, which acts as a cleanser to keep out foreign particles, keeping vision clear. Sulfur can act to keep this membrane soft, flexible, and strong. However, if sulfur becomes deficient, the membrane can become hardened, preventing the fluids and nutrients to pass through and allowing particles to build up. After prolonged periods of hardened membranes, pressure can build up in the eyes along with blurriness and a loss of focus. Vision eventually becomes impaired, resulting in severe conditions such as cataracts and even blindness. Sulfur supplementation should permit the membrane and fluids to function properly.

Sulfur assists in cellular respiratory processes that provide the cells with energy produced from oxygen. It can also balance the acid/alkaline balance of the body, help the liver secrete bile, and will not toxically build up in the body. Sulfur toxicity is unlikely—excess sulfur will be discharged in the urine or feces.

It is possible for some sulfur compounds taken as supplements to be absorbed in the upper stomach and enter the bloodstream in an undigested and in an unusable, insoluble form. If this occurs, the insoluble sulfur compound would have bypassed the enzymes that might be able to break it down. Toxic accumulations of sulfur compounds can result in joint pain and acidify the body, which can lead to even further conditions.

Some health conditions that are characteristic of sulfur deficiencies could be an inoperable enzyme that is responsible for breaking down sulfur compounds. However, if a water-soluble sulfur supplement were provided, the body would then have the proper form of sulfur. And since this sulfur would already be in the right form, it should provide immediate benefits to the body, especially since the enzymes needed to break down sulfur compounds would not be needed. Thus, as with any other mineral, sulfur should always be taken in the right form as a water-soluble sulfate, or from vegetables, fruits, and legumes.

Sulfur deficiency results in a loss of collagen, which means that cells can lose their elasticity and become stiff, which can be attributed to hardening of the arteries and hypertension. Lung tissues can also harden when collagen is lacking, resulting in various respiratory conditions.

Other symptoms of sulfur deficiency can include acne, back pain, constipation, circulatory problems, dry skin, allergies, asthma, free radical damage, infection, inflammation, nerve disorders, migraines, and various skin disorders from lack of collagen.

Good sources of sulfur usually include green leafy vegetables.

Chapter 11

The Microminerals in People

Chromium

"Chromium" comes from the Greek word for color, chroma, and was originally discovered as an element by Louis-Nicholas Vauquelin during an experiment with Siberian red lead. After mixing this with hydrochloric acid, he created chromium oxide. It wasn't until 1798 that he learned that he could isolate chromium by heating chromium oxide in an oven. Chromic oxide is the 9th most abundant mineral in Earth's crust and is used in green pigments. Some forms of chromium compounds are used to color paints. In fact, emeralds and rubies owe their unique color to chromium compounds.

Chromium has only recently been discovered for its benefits in the human body. Its ability to regulate metabolism wasn't discovered until 1969. Chromium has since been found to also play a role in regulating the insulin hormone and blood sugar levels. It is a trace element that the body only needs in small amounts to enhance the use of insulin, and it also helps the body lose excess weight by stimulating enzymes, such as phosphoglucosonetase and others that metabolize glucose (fruit sugar) for energy. Chromium also helps stabilize blood pressure and transport protein.

Chromium is one of the most important of all trace minerals but it is usually the most depleted. Richard Anderson of the United States Department of Agriculture has stated that 90% of Americans are deficient in chromium. American soils contain less chromium than European soils, and artificial and refined sugars deplete chromium from our bodies while also increasing the body's needs for it.

Extreme sugary diets that include colas, fruit juices from concentrate, candy and other forms of sugar increase urinary excretion of chromium by as much as 300% within the first 12 hours. Consumption of high-fructose corn syrup has risen steadily over the past two decades, insomuch that the rate of diabetes has increased by 45% at the same time.

One of the body's most notable uses for chromium is its responsibility in the pancreas. The pancreas is an extremely important organ that produces enzymes that are used in digestion and it produces two very important hormones: insulin and glucagon, which are both used to balance and moderate levels of blood glucose (sugar). When glucose (natural sugars) from food is being absorbed in the small intestine, it is absorbed into the bloodstream where it gets carried to the liver. If there is too much glucose already in the blood, the pancreas responds by producing more insulin. This extra insulin is meant to accomplish several things. It converts the extra glucose into glycogen for storage, increases the absorption of glucose into cells, prevents the breakdown of glycogen and fats, and increases amino acid and protein synthesis. These measures help keep the level of glucose in the blood and liver at proper levels. Chromium can also increase the number of plasma membrane receptors for insulin, which helps the body utilize this hormone.

Chromium is an essential cofactor for all the functions of insulin. It increases the effectiveness of insulin performance and glucose utilization by helping insulin perform optimally and it plays an extremely important role in enzymatic activity that metabolizes glucose. It is required for glucose to enter the cells, which makes it efficient in the metabolism of carbohydrates. When the body is deficient in chromium, it can take twice as long for insulin to remove glucose from the blood. After supplementation with chromium, some researchers have observed decreases in blood glucose levels by as much as 80-90%.

Interestingly, if blood glucose levels become too low, the pancreas will respond by producing the glucagon hormone. This hormone does just the opposite: it converts the stored glycogen back to glucose in an effort to increase the blood sugar levels. So when blood glucose levels are high, the pancreas secretes insulin in an effort to lower the levels, and if blood glucose levels are too low, the pancreas secretes glucagon in order to raise the levels. Either way, chromium's presence in the pancreas helps regulate these processes.

If the insulin-producing cells in the pancreas are inoperable or have been destroyed, insulin is unable to be produced, resulting in elevated blood sugar levels, a condition known as hyperglycemia. Type I diabetes results when the body inadvertently cannibalizes itself by producing an antibody that destroys these insulin-producing cells in the pancreas, which is usually passed from the mother to the fetus. Thus, Type I diabetics produce little to no insulin, and develop this condition during fetal infancy or childhood. As a result, these persons must take extra insulin by injection every day.

Type II diabetes tends to develop during adulthood. High blood sugar levels or failure to produce insulin to counteract these levels usually result if the body is placed under heavy stress, such as obesity or the presence of other disease conditions. Such significant stress can damage organs, such as the pancreas, and render it unable to produce hormones such as insulin. Type II diabetes is usually considered less severe than Type I and is more manageable. Affected persons are under constant monitoring and placed on a restrictive diet, or take medications designed to stimulate insulin production in the pancreas.

Another responsibility of insulin is to direct absorbed nutrients to various organs of the body, which eventually results in the normal metabolism of carbohydrates, fats, and proteins in the tissues. In healthy humans, tissues respond properly to insulin. However, it is possible for the body's tissues to become resistant to insulin. The pancreas responds by producing more and more insulin to carry out its functions in an effort to counteract this resistance, which is another characteristic of diabetes. These abnormal fluctuations of blood glucose can be attributed to low chromium levels or reduced or even nonexistent activity of a chromium-dependent enzyme.

To help insulin performance, the body will bind chromium ions to an amino acid and to niacin, which is a b-vitamin. This process occurs in tissues and results in a substance known as Glucose Tolerance Factor (GTF). In this bound form, chromium is able to participate in enhancing the insulin hormone.

Dr. Walter Mertz discovered the GTF at the Walter Reed Army Institute of Research in 1957. A short time later, chromium was identified as one of its main components and was recognized for its function in stimulating insulin performance. After experimenting with animals, Dr. Mertz recognized that deficiency of chromium could lead to diabetes. Using chromium deficient laboratory rats, he observed extremely low glucose metabolism as well as other common diabetes symptoms. Other researchers have found that glucose tolerance could be improved by supplementing with GTF. Other studies using animals lacking chromium exhibited weight loss, decreased fertility, high blood sugar, and nerve and blood tissue damage.

Dr. Mertz also noted that extra chromium resulted in less cholesterol and decreased hardening of the arteries, which is attributed to its antioxidant characteristics. Another researcher, Dr. Gary Evans of Bemidji State University in Minnesota, was the first to discover chromium's ability to decrease both blood cholesterol levels and the harmful LDL proteins also found in cholesterol. These findings were presented at the American Society for Experimental Biology in New Orleans.

Meanwhile, at the Dartmouth Medical School in New Hampshire, a prominent mineral researcher named Henry Schroeder noticed that patients who died of coronary occlusion, which is a partial or complete blockage of blood flow in an artery and can lead to a heart attack, consistently had lower levels of chromium in their blood tissues than did those who died from traumatic accidents.

Chromium is required to create muscle, and athletes can benefit from chromium's ability to burn carbohydrates and regulate the body's use of glycogen. During exercise, energy produced from these processes helps the body burn off fat and produce lean muscle tissue. A study using weightlifters showed leaner muscle gain compared to subjects that were given a placebo.

When this element is abundant in the human body, it is found in the spleen, kidneys, pancreas, heart, lungs, testes, brain, hair, and blood. It has also been shown to improve the skin. One report in Medical

Hypotheses reported giving supplemental chromium to nine patients whose acne cleared up.

Broccoli, potatoes, and green beans are vegetables that usually contain chromium. Fruits such as apples, grapes, oranges, and bananas, grown in organic soils, and various herbs like catnip, horsetail, licorice, nettle, oat straw, red clover, sarsaparilla, wild yam, and yarrow are also sources of chromium.

Cobalt

The Swedish chemist Georg Brandt first discovered cobalt in 1739. He was determined to prove that certain minerals that colored glass blue was due to something other than bismuth, which was the commonly held belief at the time. Cobalt compounds were later used as a dye to color porcelain.

Although cobalt is listed as an essential micromineral, it has long been thought that the body only needed very scant amounts. However, it is the author's opinion that cobalt should be considered in higher regard and recommended in higher amounts, especially after considering all its benefits.

The discovery and acknowledged essentiality of cobalt originally began to gain attention after observing a fatal disease in animals in New Zealand and Australia called "bush sickness." Symptoms of the disease included emaciation, anorexia, pale mucous membranes, listlessness, and dull stares, all of which were successfully treated with cobalt.

This element is the primary component in the production of vitamin B12, and in order to understand the role of cobalt, one needs to first understand vitamin B12. Researchers Murphy and Minot discovered cobalt in 1926 in liver and credited it with treating pernicious anemia, a blood disorder characterized by low red blood cells that results from lack of vitamin B12, a vitamin later discovered in 1948.

When vitamin B12 (aka cobalamin) is found in food, each particle of this vitamin is naturally too large to pass through the intestinal membranes and enter the cells. The stomach responds by producing a protein called intrinsic factor during its normal acid secretion that will bind with each vitamin B12 particle in order to protect it from being destroyed by further digestive processes. Gradually, when there are enough of these bound particles layering the intestinal membranes, a special absorption process called pinocytosis will occur, and with the help of calcium vitamin B12 will finally enter the cells.

However, people who have had large portions of their intestinal tract removed due to surgery are not likely to produce enough of the intrinsic factor protein and could result in impaired absorption of vitamin B12, which then results in pernicious anemia. Also, in persons who have a condition known as hypochlorydia, which is a lack of stomach acid production (usually a chloride deficiency from low salt intake), intrinsic factor is not produced and the vitamin B12 stands little chance of entering the cells.

Vitamin B12 is required for the formation of red blood cells and nerve cells, along with the maturation of red blood cells in bone marrow. The human liver can store a maximum of 2 mg of B12, which slowly gets released into bone marrow; excess B12 will be excreted through urine. This supply is good for up to 7 years, making deficiencies uncommon. Typically, deficiencies do not necessarily result from insufficient vitamin B12 in the diet, but rather from failure of the intestines to absorb the vitamin. This can occur from the existence of tapeworms in the intestines, a lack of stomach acid from a chloride deficiency, or from a lack of intrinsic factor production, which results from a lack of cobalt.

A single ion of cobalt is the metal component of each particle of vitamin B12, which itself activates or is a cofactor in various other enzyme processes. This vitamin is water-soluble and colored red due to the presence of cobalt. Vitamin B12 can be found either in food or the friendly bacteria found in intestines can create it by using cobalt.

Cobalt is a nutrient needed by bacteria, since all vitamin B12 is derived from bacterial synthesis. This vitamin aids in activating certain enzymes, and is also involved in the synthesis of protein. Studies using rats and pigs experiencing decreased growth have attributed this condition to a lack of protein synthesis from insufficient B12.

Some studies have shown cobalt to be an important component in the nervous system because it helps to prevent the gradual degeneration of the myelin sheath that surrounds the nerves. Demyelination results in faulty nerve transmissions and loss of functions. It is also believed that lack of cobalt and vitamin B12 lead to various neurological disorders such as mood swings and memory difficulties. In cases of extreme and prolonged deficiency of cobalt and vitamin B12, psychosis can result.

At Hadassah University in Jerusalem, Dr. Oded Abramsky, M.D. of the Neurology Department discovered that cobalt deficiencies frequently resulted in impaired reflex responses, sensory perception, muscular weakness in arms and legs which led to difficulty in walking and jerking of limbs, and even trouble speaking. It is thought that early symptoms such as these can be reversed with appropriate cobalt supplementation before severe conditions such as paralysis and mental deterioration can set in. These types of symptoms are also known to be early stages of Multiple Sclerosis.

Sufficient levels of cobalt may induce adequate erythropoieten hormone production in kidneys and allow for increased production of red blood cells. It is also believed that cobalt is essential as a cofactor in the manufacture of thyroid hormones.

Cobalt has also been used in hepatitis treatments due to its actions in synthesizing protein and fixing nitrogen during amino acid production. It is also beneficial for healthy skin, building hemoglobin by enhancing the absorption of iron. It helps transport glucose from blood into tissues, and can even substitute for manganese in enzyme activation, including antioxidant enzymes. Cobalt has also been linked to digestive disorders, poor circulation, impaired growth, and fatigue. It can even be used to fight bronchial asthma as well as increasing the performance of cellular activity and growth.

The richest sources of cobalt include green vegetables such as broccoli and spinach (spinach samples have shown 0.4 to 0.6 mcg/g). Other plant sources include various nuts and seeds, as well as grains such as oats. Legumes and grains also provide this element. The majority of cobalt—as high as 0.3 ppm—is usually stored in bones, red blood cells, and liver, with smaller amounts stored in the spleen, kidneys, and pancreas.

Copper

Archaeologists have provided evidence showing how copper has been used for almost 11,000 years. This element is simple to mine and refine and evidence shows that it was first mined as early as 7,000 years ago. The Romans obtained most of their copper from the Island of Cyprus. In fact, the word "copper" comes from the Latin word cuprum, meaning "from the island of Cyprus."

Today, large deposits of copper have been found in the United States, Canada, Peru, Chile, Zaire, and Zambia. Pure copper is a soft metal that is used to conduct electricity. It has been used in coinage for many centuries since it resists corrosion from the atmosphere and salt water. Copper pipes in plumbing systems and jewelry were some of its earliest uses.

Most people think of copper as plumbing and water pipes and remember the warnings of dangerous copper toxicity levels. What needs to be understood is that when copper is found in the same form as that found in plants (water-soluble ions), it plays a very significant role in various bodily processes, and most people are deficient in this form of copper. The National Institutes of Health examined copper levels in Americans and found 81% of the subjects in the study were deficient by almost 70% of the RDA.

The average human body fed a proper diet should have between 80 and 120 milligrams of copper, usually concentrated in the liver. It can also be found in other organs such as the brain, heart, and kidneys, although trace amounts can be found in almost all tissues. While the bones and muscles typically contain less copper, they do contain almost one-half of the body's copper reserves since copper plays a significant role in bone formation.

Hart and coworkers first discovered copper's role as an essential nutrient in 1928. This element was found to be required for the proper utilization of iron, in which Elvehjem in 1935 also found similar properties, including copper's strong presence in blood. It is here that copper assists iron in creating chromoproteins and red blood cells, both of which form hemoglobin. Copper's partnership with iron doesn't stop there. Iron also depends largely on various copper-proteins for some of its transport and storage.

Copper isn't physically contained inside hemoglobin, but a small amount is needed in order to participate in the absorption and utilization of iron to create it. In 1953, researchers Baxter and Van Wyk observed that red blood cells became impaired in maturation processes and experienced a shortened life span when copper levels were low. A copper-dependent enzyme, known as ceruloplasmin, is manufactured in the liver and oxidizes iron, which allows it to bind with the iron transport protein transferin. Symptoms of iron deficiency, such as anemia, can just as easily be a lack of copper.

All living organisms benefit from copper. One of the most important roles copper plays in the human body is to activate approximately 21 different enzymes. It is also a cofactor in hundreds of metalloenzymes. In fact, copper's presence in the body is usually inside various proteins that activate enzymes, some of which are involved in bodily processes such as the utilization of iron, energy utilization, and respiratory processes.

Generally, copper-dependent enzymes help synthesize proteins found in connective tissues in bones and circulatory vessels, and they metabolize neurological compounds found in the nervous system. Copper acts as a cofactor for the enzyme cytochrome oxidase in mitochondria, which oxidizes fats, proteins, and carbohydrates, and transfers the electrons from this process to oxygen in order to create energy. This enzyme catalyzes the reduction of oxygen to water, an important stage of cellular respiration.

One enzyme that benefits from the presence of copper is deta-9-desaturase, which assists in the proper metabolism of the essential fatty acids that provide structure to cellular membranes, such as the membrane that surrounds the nucleus. When this membrane becomes weakened, various substances can penetrate the nucleus, potentially damaging the DNA.

Many enzymes that develop and maintain the cardiovascular system are activated by copper. One such enzyme is lysyl oxidase, which is responsible for the formation of elastin. A deficiency of this polymer results in a gradual decline of structural integrity in blood vessels and a failure to convert lysyl to desmosine, one of the ingredients in elastin. Such weakened or ruptured aortic elastin can result in aneurysms or other severe conditions. Overall, copper can be considered an excellent protection against atherosclerosis, EKG abnormalities, and other blood conditions that can lead to heart attacks and strokes. Even some cases of high cholesterol can be credited as a failure to properly metabolize fatty acids, which can result when there is an absence of enzymatic activity, which again correlates with low copper levels.

When important fatty acids are missing from blood vessels, erratic blood pressure and heartbeat can result. Calcium channel blockers, such as aspirin, are used to thin the blood in an effort to control these symptoms. When these fatty acids are lacking in the walls of mitochondria where energy is created, symptoms that resemble chronic fatigue syndrome can result. Between these two enzymes—cytochrome oxidase and deta-9-desaturase—it is very possible that people suffering from low energy levels, chronic fatigue syndrome, and weakness may be lacking copper.

Many experiments using laboratory mice have shown a correlation between the presence of copper and the activation of these enzymes. In 1977, researcher Petering observed how copper deficiencies resulted in raised levels of cholesterol and other fatty substances. Later in 1987, Cunnane observed irregular heartbeat in rats fed low copper diets. Also, copper deficient animals also experience glucose intolerance, abnormal cardiac functions, and ruptured blood vessels. These researchers attributed these and other cardiovascular conditions to an absence of superoxide dismutase (SOD) enzyme activation, which is the powerful antioxidant enzyme that relies on several minerals for activation, one of them being copper. Histaminase is another enzyme that requires copper.

This enzyme is used to break down histamine. Allergies are an overproduction of histamine, which could be a copper deficiency.

Most people don't realize the many roles that copper plays in influencing mood chemistry. The copper-dependent enzyme known as dopamine beta-hydroxyl synthesizes the neurological hormone known as norepinephrine, which regulates depression and fatigue. According to researcher O'Dell (1984), copper deficiency impairs other nervous system components, such as the formation of two neurotransmitters, dopamine and norepinephrine. Other mood hormones that need copper are serotonin and a stress hormone called epinephrine. And still, copper is needed for aminoxidases to regulate the metabolism of the many neurotransmitter proteins in the brain and nervous system that help to determine our thoughts and moods.

The human body attaches copper ions to various metabolites in the body, including proteins, amino acids, and enzymes. One of the most well-known enzymes, SOD, is the fifth most abundant type of protein found in the human body. SOD relies on heavy metals such as zinc, manganese, iron, and copper to be activated. According to Dr. Joel M. McCord, one form of SOD contains zinc and copper, and the other form contains manganese and iron. This enzyme protects against oxidative damage that results from a highly reactive and dangerous form of oxygen that is known as a free radical.

According to Sherry A. Rogers, MD, the SOD enzyme also helps to protect us from developing chemical sensitivity. In order for our detoxification pathways to function, certain minerals must be present. When deficiencies are improved, many chemical sensitivities are reversed. When a 33-year old lab technician developed intolerance for public places such as shopping malls and toxic pollutants such as exhaust fumes, she experienced headaches, confusion, and fatigue, due to the high concentration of chemicals. After discovering that she had a copper deficiency, supplementation resulted in a reversal of her allergic conditions. Credit was given to copper's role in the SOD enzyme.

The role of this enzyme extends into other areas as well. With its antioxidant capabilities, it helps slow down the aging process. In most diseases, SOD levels are decreased. Some studies have shown chemically induced tumors to have low levels of both copper and SOD. Those who experience colitis have lower concentrations of SOD in the bowel, while Alzheimer's patients have extremely low levels in their brain.

Ninety-three percent of the copper found in blood plasma is fixed to an enzyme called ceruloplasmin, which participates in mobilizing iron. The other 7% of copper is bound to other substances, such as albumin and amino acids, which can eventually react with other proteins or diffuse across some membranes.

Studies using cows and sheep have shown that low copper levels result in decreased immune systems, usually by affecting the T and B cells. Studies using mice with hypocuprosis showed decreasing amounts of antibodies when copper was lacking. Most theorize that the resulting low immune system from low copper levels is largely due to its relationship with the enzyme SOD. Interestingly, copper levels in blood plasma increase during infections and liver disease.

Researchers Harris and O'Dell (1974) have shown that low copper levels can result in improper collagen formation. The lysyl oxidase enzyme requires copper in order to form the cross-linking and elastin formation in collagen. This enzyme adds a hydroxyl group to lysine residues, which provides collagen fibers with crosslinking, providing collagen with elasticity and structural integrity. Collagen strengthens tendons, cartilage, and bones. Copper also improves vitamin C oxidation, which also helps collagen formation.

Studies using laboratory rats and guinea pigs revealed some telltale signs of copper deficiency. When fed copper deficient diets, these animals experienced anemia, high mortality rates among their offspring, retarded fetal development, and a high percentage of brain damage within days after birth. It is thought that these symptoms are a result of defective red blood cells and improper connective tissue formation during early stages of development.

Both animals and humans can experience a lack of pigmentation, which is another symptom of copper deficiency. The skin pigment known as melanin is formed from the enzyme known as tyrosinase, which is activated by copper. Copper deficiency symptoms that affect the skin's pigmentation include a condition known as Menkes Kinky Hair Syndrome, which is characterized by twisted, fragile, and whitish hair without any pigmentation. Dr. Joseph R. Prohaska, associate professor of Biochemistry at the University of Minnesota, explains that this syndrome is a result of improper metabolism of copper.

When copper is deficient, the enzyme polyphenyl oxidase is either lacking or is unable to convert tyrosine into melanin. Affected persons can include albinos but it can also be manifest in other conditions such as retardation, low body temperature, loss of hair pigment, impaired keritinization of hair and wool in mammals, and ruptured aortic elastin resulting in aneurysms.

In severe cases where the body lacks copper enzymes, the body does not contain the cytochrome oxidase enzyme, resulting in gradual brain degeneration. Such cases can result in mental retardation, where the severely affected children usually do not live beyond three years old. Other enzymes that require the presence of copper include, but are not limited to, tyrosinase, dopamine-beta-hydroxylase, and ferroxidase.

A severe case of copper deficiency was recognized in 1937 in sheep. Neonatal enzootic ataxia, a condition of the nervous system characterized by demyelination of the cerebellum and spinal cord, was observed in sheep that had severely low levels of copper. This condition resulted in nerve cell death and abnormal formations of a cerebral matter known as chromatolysis. The entire nervous system was in disarray and failed to form properly. The sheep were supplemented with copper, which gradually prevented the syndrome. These conditions resembled human cerebral palsy, and were attributed to reduced enzymatic activity, namely the enzyme cytochrome oxidase, which also leads to abnormal myelin formation.

Deterioration of the myelin sheath during copper deficiencies is also similar to multiple sclerosis in humans. Two researchers, Hansen and Plumb, observed sufficient copper levels in blood and spinal fluids of multiple sclerosis patients. They noticed that there was insufficient activity of the oxidase enzyme in the blood. An interesting assessment was made by these researchers who said, "This new finding does not yet appear to have attracted comment and its confirmation and further investigation will be awaited with interest, since vital clues to the role of trace minerals in myelination are badly needed." According to researcher Voisin, it was later discovered that Australian biochemists were able to prevent a similar disease by supplementing copper in sheep. Ruth Allcroft later found comparable results in England.

Dr. Rogers explains that there are other enzyme systems besides SOD that need copper in order to detoxify foreign chemicals. The polyphenol oxidase enzyme breaks down harmful chemicals that are emitted from popular household cleaning products. Experiments using laboratory rats have shown tissue death in their livers when they were exposed to carbon tetrachloride during periods of copper deficiency. However, when copper was supplemented, they experienced an increase in chemical tolerance and were able to avoid premature death. Copper also acts as a cofactor in glutathione peroxidase and catalase enzymes, even though it is not directly used in them.

Women typically need more copper than men to mobilize iron. The amount of copper found in blood can double during late term pregnancies. Copper levels of a fetus or a newborn infant should be dramatically higher than a normal adult. Most of their stored copper is contained in the liver, allowing the child to maintain an adequate supply long after the mother's supply of copper is insufficient, or it is weaned off of the nursing mother altogether.

Copper deficiencies in pregnant women can result in congenital defects of the heart, brain cerebral palsy, and hyplasia of the cerebellum in the unborn fetus. Some forms of arthritis in newborn infants are various forms of bone spurs inside the bone growth plate, spurred on by a lack of copper. Anemia, myelin defects, lack of pigmentation and hair keratinization, and lack of white blood cells are also attributed to copper deficiencies.

Water soluble copper ions cross the blood brain barrier on their way to activating enzymes in the brain and participating in other neuro-processes. Other reports of the benefits of copper include many people who have taken copper supplements and having anti-parasitic experiences. It is unclear why those who wear copper bracelets tend to experience decreased symptoms of arthritis or Lupus. Some theories suggest that they are probably experiencing a small absorption of copper ions into their skin, which activates the SOD enzyme.

Besides those conditions already mentioned, copper deficiencies can also include sagging skin tissues, brittle hair, liver cirrhosis, hyperthyroid, learning disabilities, violent behavior, hernias, vericose veins, and Kawasaki disease. Other conditions that involve lack of copper or lack of copper-induced enzymatic activity include decalcification of bones, small skin hemorrhages, and baldness.

Foods that appear consistent in adequate copper concentrations are nuts, seeds, legumes, and fruits and vegetables.

Fluorine

Under normal conditions, the element fluorine is a pale, yellow-colored gas that is a little heavier than air and becomes a solid after it cools. In the 1670 fluorine was used in compounds for etching glass. Later, in 1886, the French chemist Ferdinand Frederic Henri Moissan successfully isolated fluorine. It is a highly reactive element that can react and bind with just about any other element and form a compound. Therefore, fluorine is rarely ever found in nature as anything other than in a compound, except in soils and plants. Although readily found in most soils, there is little record of this element providing any measurable benefit in plant growth and development.

As with any element, minerals should be ingested only in their ionic form and never as a compound. This is especially true with fluorine. When it is being referred to in its ionic state, it is known as fluoride (F-) (similar to chlorine vs. chloride).

Although fluorine has no benefits to the body, fluoride does provide some benefit to animals and people. Fluoride is not considered an essential mineral because it is not required to grow or sustain life, but if one adds disease prevention to the definition of "essential," it should be considered an important and useful mineral and could very well be listed as essential someday.

Fluoride can be found in almost all human tissues, although 95% of it is found in the teeth and bones. It is beneficial to bone collagen and teeth development, and some studies show that fluoride helps harden tooth enamel. Its other roles in the body are still being investigated.

Fluoride is absorbed through the cells of the stomach lining and the small intestine, where it enters the blood and quickly moves into teeth and bone tissue. Bone tissue is largely a crystallized structure comprised of phosphate, magnesium, boron, and calcium, commonly known as hydroxyapatite crystals. Fluoride does not accumulate in these areas. Rather, its high chemical reactivity and small radius allows it to either replace the larger hydroxyl (-OH) ion in the hydroxyapatite crystal of the bone to form fluoroapatite or its small size allows it to enter the spaces inside the crystal which increases its density, making fluoride an important component of teeth and bone structure.

Studies using rats show a strong correlation between fluoride deficiency and growth retardation, which was reversed after fluoride supplements were given. However, when it comes to understanding the role of fluoride, there is little evidence of fluoride deficiencies in people. Rather, the concern and debate about fluoride centers on conditions that result from excess exposure to fluoride compounds.

Fluoride compounds have been found in igneous rocks, sandstone, shale, limestone, seawater, and most soils. Compounds such as calcium fluoride, hydrogen fluoride, or even sodium fluoride can enter the environment from various sources. These processes include the original weathering and dissolution processes that break down rock particles into the soil which eventually liberates its ions. However, most fluoride compounds enter the environment through industrial processes.

Heavy metal manufacturers such as steel, aluminum, copper, phosphate ore, nickel, and even brick and glass industries, as well as glue and other adhesive productions, can all emit various forms of fluoride compounds into the atmosphere. Phosphate ore and aluminum manufacturers are the largest contributors to fluoride compounds being released into the environment.

Compounds of fluoride serve many different industrial purposes. Hydrogen fluoride can be either a liquid or gas and is used industrially to produce synthetic cryolite, gasoline alkolytes, chlorofluorocarbons, and aluminum fluoride. It is used to clean glass, aluminum, and bricks, and is also used in tanning leather and removing rust. Calcium fluoride is insoluble and is used as a flux in steel processing, as well as the production of glass and enamel. It is also a major ingredient in the manufacture of hydrofluoric acid and anhydrous hydrogen fluoride. Sodium fluoride is only moderately soluble and serves as a preservative in glue adhesives, wood products, glass production processes, and even pesticides. Sodium fluoride is also added to drinking water. It is true that some studies have shown a decrease in dental caries in areas treated with fluoridated water, but the toxic effects of the sodium fluoride compound should be realized.

Although fluoride compounds can enter the soil through atmospheric transport, the same processes of dissolution and microbial activities occur in the soil to break down these compounds and release the fluoride ions. Generally, when fluorine binds with another substance, it has an extremely strong binding power, and no chemical substance can free fluorine from any of its compounds, which might explain why fluorine is almost never found freely in nature. Although microbial decomposition processes can liberate the ions (fluoride) from the compounds found in the soil, this process can take many years.

Fluoride ions attach to colloidal particles to form compounds just like any other element. This process is optimal when the soil's pH level is slightly acidic—5.5 to 6.5. Fluoride has been found in oceanic plants as high as 4.5 ppm, and land plants at 0.5 to 40 ppm, depending on the soil and the local environmental and industrial processes that may have increased the plant's exposure to fluoride uptake.

With the benefits of proper fluoride in the human body centering on bone strength and teeth development, toxicity resulting from over-exposure to fluoride compounds result in various conditions that affect these same areas of the body. Fluoride compounds can accumulate in bone tissues, causing all sorts of collagen deformation and skeletal irregularities. Levels of fluoride compounds at 1 ppm or greater result in abnormal formation of collagen, the major component of skin, cartilage, ligaments, tendons, muscles, bones, and teeth. When this collagen is unable to develop normally, the skin loses its firmness and youthful elasticity and becomes wrinkled and other collagen-dependent components of the body including the ligaments, tendons, teeth, and bone structures can develop irregularly or begin to deteriorate. Arthritis and stiff joints can develop. Fluoride deficiencies or excess fluoride compounds hinder the production of collagen in the cells responsible for the formation of tooth enamel and bone density. Deformations in skeletal structure and discolored and deformed teeth can result.

Dental fluorosis is a condition that is characterized by toxic exposure to fluoride compounds. Initial symptoms of dental fluorosis are white speckles on teeth, or in more severe cases dark colored spots or stripes. Other unusual conditions include nausea, faintness, black tar-like stools, constipation, stomach cramps, tremors, skin rashes, and soreness in bones, stiff joints, and shallow breathing.

Some studies show a correlation between toxic accumulations of fluoride compounds and its effects on the nervous system. In the journal Neurotoxicology and Teratology (1995), Dr. Phyllis Mullenix, the former head of toxicology at Forsyth Dental Center in Boston, observed that animals reacted to even low doses of sodium fluoride by affecting their brain functioning and their central nervous system. Some Chinese studies show reduced IQ levels in children who were exposed to even low doses of fluoride compounds.

One of the most vivid examples of toxic poisoning from fluoride compounds was in an article in the German magazine Stern. In 1978, the article titled "Das Dorf der jungen Greise" described a village in Kizilcaoern, Turkey, as a place where the young looked and felt old. By the age of 30, the men looked very old and decrepit. They had extremely wrinkled skin, weak muscles, had difficulty walking, were hunched over, and showed little interest in women. Premature births and stillborn babies after four or five months were common.

Medical researchers from the University of Eskisehir believed that these conditions resulted from the high level of sodium fluoride in their drinking water. Samples of the drinking water by Dr. Yusef C. Ozkan resulted in 5.4 ppm sodium fluoride. The Sicilian village Acquaviva Platani experienced similar symptoms. Dr. Frada from the University of Palmero investigated and found hardening of the arteries, senility, and high mortality was rampant. The drinking water was sampled and the results showed 5 ppm sodium fluoride. Other investigations have documented high sodium fluoride levels in areas of India that resembled these conditions.

In 1979, 50 ppm of sodium fluoride was dumped into the drinking water of 50,000 people in Annapolis, Maryland. Later, Dr. Yiamouyiannis performed epidemiological studies and found that 20% of the residents suffered from either muscoskeletal, gastrointestinal, neurological, dermatological, or urological symptoms.

Other characteristics of sodium fluoride include inhibiting the function of white blood cells and impairing the synthesis of the SOD enzyme that destroys foreign agents. Other signs of sodium fluoride toxicity include wrinkling of the skin from loss of collagen. Also, when collagen is lost or disrupted, improper deposits and utilization of calcium can result. Tissues can become calcified, while at the same time bones can lose their calcium. Even as little as 1 ppm impairs the collagen-producing cells of the teeth, known as ameloblasts. Impairment of collagen will also affect the odontoblasts that form dentin. Some bony outgrowths in the spine can also occur from calcification of spinal ligaments. A study conducted in England showed that increases in sodium fluoride resulted in increases of hip fractures by 40%.

Fluorine (not fluoride) inhibits enzymatic activity, especially the enzymes required for digestion. Dr. Earl Mindell has stated that intestinal discomforts such as bloating and gas can be a result of such conditions. Decreased immune system strength, resulting in arthritis and autoimmune disorders, can also result.

Some have observed DNA repair activity declining by as much as 50% during periods of sodium fluoride poisoning. Sodium fluoride disrupts over 100 enzyme processes in the body. The DNA repair enzyme becomes inhibited and is unable to perform its functions when the cell is damaged and in need of repair. Sodium fluoride is also used as a rat poison, where its primary responsibility is to destroy enzyme functions in the rat, causing it to starve to death even though it is eating all the food it desires. Significant amounts of DNA damage have been observed in testes cells, which could explain some of the birth defects and growth deformations observed in Turkey, Sicily, and India, as stated previously.

Natural sources that consistently show high concentrations of fluorine and fluoride compounds include seawater and in rocks located in volcanic regions and high geothermal activity. Factors such as pH and the level of carbon and clay are all responsible for the retention or leaching of fluoride from the soil. After deposit from airborne transport, fluoride compounds from pollution can build up in the soil's surface until the element becomes subject to the microorganisms' dissolution processes. Fluoride is not easily leached from the soil; thus, the microbes stimulate the process for the fluoride ions to be liberated for plant uptake.

Some public water treatment systems continue to add fluoride compounds to their drinking water, while other countries have outlawed the practice. The following countries have prohibited sodium fluoride from entering public water systems: Germany, France, Belgium, Luxembourg, Finland, Denmark, Norway, Sweden, Netherlands, Northern Ireland, Austria, Czech Republic, and most recently in 2003 Switzerland. The ionic form of fluoride that is found in plants (F-) is the only form that will allow for optimal absorption in both plant and human cells. This form of fluoride can be found in plants such as fruits and vegetables grown in soils that contain fluoride.

Iodine

Named after the Greek word for violet, iodes, iodine was originally discovered in 1811 by Barnard Courtois, a French chemist, while he was busy extracting sodium and potassium from burned seaweed ash. Surprisingly, he added sulfuric acid to further process the ash, when all of a sudden a purple-colored cloud of smoke erupted. Eventually, this purple gas condensed on metal objects in the room, isolating solid iodine for the first time in history.

Iodine and iodide should not be confused. The element iodine can burn the skin, damage eyes and mucous membranes, and be poisonous if consumed. Iodide (I-) refers to its ionic state and provides many interesting health benefits for both plants and animals.

Iodine is not found consistently throughout nature. It is usually found naturally in areas close to the ocean and is more likely to be deficient in areas further inland. Mountainous areas such as the Andes, Himalayas or Alps, are not likely to contain measurable amounts of iodine. As a naturally-occurring element, iodine is typically not found in crops growing in mountains in sufficient quantities for proper human health, but is usually more concentrated in soils and plants once covered by the ocean and around coastal regions, including sea water, marine animals and plants, limestone, shale, and sandstone. This unique element has been found in small red and brown algae and plays an important role in all vertebrate animals and humans. Fortunately, microorganisms in the ocean produce a compound known as methyl iodine, which diffuses as a gas into the air where it eventually falls to Earth during heavy rains. Iodine is easily leached away in commonly flooded areas such as the Ganges. Therefore, the longer the soil is exposed to weathering, the more likely it is that iodine will be washed away through the rivers back into the ocean.

Iodine accounts for as little as 0.0004% of our body weight. Most estimates have stated iodine's amount in the body anywhere between 20 to 50 milligrams, of which around 20% is located in the thyroid, 50% in muscle tissue, and the remainder scattered throughout the reproductive organs, blood, and muscles. CM Baumann's research in 1896 first discovered iodine's significance in thyroid glands. This is the discovery that caused iodine to become listed as one of the essential microminerals.

Iodine is a necessary element with regards to human health. Its major responsibility is in the development and function of the thyroid, which is a gland positioned inside the neck between the throat and spine. This gland captures iodine traveling in the blood where it will be used to produce several different hormones, all of which have significant roles in the body. The iodine will be used to produce various hormones that will eventually be released back into the bloodstream as needed.

The thyroid is regulated by a complex process involving the pituitary gland and the brain. After the hypothalamus secretes the thyrotropin-releasing hormone (TRH), the pituitary gland responds by secreting a thyroid-stimulating hormone (TSH), which initiates the trapping of iodine in the blood, thyroid hormone synthesis, and the release of the T3 and T4 hormones from the thyroid. In liver and brain tissues, the T3 hormone binds with thyroid receptors in the nuclei of cells to regulate gene expression, while the T4 hormone can be converted to T3 by the deiodinases enzymes found in these tissues. If iodine is deficient, production of the T4 hormone is impaired.

The two hormones, T3 and T4, are produced in the thyroid when iodine is combined with an amino acid called tyrosine. These two hormones are then excreted out of the thyroid and into the blood for transport to various organs throughout the body. They help regulate many of the body's processes, such as the production of energy, growth, development, basic metabolic rate, protein synthesis, reproduction, the conversion of carotene to vitamin A, and the synthesis of cholesterol, which is a necessary ingredient in the manufacture of hormones. These hormones also have key roles in the assimilation of salts, control of digestion, body temperature, heart rate, and nervous and reproductive systems, all of which contribute to body weight.

It should be noted, however, that there is a process where the T4 hormone is converted into the T3 hormone. The mineral selenium activates one of the enzymes (iodothyronine deiodinases) responsible for this conversion. Therefore, when selenium is deficient, a noticeable decrease in hormonal synthesis can occur, which can increase the symptoms of iodine deficiency. Deficiencies of iron and vitamin A have also been shown to increase the effects of iodine deficiency.

These and other hormones created in the thyroid are also important to the growth and development of the epidermal layers of cells in the brain. It is here that they help these cells develop enough integrity to prevent toxic materials from entering the critical interior of brain cells. Thus, iodine's role in brain cells makes it critical to neutralizing and destroying harmful toxins, which allows for proper mental functioning. Also, these hormones enter cells of other tissues and bind to substances inside the cell, where they play a significant role in the cell's metabolic processes.

The most common cause of preventable brain damage in the world is iodine deficiency. Iodine deficiency disorders (IDD), according to the World Health Organization, afflicts over 740 million people throughout the world. An estimated 50 million of these people suffer from some degree of brain damage resulting from lack of iodine. Symptoms of iodine deficiency include brain damage, retardation, as well as other forms of growth and development disorders.

A study using laboratory rats showed dangerously low levels of thyroid hormones in the brain when iodine was deficient. This resulted in decreased brain function, but was eventually corrected when iodine was restored to the diet. It was observed that the rats' mental acuity was also impaired when iodine was lacking.

Iodine deficient areas are more likely to be in remote areas, which could contribute to poorer schools, nutritional habits, and social deprivation. A report studied schoolchildren who lived in remote areas deficient in iodine and compared their academic performance with children who did not lack iodine. There are many factors in determining and judging academic performance and IQ levels, and difficulty in establishing adequate control groups to perform such a test. Nevertheless, even when these factors were taken into consideration, the iodine deficient children showed decreased IQ scores, learning disabilities, and academic performance to some degree. A summary of

18 studies investigating similar conditions concluded that iodine deficiency lowered average IQ scores by almost 14 points. Regardless, it is clear that mental acuity depends partly on the presence of hormones that are produced in the thyroid, which require this element.

Mineral deficiencies in parents gradually become more severe when they are passed on to their offspring. Fetal iodine deficiency results when the mother is also deficient. Infancy is a period of rapid brain growth and development, which is heavily dependent upon thyroid hormones produced from iodine. When the expecting mother is deficient in iodine, the physical growth and mental development of the fetus becomes impaired. Infants that suffer from hypothyroidism can experience a condition known as cretinism, which is a disorder that is characterized by constipation, jaundice, poor appetite, and even impaired bone growth. The metabolic rate slows down to unhealthy rates, muscles become flabby, and the bones become weak and poorly formed. If the fetus is left without iodine altogether, mental retardation can result. A thyroid that develops abnormally from lack of iodine can cause deafness. In severe cases, infants can suffer from congenital hypothyroidism, which is characterized by slower response times and decreased mental capacity. Dwarfism can also result, which can be even more severe if selenium is lacking.

The reproductive system stores iodine and is regulated by the thyroid. Miscarriages and birth defects can be associated with a deficiency of iodine during neonatal development. Studies have shown high infant mortality rates in areas lacking iodine. Other studies have observed a reversal of these conditions once iodine was resupplied. During postnatal care, iodine requirements increase as the mother is required to pass iodine and other minerals onto her breastfeeding infant. Women who are breastfeeding and lacking iodine are not able to pass this mineral on to their infants who have very high requirements for this mineral in order to develop properly.

A study was conducted in central India with women with who had experienced two or more miscarriages or two or more stillbirths. By measuring levels of iodine in their urinary excretion, it was determined that women who continuously experienced reproductive failures unknowingly suffered from goiter, a symptom of iodine deficiency. These women experienced impairment of growth and development of their fetus when compared to women that did not experience low levels of iodine (37.9% to 16.1%). It is clear that this element has important function in the early growth and development of a fetus, and a deficiency of this element has been overlooked.

When insoluble iodine is found in extremely high concentrations, a condition known as hyperthyroidism usually results, otherwise known as Grave's Disease. This results in an overactive thyroid, characterized by an abnormal increase in thyroid secretions. This condition is also characterized by increased heart rate, raised blood pressure, intolerance of heat, excessive sweating, most of which result in weight loss. Persons going through this condition can show signs of nervousness, short tempers, irritability, increased appetite, frequent bowel movements, and difficult sleep patterns such as insomnia.

Other observations have shown that an excess of iodine compounds unable to be absorbed by the body can cause or aggravate acne in adolescents. Some researchers suggest that this is caused when the body tries to excrete the insoluble and unusable iodine through the pores, thus irritating the skin.

During conditions where there is insufficient iodine, thyroid activity slows down. This condition is known as Hashimoto's Disease, or hypothyroidism. Some sufferers have reported enhanced sensitivity to cold, especially in the hands and feet. No matter how many layers of clothes they put on, they never seem to get warm. Experiments in this manner have shown symptoms of lethargy, exhaustion, tiredness, depression, and even low sex drive. Thus, inadequate amounts of iodine can affect our personalities a great deal. Disease conditions can also occur when a lack of iodine causes the thyroid gland to absorb sodium fluoride compounds instead.

Circulation of the blood is also affected by iodine. Therefore, an increase in oxygen and other elements being transported throughout the body can be enhanced with a proper amount of iodine. Weight gain, hardening of the arteries, high blood cholesterol, breast lumps, constipation, puffy face, and even brittle nails, hair loss, dry skin and dry hair are also common symptoms of iodine deficiency.

In an article published in the Western Journal of Surgery, Obstetrics, and Gynecology, the significance of iodine was clearly established. The study examined three women who were given iodine and maintained proper metabolic rates during pregnancy. If their metabolism was high, iodine actually lowered the rate to normal, and if their metabolic rate was too slow, the iodine supplement raised the metabolic rate. Clearly, iodine's role as a harmonic balancer of the basic metabolic rate is understood. It is estimated that approximately 11 million Americans suffer from either hypothyroidism or hyperthyroidism.

In areas of the world where iodine is deficient, people are likely to suffer from prolonged iodine deficiency. This results in unusually low metabolic rates, which signals the thyroid to increase output of the hormone thyroxin in an effort to boost metabolism (this balancing act is determined and regulated by the thyroid). However, if iodine is not supplied soon, the overactive thyroid can become enlarged—a condition known as goiter. In some cases, as little as one millionth of an ounce of iodine that is deficient for an extended period of time is usually enough to result in enlargement of this gland.

Goiter results when the thyroid gland becomes swollen and enlarged due to an extreme and prolonged lack of iodine, although this condition is rare, due in part to the consumption of "iodized salt." As early as 1850, iodine was being used to prevent goiters. During the 1920s, goiters were relatively common, especially in the Southern United States, the Great Lakes region and the Swiss Alps, where iodine is almost non-existent in their soils. Measuring the public's iodine levels has usually involved urine samples and measuring thyroid hormone levels. However, even today some rare cases of goiter can still be seen in the South, as well as areas in Texas and California, and some areas of Canada. Unfortunately, goiters are still common throughout Africa. Iodine is usually found in high amounts in ocean water. Interestingly, some physicians during the time of Hippocrates realized that something inside seaweed and seafood prevented goiter.

Sodium iodide was added to regular table salt in 1924. Soon afterward, cases of goiter decreased dramatically, even though sodium iodide is a compound and not a water-soluble form of iodine, it still proved useful in abolishing goiters.

There are other factors that come into play when discussing thyroid problems. Before a particular food gets labeled as being a "goitrogen" (something that blocks iodine absorption), some elements such as selenium and copper are also required for proper utilization of iodine. Even a lack of vitamin A and iron can cause iodine deficiencies to worsen.

In rare circumstances, radioactive fallout usually results in a heavy increase of radioactive iodine released into the air. Once this air is breathed, this dangerous form of iodine usually finds its way into the thyroid. In such cases, if the thyroid gland is lacking the correct form of iodine, the radioactive form of iodine builds up to extreme levels, quickly causing thyroid cancer. During the nuclear power plant disaster in Chernobyl, Ukraine, people were quickly supplemented with the compound potassium iodide from the Polish government in an attempt to prevent the radioactive iodine from gaining position in the thyroid. When the body is already properly supplied with plenty of water soluble iodide, emergency remedies such as these become unnecessary.

Common foods that seem to consistently have ample amounts of iodide include kelp and dulse seaweed since ocean water is a good source of iodide. Iodized salt also contains iodide, but this product should be kept at a minimum due to its compound form with sodium. Rather, getting iodide from land and marine crops such as green vegetables or even sea vegetables such as seaweed are better choices. These foods should be eaten fresh, since frying has shown to reduce the content of iodide by 20%, grilling by 23% and boiling by 58%. Other plant sources of iodide include fruits such as pineapples and grapes, and vegetables such as asparagus, garlic, squash, chard, and turnips. Beans and sea salt also contain iodide.

Chapter 12

The Microminerals in People (cont'd)

Iron

Iron is abundant and comprises 5.6% of Earth's crust and nearly the entire mass of Earth's core. It has been used for almost 5,000 years to make tools, weapons, and other heavy metal objects. Iron and carbon are combined to produce steel, and when chromium is included in the mixture, the steel alloy is able to resist rust.

Iron is a well-known but also misunderstood mineral that performs very important functions in the body. It is involved in biochemical reactions such as transporting oxygen to cells all over the body. It also acts as a cofactor and activator of hundreds of enzymes, including a healthy output of pancreatic enzymes that aid in digestion, elimination, metabolism, circulation, and other important functions.

One of iron's biggest contributions is found in the blood. Interestingly, its role in human blood is similar to magnesium's role in chlorophyll in plants. It participates in the entire process of respiration to produce energy. Iron has been called the "energy giver" since it attracts and carries oxygen. This transport of oxygen occurs in healthy, iron-rich blood.

Healthy blood requires more than just iron. Iron combines with copper and manganese to produce vital blood proteins known as hemoglobin and myoglobin. These two proteins contain a red iron-rich compound known as heme, and they participate in the storage and transport of oxygen throughout the body. Hemoglobin is found in red blood cells and is the most abundant of these proteins, making up about two-thirds of the body's total iron. Each hemoglobin molecule can carry up to four molecules of oxygen from the lungs to the rest of the body. Myoglobin transports iron into muscle cells for short-term storage of oxygen, which provides the body with an ability to balance the supply of oxygen to meet the demands during muscular exercise.

Hemoglobin, which carries oxygen to every cell in the body, and myoglobin, which stores oxygen in muscle cells, are two sources of iron that store oxygen in the blood. These sources are known as "functional" sources, and comprise about 70% of iron's usefulness; the other 30% is used for storage. Healthy bodies will usually contain between 3 and 5 grams of iron, 65% of which is located in hemoglobin.

Iron is essential for maintaining high levels of athletic performance. Since iron carries oxygen into muscles, low levels of iron in the blood could result in fatigue and early exhaustion. Young women who frequently diet and participate in strenuous activities are the most susceptible to iron deficiencies. Investigations have tested female college students and found that 31% were experiencing low iron content. Some researchers have observed female athletes benefiting from additional iron during athletic performance, even when they tested as having normal iron levels. One observation of high school cross-country runners discovered that 45 percent of the women and 17% of the men were low in iron. Athletes can benefit from adding water-soluble iron supplementation to their daily regimen to increase endurance, energy, and to keep their number of red blood cells high.

Another responsibility of iron is to strengthen the immune system. It is required for various immune responses, such as the differentiation and proliferation of T-lymphocytes and the activation of iron-containing enzymes that are used to destroy infectious pathogens. During periods of infection, the body reacts in a very interesting manner. During an acute inflammatory response, iron levels in the blood will decrease, in order to allow ferritin, a protein that stores iron, to increase, which suggests that the body is preventing the infectious pathogen from using or benefiting from iron's presence in the blood.

White blood cells need iron to produce special reactive forms of oxygen known as superoxides, which destroy bacteria. T-lymphocytes are cells in the blood that act like antibodies by attacking infectious agents, such as viruses. The production of these disease-fighting cells requires quick DNA synthesis. Since iron is an integral part of an enzyme that synthesizes deoxyribose, a DNA building block, DNA synthesis slows down when iron is low. When iron is lacking, a decrease in red blood cells (anemia) can occur.

While recognizing iron's critical role in blood, it should be understood that when iron is lacking for an extended period of time, the number of red blood cells considered normal (25 trillion) can drop to less than 15 trillion, resulting in a severe condition known as anemia. Excess fatigue and shortness of breath, which stems from insufficient oxygen being supplied to the cells, are characteristic of this condition. Therefore, people suffering from iron-deficient anemia report both an inability to exercise and muscle weakness. Other symptoms affected by anemia include brittle fingernails and toenails, and hair that usually becomes dry and lacks integrity. The skin can appear pale, pasty, and gray, and result in premature wrinkling. Although anemia can be attributed to other deficiencies, such as vitamin B12, folic acid, or copper, iron-deficient anemia can be overcome with proper supplementation using water soluble iron, or a dietary change that included a wide variety of dark green plants that have absorbed plenty of iron from the soil.

An iron deficiency can interfere with proper brain functioning. People may be surprised to learn that iron is essential in the functioning of neurotransmitting chemicals such as dopamine, serotonin, and norepinephrine, which help conduct electrical impulses between nerves in the brain. Iron is highly concentrated in dopamine pathways, which are major neurotransmitters in the brain. Enzymes that metabolize dopamine, serotonin, and norepinephrine all require iron in order to be activated. Studies involving animals have shown that iron deficiencies can lead to learning disabilities and gradual behavioral impairment because dopamine was lacking iron.

According to the Archives of Pediatric and Adolescent Medicine, children with Attention Deficit/Hyperactivity Disorder (ADHD) appear to have an iron deficiency. In 2004, a small team led by Dr. Eric Konofal at Hopital Robert Debre in Paris examined iron levels in 53 children with (ADD). The researchers measured the severity of the ADHD symptoms by looking at ferritin levels in their blood. After examination, they found that 84% of the children with ADHD had decreased ferritin levels compared to only 18% in the control group. Dangerously low ferritin levels were observed in 32% of the ADHD children. They concluded that the lower the ferritin levels, the more severe the ADHD symptoms, since iron contributes to the normal functioning of the dopamine neurotransmitter. Therefore, iron supplementation may be able to help dopamine activity in those who have ADHD.

In the Journal of Orthomolecular Medicine, Dr. Merlyn Werbach explained how iron deficiencies are now being researched for contributing to aggressive behavioral syndrome. Adolescent males experiencing aggressive behaviors have been shown to have iron deficiencies. In a study of incarcerated adolescents, iron deficiencies were almost twice as prevalent compared with those who were not incarcerated.

Other studies show a correlation between iron deficient anemia in school-age children and impaired intellectual development, scholastic achievement, and behavioral disorders, although other mineral deficiencies may also be present. Studies observed how anemic children tend to explore their surroundings less than healthy children, which may help to explain the delays in their development. Also, studies using iron-deficient animals have shown decreased optic and auditory nerve impulses to the brain, which is thought to be attributed to impaired nerve myelination. Other studies show a strong correlation between iron supplementation and increased cognitive development in children over two years of age. Researchers theorize that iron deficiencies can affect neurotransmitter synthesis.

Women typically require more of the blood minerals, such as iron, potassium, copper, manganese, and cobalt, than men, due to their blood loss during menstruation. During pregnancies and breast-feeding, their need for these elements increases due to the needs of the fetus and infant. Some studies report infants born with low iron display irritability and lack of interest in their surroundings. Epidemiological studies show that premature birth, low birth weight, and even various forms of maternal mortality are all symptoms that arise during periods of low iron content in pregnant women. Researchers suggest that preventing neonatal anemia is an important component of fetal development. Without enough iron, one can only imagine all the other possible mental deterioration and behavioral disorders that could result.

In order for iron to be utilized optimally, other nutrients such as copper, manganese, cobalt, and vitamin C need to be present. The B-complex vitamins also assist iron. According to the University of Maryland Medical Center, Vitamin B9, also known as folic acid, works closely with Vitamin B12 to help iron work properly in the body, such as making red blood cells, white blood cells, platelets, new genetic material (DNA), and aiding in normal growth. Many studies report that folic acid is also essential for brain function as well as intellectual and emotional health. It is also essential when cells and tissues are growing rapidly, such as during infancy, adolescence, and pregnancy, which is when it helps iron to develop the fetus.

The British Medical Journal reported in 2009 that healthy amounts of folic acid appear to decrease the number of babies who are born with congenital heart disease, which is the most common of all birth defects. The researchers who conducted the experiment concluded that it is important for women to get enough folic acid before and during a pregnancy to prevent birth defects that involve a baby's brain or spine. Clearly, human develop and cognitive health rely on nutrients such as iron and some vitamins.

Mild iron deficiencies usually manifest in symptoms long before anemia develops, including fatigue, decreased cognition, impaired memory, anorexia, depression, learning problems in children and adolescents, impaired sense of alertness, and even dizziness. Observations have also shown that insufficient iron results in a symptom known as “pica,” which tends to drive both adults and children to consume non-food items such as ice (pagophagia), dirt (geophagia), or even lead paint.

Water soluble iron seems to keep the body free of toxic accumulations of insoluble minerals, such as lead, which can cause lead poisoning. Some studies show a correlation between iron deficiencies and increased levels of insoluble lead compounds in the blood of young children. Investigations have concluded that when iron is lacking, an increase in lead absorption occurs through the intestinal lining of animals and people.

Iron has many other benefits that should also be mentioned. Amino acids require iron in order to produce blood sugar (glucose). Cytochrome P450 is an enzyme system that needs iron to help the liver break down and remove toxic chemicals such as drugs, pollutants, and other waste products from the cells. Peroxidases and catalase are two heme-containing enzymes that break down hydrogen peroxide into water and oxygen, thus preventing cells from accumulating this toxic form of oxygen. During this enzymatic process, some white blood cells will gather together harmful bacteria and expose them to the hydrogen peroxide to kill it.

Ribonucleotide reductase is an iron-dependent enzyme that is required for DNA synthesis, which makes iron critical for various reproduction, immune, healing and growth functions. Other iron-containing enzymes initiate production of collagen and elastin, which are the structural proteins required to form and hold cells and tissues together. Enzymes that do not contain heme, but still contain iron, such as NADH dehydrogenase and succinate dehydrogenase, also participate in energy metabolism.

Iron helps oxidize carbohydrates to produce energy that is required to preserve tissue functioning. Heme-containing cytochromes and other enzymes burn fat and carbohydrates to produce ATP, the cell's chemical energy. Cytochromes also transport electrons during the production of ATP. These cellular processes require iron to produce carnitine, which is used to carry fats into the cells to be oxidized.

Some people suffer from a neurological disorder known as Restless Leg Syndrome (RLS), an uncomfortable condition characterized by an urge to move their legs during sleep or during periods of rest. Although not yet labeled as an iron deficiency, RLS tends to occur in people who are lacking iron, and iron supplementation tends to decrease the symptoms. Magnetic Resonance Imaging (MRI) has observed low iron levels in brains of those who are afflicted with this disorder. Studies show decreased ferritin levels when transferrin levels were increased in the cerebrospinal fluid of those suffering from RLS. This could imply that low levels of iron in the brain lead to these types of disorders, although researchers are still trying to explain specifically how low iron concentrations lead to such conditions. However, some research suggests that activity from the iron-dependent enzyme tyrosine hyroxylase affects the synthesis of the neurotransmitter dopamine.

Dr. Barbara Phillips of the University of Kentucky reported at an annual meeting of the American College of Chest Physicians that people who suffer from RLS also tend to suffer from depression and anxiety. The researchers found that symptoms of sleep apnea, insomnia, and difficulty falling asleep were also common in RLS patients. Dr. Phillips stated, "The brain content of iron is different in RLS…Iron and dopamine stores are low…Treating iron deficiency can correct the symptoms."

With iron's role in the cardiovascular system, it should come as no surprise that according to a medical study reported in the journal Neurology, people who suffer from RLS are twice as likely to suffer a stroke or heart disease. Interestingly, the risk of cardiovascular problems was greatest in those who experience severe and frequent symptoms of RLS.

A sound understanding of iron's role in the human body makes it easier to accept other indications of iron deficiencies. These include irregular heartbeat, heart failure, susceptibility to infections such as the common cold virus, and even fibrosis of the pancreas. Iron deficiencies also contribute to constipation, fragile bones, hair loss, dysphagia (difficulty swallowing) and angular stomatitis, diabetes, pale skin, and impaired growth.

When iron is consumed in any other form besides water-soluble ions from sources such as plants, the risk of iron toxicity is greatly enhanced. Iron compounds are not efficiently absorbed or excreted from the body like water soluble ions. When iron (or any other mineral) is ingested in a compound form, it is likely to be too large of a molecule to pass through the cells' ion channels, which can result in toxic accumulations in tissues. Some research suggests that toxic accumulations of insoluble iron in tissues such as the cardiovascular system raise the risk of high blood pressure and heart problems. Other research suggests that women can experience increased risk of heart disease following menopause due to the toxic accumulations of iron compounds that remain collected in their tissues and not excreted from the body during menstruation.

Toxic levels of iron accumulation are usually the result of people consuming insoluble metallic iron. Examples include iron shavings getting into food via the cooking process, steel barrels used in the fermentation of beer, or consuming particles larger than an ion, such as colloidal or chelated particles of iron found in many supplements. Common among Europeans and other developed nations is a condition known as hemochromatosis, which occurs when insoluble iron is deposited in the liver and other tissues. Such dangerous forms of iron can result in liver cirrhosis, arthritis, heart muscle damage, or even diabetes, and are not to be consumed since they are not in the same form as the iron found in plants.

The iron found in plants today came from the same meteorites that bombarded Earth and delivered iron, nickel, phosphorus, and all the other minerals that spawned our planet. All of this matter came from the original nebula that compressed together 15 billion years ago and eventually formed our galaxy.

Plant sources of iron include dark green and leafy vegetables, potatoes, and beans. Apricots, prunes, and most other fruits are also good sources.

Manganese

Carl Wilhelm Scheele first proposed the existence of manganese in 1774, but it was eventually discovered by the Swedish chemist Johan Gottlieb Gahn. Manganese is a heavy metal and almost 90% of all industrial manganese is used in the production of steel alloys. Zinc compounds are used in dry cell batteries, to remove green color in glass that results from iron contaminants, and in black paints to stimulate drying.

Manganese is widely abundant in surprisingly high concentrations throughout Earth in igneous rocks, shale, limestone, sandstone, and soil. Both fresh and ocean water contain ample amounts of this element, while both marine and land plants and animals usually contain only enough parts per million for it to perform its roles.

The word "manganese" is derived from the Latin word for magnet and from the Greek word for magic, which might explain why this element is misunderstood and its full range of benefits on the human body remains to be seen. Even though the role of manganese in plants is well established, its role in humans is still being researched. It is classified as an essential micromineral and was first recognized by two researchers, Orent and McCollum, in 1931. An average human body contains approximately 10-20 milligrams of manganese, most of which is contained and serves functions in pancreas, liver, bones, and kidney tissues. The far-reaching capacities of all of its various functions make studying manganese more difficult and more is being learned about it every day. What is known so far is that manganese is an essential micromineral for all living organisms.

Like other metallic minerals, manganese activates many enzymes and it acts as a cofactor for many other enzymes. The metabolism of glucose, production of energy, and participation in the SOD enzyme are some of the largest enzymatic processes that involve manganese. In fact, whenever the SOD enzyme is found to require manganese, it is referred to as manganese superoxide dismutase (MnSOD). Some enzymes are completely dependent upon manganese to be activated, while other enzymes such as SOD simply need manganese to be a part of the overall process. Other metallic minerals, such as magnesium, can occasionally act as a substitute if manganese is lacking.

Some of the large enzyme systems that can be activated by manganese include kinases, hydrolases, transferases, and decarboxylases, although magnesium can be substituted in these enzymes with little or no loss in activity. Some enzymes are activated by manganese only, such as glycosyltransferases and xylosyltransferase, while other enzymes such as pyruvate carboxylase, glutamine synthetase, and arginase require manganese as well as other minerals. This list of manganese-dependent enzymes may not be long, but the list of other enzymes that can simply be activated by manganese is rather lengthy.

SOD is a very important enzyme. It degrades a dangerous form of oxygen called superoxide, commonly known as a "free radical." In this role, manganese acts as an antioxidant. Two doctors from the University of Wisconsin observed 47 women over a four-month period. They reported in the American Journal of Clinical Nutrition that SOD activity in white blood cells decreased when manganese was deficient. Proper supplementation eventually resulted in a healthy increase of this enzymatic activity in the white blood cells.

There are other enzymes and substances scattered throughout the body that benefit from manganese. One enzyme located in the brain synthesizes an amino acid known as glutamine, which helps remove ammonia, a toxic result of nitrogen metabolism. Collagen is used to heal wounds, and manganese is needed to activate the prolidase enzyme, which produces the amino acid praline in order for collagen to form in skin cells. A condition known as prolidase deficiency, characterized by abnormal wound healing, results from impaired manganese metabolism.

Manganese develops the tendons and ligaments found in our joints by activating the enzyme that produces mucopolysaccharides, which comprise collagen. According to Dr. George C. Cotzia, who spoke at the First Annual Conference on Trace Substances in Environmental Health at the University of Missouri, a manganese-dependent enzyme forms the material of mucopolysaccharides. This material creates cushion-like substances in joint fluids, which makes the fluid strong and flexible. When these substances are weak or missing, the tissues in the joints eventually break down because the fluids are breaking down. As a result, bone and cartilage begin to wear and tear because this lubricating and cushioning ability has eroded, causing the joint pain associated with rheumatoid arthritis. Repetitive motion of these damaged joints can result in carpal tunnel syndrome. Research continues to provide evidence that manganese deficiency results in an erosion of the mucopolysaccharide material. Manganese is also the preferred cofactor in the enzymes that are responsible for the synthesis of proteoglycans, which are essential components of cartilage and bone formation.

The mucopolysaccharide material is what forms collagen, the flexible material in our joints, tendons, ears, skin, and other areas of the body. It is thought that deafness, if it is attributed to damage of the cartilage in the ear, could be a result of manganese deficiency. In areas where manganese deficiencies are common, children's development of cartilage is impaired. In bones, collagen is the mesh framework on which calcium, boron, magnesium, and other bone strengthening elements get deposited. Therefore, like a domino effect, loss of collagen can eventually result in bone loss.

Animals that suffer from manganese deficiency tend to show signs of skeletal abnormalities. Some studies using laboratory mice show how manganese is an important mineral in bone formation. Another study observed low blood levels of manganese in women who were suffering from osteoporosis.

In various animal studies, bones that lack sufficient manganese grow short and stubby. This is where the role of collagen becomes important. Manganese is also responsible for activating the enzyme glycosyltransferases, which produces the molecule that forms collagen. Detecting a manganese deficiency can be difficult since the symptoms are not always visible immediately. Rather, it can take years before clear signs of a mineral deficiency will be seen.

Manganese has important characteristics in the structural integrity of cells. Abnormal cellular functions and structure in mitochondria can occur when manganese is deficient, probably because the manganese SOD enzyme is the main antioxidant enzyme of mitochondria. Mitochondria use up to 90% of the oxygen in cells, making them prone to oxidative stress and vulnerable to free radicals. During the natural synthesis of ATP, a very highly reactive form of oxygen known as a free radical is created inside mitochondria. Fortunately, the MnSOD enzyme is supposed to convert them into hydrogen peroxide, which will eventually be reduced to H2O during other enzymatic processes.

Using laboratory mice, researchers Bell and Hurley observed how low manganese levels resulted in weakened cell membranes in the organs that commonly contain manganese—the pancreas, kidneys, liver, and heart. Much of the influence that manganese has on the permeability of cell membranes is from activating enzymes that are involved in the metabolism of fats and cholesterol. Since manganese protects cells from free radicals by activating the SOD enzyme, the integrity of the cell membranes will be maintained. If the fatty acids and cholesterol balance become impaired due to manganese deficiency, the permeability of the cell's membranes will be affected.

The free space between cells of the arteries contains glycoproteins, which are structural components that regulate the arteries' permeability and preserve the blood plasma. As an activator of enzymes, manganese can affects these glycoproteins in various ways. For example, prothrombin is a glycoprotein that is usually thought to be regulated by vitamin K. However, manganese is also required for its synthesis, and when manganese levels are low, vitamin K's response to blood clotting slows down. These key roles of manganese in the metabolism of fatty acids and proteins provide numerous examples of how this element is instrumental in the health of the arteries. Blood clotting, cholesterol synthesis, and fat synthesis are all processes that are affected when manganese is deficient. When these processes are impaired, hardening of the arteries can result.

Some studies have observed this mineral's role in activating the enzyme glycosyltransferases, which has some responsibility to biosynthesize plasma proteins in the liver. Some have suggested that manganese deficiency will impair this process, which could result in deformed protein formation and abnormal protein secretion from the liver. Many studies have shown this imbalance to result in a toxic accumulation of liver fats.

There are many other biochemical processes in organs such as the liver that rely on manganese, including the synthesis and utilization of carbohydrates, proteins, and fats. The presence of manganese inside the cells has long been known to be one regulator of carbohydrate metabolism. Therefore, changes in manganese levels can result in abnormal variations of this metabolic control. One example is the loss of glucose utilization. When this occurs, some studies show extreme abnormalities in the pancreas, and when the pancreas suffers, so does insulin production. A study performed in 1990 that used laboratory rats with low manganese levels showed a marked decrease in insulin receptors per cell, compared to other rats that had higher levels of manganese.

There are other enzymes that depend on manganese, pyruvate carboxylase and phosphoenolpyruvate carboxykinase (PEPCK). These enzymes are responsible for gluconeogenesis, which is the production of glucose from products that do not contain carbohydrates. Another manganese-dependent enzyme known as arginase is needed by the liver during the urea cycle, where ammonia is detoxified after amino acids are metabolized.

The role of manganese in the liver does not stop there. There is significant data on its control of pancreatic exocrine and endocrine metabolism. Observations in animals experiencing manganese deficiencies have shown symptoms that mimic diabetic glucose intolerance. Research suggests that this results from improper glucose metabolism and the degradation of the pancreas. Many elements affect the absorption and utilization of other elements. If manganese deficiency results in the aforementioned conditions, the symptoms could also be the result of improper absorption of other elements. This critical understanding of manganese and other elements in general should further our understanding of diabetes.

The brain is another organ that benefits from manganese. Studies show that laboratory rats are prone to convulsions when manganese levels were low. Other studies show that people with convulsive disorders also tend to have low manganese levels. Researcher Tanaka noticed that children with convulsive disorders showed 1/3 less manganese levels than neurologically stable children. Clinical supplementation of manganese marked a decrease in seizures.

There are also studies that document how conditions such as epilepsy consistently show low levels of manganese. A study by Papavasiliou involved 52 epileptic adults and their manganese content. Patients with the lowest levels of manganese had the highest number of seizures. Carl examined 44 epileptic patients and documented that whole blood levels of manganese were usually lower than normal adults. He also noticed that patients who had unexplained epilepsy consistently had lower manganese levels when compared to patients who were able to attribute their seizures to brain damage from trauma.

Laboratory rats are more likely to experience epileptic seizures during periods of manganese deficiency, and rats that were genetically prone to these seizures have also shown to be lacking manganese. Animals with early exposure to manganese deficiencies in utero had higher susceptibility to seizures than animals with similar deficiencies postnatally. Interestingly, epileptic seizures can result in high levels of manganese in the liver, although evidence isn't clear that would point to a relationship between seizure frequency and levels of manganese.

Manganese has been called the "brain mineral" since it assists mental functions. Neurological disorders that might be attributable to manganese deficiency include multiple sclerosis, as well as behavioral disorders such as schizophrenia. Studies have measured unusually high copper levels in patients with schizophrenia, although it is most likely an insoluble form of copper that has accumulated, or the body is lacking other minerals that assist in utilizing it. Manganese and zinc can both assist the body to excrete insoluble copper. Many researchers around the world have reported success in treating schizophrenia with water-soluble manganese supplementation.

Manganese can be both extremely useful and beneficial if it is found in its ionic state, or it can be extremely toxic if it is not. Water-soluble manganese, like any other element, is non-toxic. However, insoluble metallic manganese can be problematic. Manganese toxicity does not come from eating foods, but oftentimes results from inhaling insoluble forms of metallic manganese. Inhaled manganese dust is transported straight to the brain before it has a chance to be collected in the liver.

This can become problematic because this form of manganese is not water soluble. Chilean miners mining for manganese who inhaled toxic levels of manganese dust ore often fell victim to early stages of neurological conditions, such as extreme irritability and hallucinations. These psychiatric and neurological changes gave these disorders the nickname "manganese madness," also characterized by violence, aggression, criminal activity, and states of unusual mental excitement. Gradually, this condition resulted in neurological impairment, with symptoms similar to Parkinson's disease, such as tremors, spasms, and difficulty walking.

L.A. Gottschalk, et al researched manganese levels in violent male offenders. They consistently found higher levels of manganese in hair samples, suggesting once again that excess insoluble manganese could be associated with aggressive behavior. Other studies show unusually high levels of insoluble manganese exist in overly excited and extremely hyperactive children, while men who have a history of childhood hyperactivity tend to have higher rates of antisocial behaviors and illegal drug use. Laboratory rats tend to experience increased hyperactivity, followed by increased tendency to fight, also when afflicted with insoluble manganese toxicity.

Some researchers suggest that manganese acts to help the nervous system by stabilizing nerve impulses and transmissions. Multiple sclerosis is a condition where the myelin sheath that protects the nerves breaks down. Many have suggested that this condition could be treated with manganese supplementation. A lack of manganese is also thought to contribute to the autoimmune disease known as myasthenia gravis, a disorder that affects the muscles.

Studies of animals experiencing manganese deficiencies show impaired reproductive development. In fact, this element's role in reproduction was one of the first signs of deficiency ever documented. Guinea pigs, rats, and baby chicks have all been shown to suffer from irreversible congenital defects, resulting in loss of equilibrium. Female rats under observation displayed offspring with ataxia, impairment of estrus (no second generation reproduction), and many died shortly after birth. Failure to reproduce has also been documented in other animals, including cows and birds. Researcher Leach examined manganese-deficient chickens. Results showed decreased egg production, poor shell quality, and impaired hatchability. He also observed rabbits and rodents suffering from testicular degeneration when lacking manganese.

Other animal studies show a wide range of symptoms when manganese levels were low. Growth, reproduction, and skeletal framework become impaired, while glucose tolerance and carbohydrate and lipid metabolism are also affected. One long-term study observed a decline in growth that resulted from bone demineralization in a child who was fed a diet that lacked manganese, which was reversed after manganese supplementation. Another study observed that young males experiencing low manganese levels developed a mobile skin rash and abnormal cholesterol levels, followed by increased levels of calcium and phosphorus in their blood, suggesting that these minerals were being leached from bone crystals.

Other developmental symptoms of manganese deficiency include improper skeletal development, stunted growth, and lack of reproductive function. Dr. Todd states that manganese deficiency can also be attributed to poor equilibrium resulting from poor middle ear formation, as well as asthma, sterility, and impotence. Many of these birth defects from manganese deficiency are attributed to a decrease in enzymatic activity and the body's inability to metabolize the mucopolysaccharides.

Plant sources of manganese include pineapples, blueberries, and potatoes. Spinach, peas, and rice, and various nuts and seeds such as peanuts, almonds, and pecans are also good sources. Overall, manganese is an unsung hero. Many people have never even heard of this element or know of its wide range of benefits in the human body.

Molybdenum

Molybdenum is closely related to lead. In fact, while examining a lead compound, the Swedish chemist Carl Wilhelm Scheele in 1778 was the first to discover molybdenum, and it wasn't until 1781 that Peter Jacob finally isolated it. Molybdenum is named after the Greek word for lead, molybdos. It is a heavy metal that is used in various industrial and manufacturing processes such as strengthening alloys that are used in the aircraft and the nuclear power industries and coating pistons in some luxury automobiles. Molybdenum has even been used as a catalyst for petroleum. However, in the natural world, environmental carbon, nitrogen, and sulfur cycles all benefit from the enzymatic processes that are activated by molybdenum.

This trace mineral was once classified as "toxic" because miners inhaling it became very ill. This is true if it is found in a compound or an insoluble metallic form that is not found in plants. But when molybdenum is ingested as water-soluble ions, it becomes very useful and provides many different benefits.

In plants, molybdenum participates in many enzymes and many metabolic processes. These molybdenum-dependent enzymes activate processes such as nitrogen fixation and other oxidation-reduction processes. Likewise, molybdenum plays an extremely vital role in human enzymes.

Although molybdenum is not needed in high amounts to provide health benefits, trace amounts of this element can still be found in all body tissues. There are over 40 enzymes, also known as molybdoenzymes, in all animal organisms that play a key role in oxidation-reduction reactions, as well as the metabolism of carbon, nitrogen, and sulfur. Three of these enzymes need molybdenum as a cofactor: 1) xanthine oxidase, which metabolizes the breakdown of various nucleutides to produce uric acid and mobilize iron from liver reserves, 2) aldehyde oxidase, which assists in fat oxidation, and 3) sulfite oxidase, which catalyzes sulfite into sulfate. Molybdenum can therefore be considered an antioxidant in the blood through its activity in these enzymes. These three enzymes share a common cofactor called molybdopterin, which are molybdenum ions bound by two atoms of sulfur.

Interest in molybdenum as an essential nutrient began when this element was discovered to activate the enzyme sulfite oxidase. This enzyme produces uric acid by breaking down tissue purines (building blocks of RNA and DNA), helping to turn nitrogen waste into uric acid, which is then easily flushed from the liver out of the system.

The sulfite oxidase enzyme has been isolated from the liver of humans and a lack of this enzyme has been detected in young infants, with fatal results by ages 2-3. Dr. John H. Enemark, professor of chemistry at the University of Arizona, states that sulfite oxidase is required for normal neurological development in children. Some research concludes that a lack of this enzyme results in neurological abnormalities such as mental retardation.

Molybdenum is also required for the xanthine oxidase enzyme, which helps remove iron from the liver. When iron is stored in the liver, this enzyme releases it, allowing it to carry on its own functions, such as working with potassium to carry oxygen to body's cells and tissues. This is one way a molybdenum deficiency can result in anemia and liver problems.

When molybdenum is lacking, tissue activity of this enzyme decreases, which is identified by a low production of uric acid, a condition known as xanthinuria. Some observations show that xanthine oxidase activity slows down when protein intake is low and activity increases when protein is high. Other cases observed decreases in enzymatic activity when vitamin E was low and in rare cases of hepatoma. However, studies have not yet conclusively shown that a change in molybdenum intake is sufficient alone to alter the activity of this enzyme, at least not significant enough to allow diagnostic conclusion.

Another enzyme that seems to require the presence of molybdenum is aldehyde oxidase. This enzyme resembles xanthine oxidase in that it has similar tissue distribution and even shares some properties, although its exact functions in the body are still being identified. What is known so far is that it is necessary for the oxidation of fats.

Dietary molybdenum deficiencies in humans are rare. Only one medical case has been recorded so far of an actual molybdenum deficiency, which occurred in a patient with Crohn's disease. After a prolonged period of time, this patient developed irregular heartbeat and difficulty breathing, headaches, night blindness, and eventually became comatose. The patient also suffered from low production of uric acid and an improper sulfate/sulfite balance. This was evidenced by a decrease in uric acid and sulfate excretion and an increase in sulfite accumulation in his body. After molybdenum was added to his diet, these conditions improved.

However, many medical cases have shown impaired enzyme activity during periods of molybdenum deficiency. One symptom includes brain damage, which can be attributed to a lack of activity in the sulfite oxidase enzyme. It is not entirely clear, yet, whether damage to the brain is a result of the lack of sulfur production or an accumulation of a toxic substance. This may help explain the eventual comatose condition of the patient with Crohn's disease. Regardless, molybdenum's role in these enzymatic processes is clear.

In a study conducted in the northern region of China known as Linxian, the rates of esophogal and stomach cancers averaged over 10 times higher than in other areas of China, and over 100 times higher than the United States. Researchers attributed the high incidence of cancer to the soil's lack of molybdenum and other minerals, causing molybdenum to be deficient in their diets. If molybdenum is lacking in soils, plants are unable to complete one of their metabolic processes that prevents the conversion of nitrates to nitrosamines (toxic carcinogens), resulting in higher exposure to this toxin. A five-year study was completed to determine if adding insoluble molybdenum supplements was enough to reverse the high cancer rates. Results showed that it was unable to decrease the high cancer rates, suggesting that if this element was indeed largely responsible for the high cancer rates, molybdenum needs to be present in the soils and in the right form to inhibit the original production of these carcinogens in the first place.

Molybdenum performs other interesting functions in the body that are not well-known. One of those includes helping the body maintain a proper pH level. This is important because it also helps the body utilize other minerals, including copper, sulfur, iron, calcium and magnesium. Molybdenum also promotes a general state of well-being, is useful in preventing MSG sensitivity, and increases libido. It is instrumental in proper fetal development and protein formation. Some research shows molybdenum's role in the formation of strong bones and teeth, since it is a constituent of tooth enamel and enhances the effects of fluoride.

Most molybdenum deficiencies are being attributed to lack of enzymatic activity, such as sulfite oxidase, which results in toxic accumulations of sulfites (food and drug preservatives) or from regular consumption of refined foods. Deficiency symptoms can also include mental retardation, weight gain, abnormal appetites, impaired reproduction, irregular heartbeat patterns, increased breathing rates, and vision problems such as cataracts. A deficiency of this element can even increase susceptibility to stomach and esophageal cancers. Molybdenum also participates in enzymatic activities that are involved with fats, proteins, and carbohydrates.

Molybdenum can be found in fruits and vegetables that are grown in mineral rich soils. Broccoli, spinach, beans, buckwheat, peas, and various nuts and seeds are all well-known sources.

Selenium

The Swedish chemist Jons Jacob Berzelius inadvertently discovered selenium in 1817 while studying sulfuric acid. It was originally thought to be the element tellurium, until he realized that he had just discovered a new element. Today, selenium is usually obtained during copper refining processes.

An interesting characteristic of selenium is its ability to conduct electricity. When low light is shined on selenium, its ability to conduct electricity is low. If the light is brightened, selenium can conduct electricity much better. This unique property of selenium makes it a useful component of photocells, electric security eyes, and light meters for cameras and copiers. This element can even produce electricity from sunlight, making it a valuable tool in solar panels. It is used in making semiconductors, electronics, and products that convert alternating current electricity into direct current electricity. It can be added to steel and is even used as a dye in red-colored glasses.

Selenium is a scarce mineral that chemically resembles sulfur. It is found throughout Earth's crust in rocks, sand, and soil, which implies that it can be found in vegetation. Some areas of Earth are naturally rich in selenium, due to volcanic activity that deposited large amounts of selenium into the soil. Dr. Richard Passwater, author of Selenium as Food and Medicine and Director of Research at the Solgar Nutrition Research Center in Maryland, explains that the selenium content of soils is already low and is being eroded away even further through modern agriculture.

Animal cells grow abnormally if selenium is deficient. Before the Food and Drug Administration allowed selenium to be put into animal feed, farmers in many parts of the United States suffered annual losses when trying to raise livestock on selenium-deficient soils.

Selenium can be found in all tissues of the body, especially in muscles, kidneys, liver, pancreas, testes, and the spleen. Sperm cells naturally contain large amounts of selenium, making men more likely to need extra selenium than women, and deficiencies can lead to infertility in males.

Like other minerals, selenium was once listed as "toxic" until it was actually researched for its benefits. Most elements that are currently listed as essential were accepted much earlier than selenium. It wasn't until 1957 that researchers C.M. Katz and Dr. Klaus Schwarz recognized selenium for its health benefits and added it to the list of essential minerals. Shortly after, university research opened up the investigation of selenium in the late 1960's. Interestingly, in just over 20 years selenium went from being labeled "toxic" to being classified as an essential mineral. Researcher Mertz explains that it usually takes anywhere from 30-40 years on average for the scientific community to recognize and accept the discovery of a new essential element.

Selenium consumed from anything other than plants is unlikely to be found in its ionic form. Many times minerals such as selenium found in animals are no longer in their ionic state. Rather, their bodies have bound the selenium to other products, similar to sulfur. After selenium is consumed as an ion in animals, the body uses it to bind with other products such as the amino acids cysteine and methinine to form selenocysteine and selenomethionine. The selenium found in various proteins such as glutathione peroxidase in animals has already been bound to amino acids.

Selenoproteins are proteins that contain selenium and are found in muscle tissue, plasma, and lined along the inner wall of blood vessels. Some of them transport substances, while others act as antioxidants. It is thought that selenium is an effective antioxidant by itself and it probably interacts with every nutrient one way or another that has antioxidant responsibilities.

The National Cancer Institute states that free radicals in humans are oxygen molecules that have an incomplete outer electron shell, making them highly reactive and dangerous. When these oxygen molecules become electrically charged, or "radicalized," they try to steal electrons from other molecules, which can damage cells, DNA, and other molecules. Antioxidants destroy these free radicals by neutralizing their electrical charges. Antioxidants, such as various vitamins, minerals, and enzymes, are found in fruits and vegetables, as well as various nuts and grains. Beta-carotene, vitamins A, E, and C, lutein, lycopene, and the minerals manganese, zinc, and selenium are all known to be effective antioxidants, or they activate enzymes that perform antioxidant activities.

Selenium is heavily involved in enzymatic activities. Four of these enzymes are antioxidant enzymes which prevent cellular damage by breaking down harmful oxygen products such as hydrogen peroxide and lipid hydroperoxides into water and alcohols. Stabilizing these free radicals may prevent some of the damage they inflict on cells. Other enzymes work to produce vitamin C, which is important for regulating cell growth and viability. A small group of molybdenum-dependent enzymes need selenium as a cofactor, while other enzymes play a role in the thyroid and immune system.

Selenium is a major component of many thyroid hormones and thyroid enzymes, which is needed to facilitate the action of some medications. Some pharmaceutical medications that rely on thyroid enzymes can go unutilized if selenium is absent.

In 1965, Dr. Raymond Shamberger was recognized as the first researcher to study the effects of selenium on cancer. He was one of the first to examine the antioxidant effects of selenium by using it to counteract free radical damage in animal skin cancer. In his experiments, animals were supplemented with selenium and then heavily exposed to ultraviolet light. He observed a decrease in skin cancer, which resulted in various other forms of anti-cancer research. This was one of the first trials that sparked an interest in studying selenium's influence against cancer.

There is a large amount of research data showing selenium's ability to protect against various forms of cancers in animals. Over 100 documented studies have been conducted, and in two-thirds of these selenium was shown to dramatically reduce tumor incidence. According to these observations, selenium was formed into a methylated compound after consuming large doses of ions. Some of the studies showed, however, that selenium deficiency did not necessarily make animals more susceptible to developing cancerous tumors, such as spontaneous, viral, or chemically-induced. Although there is significant amount of data regarding selenium's effects on animals, what about humans?

As early as the 1980s, selenium's role against certain forms of cancer was being researched in China. At the Cancer Institute of the Chinese Academy of Medical Sciences in Beijing, Dr Shu-Yu Yu, et al coordinated research with a nutritional supplement company. They began an experiment using a double-blind, placebo-controlled study of 226 people who had hepatitis B and were prone to getting liver cancer. After they ingested 200 mcg of selenium or the placebo every day for four years, there were five cases of liver cancer in the placebo group and zero in the selenium group.

Later, Dr. Yu performed another experiment with Dr. Larry Clark, senior epidemiologist at Cornell University, now at the University of Arizona, using 2,474 high-risk family members of someone who had already developed liver cancer. Again, some of the recruits were given a placebo and the some were given the 200 mcg selenium supplement. Although not quite as successful, the results are still worth considering.

It was reported that 13 out of 1,030 members of the placebo group developed liver cancer, while only 10 of 1,444 members of the selenium group developed liver cancer. Statistically, this represents a 45% difference.

Later, Dr. Clark decided to experiment using dermatology patients who had various forms of skin cancer surgically removed. Coordinating with dermatology clinics, he used 1,312 patients from 1983 to 1991 and proceeded with a double-blind, placebo-controlled experiment using 200 mcg of selenium. The patients averaged 114 ng/ml of selenium in their blood, while the blood content of the selenium group rose to 190 and remained there during the study. The selenium-controlled group experienced a 37% decline in overall cancer, while the placebo group had double the rate of mortality from cancer. Although researchers have observed skin cancer in animals decline after supplementing with selenium, skin cancer in humans does not seem to be affected.

Cornell University in New York is widely touted as having the longest history of selenium research in the world. Dr. Larry Clark, now at the University of Arizona, piloted a study with Dr. Bruce W. Turnbull and Dr. Gerald F. Combs, Jr., both of Cornell, in conjunction with Dr. Elizabeth Slate and Dr. David S. Alberts, MD, also from the University of Arizona. Their results were published in the Journal of the American Medical Association January 1st, 1997.

The objective of the investigation was to determine whether a selenium supplement would decrease the incidence of cancer. The study involved 1,312 men and women from low-selenium areas of the United States taking selenium supplements for 10 years. It was observed that the subjects experienced 41% less cancer than the group taking a placebo. Although this study found that skin cancer did not decline, prostate, esophageal, colorectal, and lung cancer declined by 71%, 67%, 62%, and 46%, respectively, when compared to the placebo group. Combs noted that "Overall, the selenium-supplemented group experienced 18% less mortality than the placebo group, and almost all of that difference was due to some form of cancer."

Dr. Combs, a nutritional biochemist and professor of nutritional sciences, explains, "Although more than a hundred of animal and dozens of epidemiological studies have linked high selenium status and cancer risk, this is the first double-blind, placebo-controlled cancer prevention study with humans that directly supports the thesis that a nutritional supplement of selenium, as a single agent, can reduce the risk of cancer" (Lang, Selenium Supplements Can Reduce Cancer Rates, 1997).

The researchers concluded their study by saying: "The results of this randomized controlled trial do not support the hypothesis that selenium supplementation reduces the risk of basal cell carcinomas or squamous cell carcinomas of the skin, showing no statistically significant treatment effect on their incidence. However, selenium supplementation was found to be associated with significant reductions in secondary end points of total cancer incidence (all-sites combined), lung, colorectal and prostate cancer incidences, and lung cancer mortality."

One big question still remains—can selenium reverse pre-existing cancerous tumors? Various independent studies are currently trying to answer that question, but it should be mentioned that these researchers stated "supplementation with selenium inhibits tumor growth and stimulates apoptosis in cultured tumor cells. These observations support the hypothesis that selenium supplementation inhibits the late stage promotion and progression of tumors."

The research teams from Arizona and Cornell Universities reported in 1991 that selenium deficiencies in the blood corresponded to an increase in neoplastic polyps in the colon, which usually precedes colon cancer. Also, in 1995, Cornell University observed animals that were fed high selenium diets tended to experience half as many tumors as the animals fed what was considered normal selenium amounts.

Many cancer patients have lower selenium levels in their blood, making these forms of experiments easily criticized by saying that the cancer came first and caused the selenium deficiencies. However, according to Dr. Patrick Quillen, PhD, R.D., author of Healing Nutrients, blood samples were taken from 10,000 Americans by Cornell University and then frozen. For the next five years, blood samples from anyone who developed cancer were examined for their selenium content. Those who developed cancer tended to have the lowest amount of selenium in their blood when the samples were first taken. In fact, they experienced twice the rate of cancer incidence than those who had adequate levels of selenium.

Geographic studies consistently show trends for populations who live in areas with high selenium in the soil tend to have lower mortality rates when compared to those who live in low selenium areas. It is widely known that the Midwestern United States, especially Nebraska and North and South Dakota, have high levels of selenium in their soil, which increases the rates of selenium intake by these residents. Also, residents of the Pacific Northwest and the Southeastern coast of the United States tend to have the lowest selenium intake. However, even this low intake is still 4 or 5 times higher than residents of New Zealand, and 10 to 20 times higher than most areas of China.

Other geographic studies show a relationship between environmental selenium content and cancer incidence. In counties with normal or high selenium concentrations, cancer rates tend to be significantly lower for lung, colon, rectum, bladder, esophagus, pancreas, breast, ovary, and cervical cancers, when compared against counties with low selenium. These types of studies seem to be very consistent. To date, no study has proven otherwise.

The effect of selenium seems to be more pronounced on men than on women. A Harvard study of 62,000 female nurses found no relationship between selenium levels measured in toenail clippings and total cancer risk. However, another study using 50,000 male participants found a significant relationship between selenium levels measured in toenail clippings and cancer risk. It was observed that in men who had normal selenium levels, the risk of prostate cancer was only 35% of those men who had only half as much selenium. Similar findings have also been shown in Japanese studies. However, Dr. Combs mentions that these types of findings may imply that selenium levels in toenails are an accurate representation of metabolic status of selenium in the rest of the body. "There is no evidence for that," he says.

According to research done by the National Institutes of Health, there are two major reasons why selenium affects cancer. It is thought that selenium's major role as an antioxidant makes it effective in protecting the body from free radicals. Also, selenium seems to be able to slow tumor growth.

Selenium also affects cardiovascular and reproductive areas of the body. Pregnant women occasionally develop a condition known as pre-eclampsia, characterized by high blood pressure, decreased kidney function, and a decline in blood flow to the placenta, all of which complicate pregnancy. European researchers at the University of Surrey in Guildford, UK, determined that this condition is probably caused by a lack of selenium, due to selenium's antioxidant effects in neutralizing oxidants that develop from a malfunctioning placenta. They reported that women who were low in selenium were four times as likely to develop pre-eclampsia. Their findings can be found in the November, 2003 issue of the American Journal of Obstetrics and Gynecology.

Selenium is often credited with strengthening the immune system. Being an effective antioxidant makes selenium capable of combating infections, such as inhibiting the replication of viruses. Some studies show increased immune response to infectious organisms when selenium levels increase, and that selenium aids the expression of cell-signaling molecules known as cytokines, which help govern the response time of the immune system. High levels of selenium also increases the cytotoxicity of killer T-cells and makes them more responsive against infections. Selenium maximizes the activity of antioxidant enzymes, improves the immune system, affects the metabolism of dangerous carcinogens, and prevents tumor growth. Selenium also seems to be able to prevent certain types of cancerous tumors by enhancing immune cell activity and decreasing the development of blood vessels to the tumor.

Selenium can inhibit the progression and replication of some viruses. In studies performed using selenium-deficient mice, a harmless virus called coxsackievirus eventually mutates into a more progressive form that inflames the heart muscles and creates a condition known as mycarditis. Keshan disease is the cardiovascular condition associated with this viral inflammation of the heart, and this virus has been isolated in patients suffering from this condition. The glutathione peroxidase enzyme is known to help inhibit this virus and prevent myocarditis, even after it mutates. When selenium content is low, the activity of this enzyme will decrease, which furthers the chance that this virus will mutate into its more dangerous form. According to Dr. Todd, selenate is the active metal ion in the glutathione peroxidase enzyme system. On a side note, this enzyme system tends to become inoperable during the development of cataracts, suggesting that selenium deficiencies could also result in impaired vision. Interestingly, healthy optical tissues contain some of the largest concentrations of vitamin C.

One of selenium's most significant contributions to the human body is its effect on the HIV virus. A report by the University Of Georgia School Of Pharmacy in August, 1994 concluded that low selenium levels contribute to the proliferation of the HIV virus into full blown AIDS. They concluded that HIV patients actually die due to symptoms of selenium deficiency, such as liver cirrhosis or cardiomyopathy. The HIV virus progresses more rapidly toward developing AIDS when selenium levels are low. Patients who have had the HIV virus for as long as 20 years and have not developed AIDS tend to have adequate selenium levels in their blood.

Increased mortality rates from the HIV virus have also been associated with selenium deficiencies. In 1997, researchers at the University Of Miami School Of Medicine Center for Disease Prevention reported in the Journal of AIDS that HIV-1 infected patients were 20 times more likely to die if they were experiencing a selenium deficiency. The HIV virus gradually decreases the immune system while free radicals are given free rein to inflict damage. It is believed that selenium can increase the activity of T-cells, which provides the body with increased resistance to viruses, including HIV. With its antioxidant responsibilities, selenium can limit damage from free radicals in HIV-infected cells, which could prevents the replication of the virus.

The National Institutes of Health reported findings of an examination that was performed using 125 people who were HIV-positive. They found that those who had very low selenium were more likely to die. Another group studied 24 children for five years and found that anyone who lacked selenium suffered death at an earlier age. It is thought that selenium's ability to control the proliferation of this virus is due to either its antioxidant effects or its actions in gene regulation, which affects HIV replication. It seems that selenium and the HIV virus are constantly at battle with one another for territory in the body. If selenium levels are high, the virus is much more likely to experience a delay in the disease's progression; likewise, when selenium levels become low, the virus is able to proliferate at a much faster pace. These types of studies suggest that when selenium is deficient, the proliferation of viruses such as HIV increase.

Selenium and vitamin E work together as antioxidants by participating in the glutathione peroxidase enzyme. This enzyme is a very powerful enzyme that wipes out renegade cells and the free radicals inside. Vanderbilt University reported that pigs lacking both selenium and vitamin E resulted in a thickened heart wall and an inoperable left chamber of the heart, which led to blood pooling in other areas of the body, including the liver and lungs. It was also noted that glutathione peroxidase activity in the heart was measured at only 30% of normal activity levels.

Over thirty years ago, Dr. Passwater investigated selenium's involvement with cancer. In an effort to extend lifespan, he created a range of supplemental antioxidants that included selenium, vitamin E, and amino acids that extended the average lifespan by 20-30% and up to 10% in mice. When these mice were given age-accelerants and his supplements, it was found that they lived 175% longer, showing that antioxidants such as these help lengthen the lifespan by suppressing or slowing down the aging process and vulnerability to disease. Aging is thought to be primarily an oxidative process, and selenium deficiencies can allow the oxidative processes to accelerate, making selenium effective in slowing down premature aging.

According to the National Institutes of Health, surveys suggest that higher free radical activity results in higher rates of heart disease. The oxidized form of low-density lipoproteins, often referred to as bad cholesterol, tend to build up in arteries, causing plaque formation and resulting in high blood pressure and cardiovascular conditions. Selenium is one of the antioxidants that limits the oxidation of these bad fatty acids.

One of selenium's roles as an antioxidant involves its ability to prevent lipids and fats from becoming rancid, which is a damaging process known as peroxidation. If peroxidation occurs, it can be seen as age spots or liver spots; the brown peroxidized lipid is called ceroid lipofucsin. High consumption of commercial vegetable oils, margarine, and other cooking oils during periods of selenium deficiency can quickly result in heart attacks or cancer, since the cooking process quickly converts these rancid fats into damaging free radicals. All fats and oils will melt at body temperature. However, if these synthetic fats and oils become commercially hydrogenated, they convert to a new compound and no longer melt. Any oil that will not melt in the body becomes rancid, and rancid fats act as free radicals.

Selenium and vitamin E are both helpful in protecting the body from these types of free radicals. Some have observed that when these hydrogenated fats are consumed, oxidative damage such as age spots and rapid aging become noticeable. Also, heavy consumption of these fats coupled with a selenium deficiency can result in elevated body temperature in an attempt to make the fats liquefy. Hydrogenated products can result in difficulty sleeping and night sweats. Fluctuations in body temperature and irregular heart patterns can also be a result of heavy oxidative damage.

A Chinese study reported how heart cells in rats growing in a controlled culture increased their frequency and amplitude of contractions, and the cells continued to promote the synthesis of nucleic acids (RNA) and enhanced membrane stability after selenium was added. It is thought that selenium can help maintain the physical integrity of heart tissue even during a gradual loss of blood flow, as in cases of heart attacks or restricted arterial passages.

Clotting is a major function of blood, and in order for blood to clot, the clumping of platelets must first trigger it. Research shows that selenium regulates platelet formation. During a four-week observation, platelet glutathione activity increased after men were supplemented with selenium. If selenium can improve platelet formation, blood clotting will increase, which will protect against some cardiovascular conditions. N. W. Schoene and coworkers observed similar findings on the role of selenium and blood clotting while experimenting with laboratory rats.

An interesting characteristic of selenium is its role in the thyroid, and a selenium deficiency is believed to affect the function of iodine. The production and utilization of thyroid hormones is dependent upon iodine and three selenium-dependent enzymes that regulate thyroid hormones.

Arthritis sufferers tend to have low activity of the glutathione peroxidase enzyme and large amounts of free radicals. Selenium levels could be associated with this low enzymatic and high free radical activity. Studies have shown that arthritis patients tend to have low levels of selenium. According to the Rheumatism Research Unit in Denmark, low activity of the glutathione peroxidase enzyme usually results in high levels of free radicals, resulting in rheumatoid arthritis.

Osteoarthritis is characterized by a degeneration of articular cartilage between joints, which is commonly found in low-selenium areas of China, North Korea, and eastern Siberia. In severe cases, joint deformities and dwarfism occur when cartilage formation is deformed. However, it is still unclear if selenium supplementation can reverse this condition because other factors such as iodine deficiency, parasitic fungi, and polluted water are also suspect.

At the Dartmouth Medical School, Dr. Henry A. Schroeder of the Trace Mineral Laboratory reported that selenium is effective in removing heavy metal toxicity such as insoluble cadmium from the body. The body can only use cadmium if zinc is present. At the University of Wisconsin, Dr. W. G. Hoekstra, et al discovered that mercury found in tuna was less likely to have toxic effects if selenium was present.

Eating plenty of natural sources of selenium will prevent deficiencies. The ionic form of selenium that is absorbed into plants is properly referred to as selenate. Selenate can be derived from food sources that are grown in mineral-rich soils that contain high amounts of selenium. Fruits and vegetables such as broccoli grown in these soils will contain selenate. Scientists at the United States Department of Agriculture observed that high amounts of selenate in broccoli may help prevent breast and prostate cancer. If mineral analyses of fruits or vegetables do not show high selenate, it is due to a lack of selenate in the soil, not because the plant failed to absorb it. Plants are not always selective about what ions they absorb; any ionic form of an element within reach of roots will be absorbed.

Nuts, such as Brazil nuts, walnuts, and other legumes usually tend to show high levels of this mineral. Corn and grains such as wheat can also yield adequate amounts, although sometimes their selenium can be found in an amino acid known as selenomethionine, which can be stored in tissues. Animals that eat these natural sources of selenate tend to have high amounts in their muscles. Processing grains to produce flour and bread removes its minerals content, including selenium, by up to 75%.

Selenium is absorbed by the body's cells through passive diffusion, and competes with sulfur for absorption through the ion channels. It is not known if there are any antagonisms or other elements that may inhibit selenium absorption.

Failure to absorb selenium is widely known to be a major cause of selenium deficiency, usually seen in chronically ill persons. Parasites in the intestinal tract can impede the absorption of selenium. Symptoms of selenium deficiency can include muscle weakness and deterioration, as well as inflamed and damaged heart tissue. People who have gastrointestinal disorders such as Crohn's disease, or who have had large portions of their intestinal tract surgically removed, are in danger of improper mineral absorption. Those on special medical diets should have their mineral levels monitored occasionally.

According to Dr. Gerald Combs of Cornell University, it is wrong to conclude that vegetarians are getting the wrong form or the wrong amount of selenium when compared to meat eaters. The selenium in plant amino acids consumed by vegetarians is far more likely to be utilized by the body. Many minerals found in plants become utilized and converted into a compound form once an animal consumes it. He explains, "The result will be that vegetarians should show relatively higher tissue selenium levels at any given level of intake, while non-vegetarians will tend to retain somewhat less selenium and show lower tissue levels."

This is a direct result of selenium already having been utilized and converted by the animals being eaten, making that form of selenium less usable by the human body. This would help to explain why people living in geographic areas of the world that have high selenium in their soils tend to have fewer cases of selenium deficiency. Minerals should always be consumed in their ionic form, such as are found in plants.

Selenium can be used to treat other conditions such as dandruff, hot flashes, and help keep skin youthful and elastic. Other symptoms of selenium deficiency include anemia, cirrhosis of the liver, irregular heartbeat, infertility, nerve disorders such as muscular dystrophy and multiple sclerosis, pancreatic atrophy, premature aging, sickle cell anemia, and sudden infant death syndrome (SIDS).

Zinc

For over 2,500 years, zinc compounds have been used to produce brass. Brass is a heavy metal alloy made from zinc and copper and was used by the Romans to produce coins, kettles, and other decorative products. Brass is still used today to manufacture many other types of items, such as musical and medical instruments, as well as plumbing systems and electrical parts.

It wasn't until the 15th Century that zinc was first processed in India although the rediscovery of this element in 1746 is credited to the German chemist Andreas Sigismund Marggraf. Today, the compound zinc oxide is widely used in a chemical process known as galvanization, which is a protective layer of zinc that is used to prevent corrosion (oxidation) on other metals, such as iron. Zinc compounds are also used in the manufacture of cosmetics, paints, rubber, ink, soap, and pharmaceuticals, along with producing batteries and die-castings.

Jules Raulin, a French chemistry professor who taught at the University of Paris, was the first to research zinc as a nutrient. In 1869, his experimental doctorate thesis involving the bacteria Aspergillus niger was the first evidence of zinc's role in living organisms. His experiments showed how zinc was essential to the growth and development of mold. Today, the distinguished Raulin Award is given to recipients who have made an outstanding research contribution over a lifetime in the field of trace elements that have significant impact on human health and disease.

The "rediscovery" of zinc captured the attention of researchers all over the world. In 1877 zinc was discovered in human liver. Later, in 1934, Gabriel Bertrand conducted laboratory experiments using rodents and documented zinc's role in their growth and development. One year later, researchers Hart, Stirn, and Elvejehm also provided evidence on zinc's function in rats. But it wasn't until 1974 that zinc became recognized as an essential human nutrient. It is now known that zinc is a required trace mineral that is needed to perform a wide range of metabolic processes in mammals. The role of zinc in the human body is so widespread and critical that it can be found in almost all of the body's tissues and fluids. Dr. Earl Mindell suggests that zinc can be thought of as a traffic policeman, since it is involved in, directs, and regulates many of the body's processes.

Zinc is present in almost all human tissues, comprising approximately 2 grams of total zinc content, which is usually more than most other trace elements. It is largely concentrated in the liver, skin, kidneys, bones, pancreas, and muscles, as well as reproductive fluids and organs. Other organs and tissues with zinc include the eyes, hair, prostate, semen, and nails.

Researcher O'Dell has observed early signs of zinc deficiency that can include a dehydrated appearance, unusually high hematocrit in the blood, and even diarrhea. Using chickens in his examination, he noted how zinc deficiencies caused a shift in the water balance of their bodies. The water was shifted from extracellular spaces to intercellular compartments. The total extracellular water concentration went from 29.4% to 19.6% of body weight, while the plasma volume dropped from

6% to 3.4%. Some researchers suggested that there was a corresponding increase in sodium levels into tissues during these low zinc periods, which would create an abnormal sodium/potassium balance, probably resulting from increased cellular membrane permeability or even a defective sodium pump.

Zinc participates in the metabolism of proteins, amino acids, nucleic acids, lipids, and carbohydrates through its involvement in enzymes. In fact, zinc is widely known to participate in more enzymatic processes than any other element, including manganese. Zinc activates over 90 zinc-dependent enzymes, while acting as a cofactor in over 100 other enzymes, and is found in over 200 zinc proteins. Zinc's involvement in SOD, the enzyme that dismantles a dangerous form of oxygen, makes zinc one of the most effective antioxidants. This powerful antioxidant enzyme will not function without the presence of zinc and copper ions.

Zinc acts as both the activator of enzymes and as a molecule in other enzymes that need it to help stabilize their structure. In fact, zinc is so effective at binding enzymes to their substrates and protecting their structural shape and arrangement that even if zinc becomes deficient later, some enzymes would still be able to perform limited functions.

Zinc's involvement with enzymes includes large enzymatic processes such as carbohydrate metabolism, nucleic acid metabolism, and even protein synthesis. It is thought that zinc's involvement with protein includes the transcription and translation of genetic material, which might explain its critical role in cellular division and differentiation. It has also been shown that zinc aids in the synthesis of both DNA and RNA. Therefore, some of the enzymes that benefit from zinc include those involved in the structures and production of RNA, DNA, and ribosomes. Moreover, some gene activators that govern how genetic information is expressed will use proteins that contain zinc to attach to DNA molecules. Dr. Todd has stated that certain neurological functions, such as memory, require RNA.

Two critical genetic enzymes that need zinc are the RNA polymerase enzyme and the thymidine kinase enzyme. When zinc is deficient, these enzymes become dysfunctional or become inoperable, resulting in reduced synthesis of DNA, RNA, and protein. These abnormalities eventually impair cellular division, growth, and repair; some have suggested that dwarfism is likely a zinc deficiency. Other enzymes with similar functions that require zinc include lactic dehydrogenase, alkaline phosphatase, and carbonic anhydrase (0.3% zinc).

Many minerals such as zinc are also responsible for cell division and healthy cell membranes. Researchers O'Dell and Bettger suggest that zinc's functions in cell membranes include functional and structural support. Decreased growth has consistently been shown to be a symptom of zinc deficiency, and is most likely attributed to depressed nucleic acid biosynthesis. Studies using zinc supplementation on children who were experiencing growth delays have observed increased growth rates after zinc was added to their diets. Others suggest that zinc influences cell signals that govern the insulin-like growth factor-1, a hormone responsible for regulating growth rates.

Cell division with regard to zinc levels is not limited to growth and development following birth because zinc levels also influence growth and development during pregnancy. At the University Of Washington School Of Public Health in Seattle, Dr. Lowell E. Sever was one of the first researchers to examine the connection between zinc levels and deformities. In studies conducted in Denver and Baltimore, zinc deficiencies often resulted in birth defects such as cleft lip, Down's syndrome, spinal bifida, club limbs, and hiatal and umbilical hernias. Such abnormalities were observed in Turkey, Iran, and Egypt. Complications with deliveries, low birth weight, and learning and delayed sexual development are also attributed to zinc and other mineral deficiencies.

Other enzymatic activities require zinc, such as digestion and blood sugar regulation. Thymidine kinase is an enzyme that requires zinc for protein synthesis. Another enzyme known as carboxypeptidase is located in the pancreas and needs zinc to break down amino acids in an effort to synthesize proteins. Interestingly, the pancreas is also the site where the insulin hormone is made from various products, two of which are the minerals zinc and sulfur.

Along with activating enzymes, zinc also plays a critical role in hormonal activities. Generally, zinc helps produce, store, and secrete various hormones, as well as enhancing the effectiveness of receptor sites and organ responsiveness. Some studies show diminished male and female reproductive performance when zinc levels were low. Testosterone, insulin, and adrenal coricosteroids all benefit from the presence of zinc.

Zinc is found in its highest levels for men in the prostate gland; up to 1 mg of zinc can be lost in every semen ejaculation. Studies using male subjects have shown corresponding drops in testosterone levels during periods of zinc deficiency. Testosterone is thought to regulate zinc metabolism in the prostate, while at the same time zinc is thought to help metabolize testosterone in the prostate. Zinc has even been shown to reduce the size of the prostate gland. However, when zinc is deficient, low sperm count, even impotence in prolonged deficiency cases, may result. Impotence can be attributed to the loss of zinc through diuretic treatments. Some therapists have used zinc successfully in such cases.

Dr. Isadore Rosenfeld, M.D., a clinical professor of medicine at New York Hospital/Cornell University Medical Center, once stated that for many years men have eaten oysters to increase their masculinity, although at the time it was relatively unclear as to why oysters were providing such results on their sexual performance. It was later determined that oysters are an excellent source of zinc.

During fetal development, the growth and development of both primary and secondary sex organs in males, along with all stages of development of female organs, can be impaired during periods of zinc deficiency. Testicular hypofunction, which affects the production of testosterone by the Leydig cells, is the primary abnormality that is experienced in males.

This mineral is essential to the normal sexual development and maturation in children. It is thought that as children grow into adolescence, their zinc levels are supposed to increase. However, these levels decline due to poor dietary habits, resulting in an impaired ability to utilize proteins for growth, such as those in children experiencing retarded growth.

Research conducted by the federal Human Nutrition Research Center in Grand Forks, North Dakota showed that zinc improved the memory of 209 seventh-graders who participated in a study. These students supplemented their diet with 20 milligrams of zinc per day in a glass of orange juice. Students who consumed the juice supplemented with zinc decreased their reaction time on a visual memory test by 12%, compared to only 6% in students who consumed juice without zinc. Interestingly, the students who took the zinc also scored higher on a word recognition test and on a task that involved sustained attention and vigilance.

Dr. James G. Penland, the project's lead researcher, noted that these results were achieved using students who were not considered zinc deficient. If results such as these are possible by increasing the amount of zinc, perhaps they may convince authorities to review recommended zinc intake guidelines for young adults. "Adolescence is a critical period of rapid growth physically, emotionally, and mentally. That coupled with the fact that zinc is one of the nutrients that adolescents do not consume in recommended amounts led us to this study."

A study using laboratory rats, calves, and lambs showed conclusive evidence that development of male reproductive organs is diminished when zinc is deficient. In lambs, testicular development was greatly depressed, and spermatogenesis ceased within 5-6 months after zinc levels dropped.

Zinc is a major factor in the production of insulin. Along with chromium, zinc's presence in most of the body's tissues also helps insulin interact with tissues to utilize blood sugar. During early stages of insulin dependency, diabetic patients tend to have low levels of zinc, and the level of zinc is significantly reduced in the pancreas. Laboratory rats secrete lower amounts of insulin when zinc is deficient. Other experiments show adrenal hypertrophy, with symptoms such as weakness, anorexia, nausea, irritability, vomiting, depression, lack of resistance to cold, and inability to respond physiologically to stress, in pigs and rodents when zinc levels are low. Adding zinc to insulin treatments could magnify its potency and result in normalized blood glucose. The complete role of zinc in the pancreas, insulin, and glucose levels needs further examination.

Zinc also plays a major role in strengthening the immune system by increasing resistance to disease. It stimulates the T-lymphocyte cells, which respond to infections in the blood, thus increasing the white blood cell and antibody count. During periods of zinc deficiency, studies using laboratory mice showed extreme decreases in immune system response, and rodents and pigs experienced reduced functioning of the thymus.

In 1978, researcher Chesters observed a complete loss of lymphoid tissues, including tonsils, lymph nodes, and thymus in patients who suffered from acrodermatitis enteropathica, an inherited disease that is characterized by a zinc deficiency. In 1986, Dr. Hambidge explained how zinc deficiency results in a wide variety of immune system incompetencies, largely related to the production of thymus hormone production, lymphocyte function, and neutrophil function.

Scientists in Italy believe that zinc deficiency, rather than a malfunctioning thymus gland, is responsible for low immune strength in the elderly and in cases of Down's syndrome. The thymus gland is the site where T-cells mature as they are produced and secreted from bone marrow. This gland also produces a hormone called FTS that helps boost the immune system. Studies show that low immune strength in the elderly, as well as in children suffering from Down's syndrome, likely results from a zinc deficiency. Zinc deficiencies in the womb lead to increased susceptibility to infections in neonatal development and newborn infants.

Zinc's presence in all the fluids in the body, including saliva, optical fluids, mucous, lungs, and urine provides some defense against infectious pathogens trying to enter the body. Although zinc appears unable to destroy infectious pathogens on direct contact, it does appear able to initiate antibody response while preventing bacteria and viruses from reproducing. This might explain zinc's success with healing ulcers that originate from bacterial infection.

HIV and AIDS patients tend to have low levels of zinc and experience extremely low immune system strength. These two diseases are known as "opportunistic infections," which refer to a person's susceptibility to the disease after prolonged zinc deficiency. Supplementation with zinc has resulted in increased white blood cell count and improved weight in HIV patients. Zinc could also provide support against autoimmune disorders, such as rheumatoid arthritis, a condition where the body attacks its own tissues.

Infectious pathogens appear to have an easier time infecting people who lack zinc. Diarrheal diseases caused by infectious pathogens, such as the E. coli bacteria as well as other toxins, become more likely when zinc is unable to ward them off. Other infections, such as pneumonia and malaria, are reduced in their ability to infect their host when zinc is supplemented. A research study in Papua New Guinea resulted in a 38% decline in hospital visitations from malarial infection in preschool children who began supplementing with zinc. Surprisingly, the total number of malarial infections declined by almost 70%.

During the Civil War, zinc supplementation was used to help stop infections. Throughout the 19th century, surgeons used zinc as both an antibiotic and an antiseptic. Today, some people use zinc to destroy molds and fungal growths located outside the body. When zinc is present in saliva, it prevents bacterial replication in the mouth, which produces the acid that dissolves tooth enamel. If zinc is present in sweat, it is possible to not have body odor since zinc kills bacteria that causes body odor.

Zinc is a mobile element inside the human body. It can be remobilized after being deposited inside bodily fluids and tissues. Thus, there is no "store" of zinc per se, but rather the ability of the body to reutilize this element when called upon. Bone resorption and tissue catabolism are two functions that require the remobilization of zinc through the blood. Even when zinc levels are low, the level of zinc and activity of its enzymes in blood can be maintained over long periods of time, such as several months, indicating that the zinc that is present will be used again and again for various functions.

Zinc is essential for repair and growth of tissues. Some people who supplement with zinc have experienced faster healing and recovery from wounds and injuries. Animals suffering from various incision punctures and burns experience delayed recovery when they lack zinc. Studies show how zinc deficiency results in longer bleeding times, which is characterized by a failure of the blood to clot normally, most likely from a defective platelet condition. Studies also show that common cuts, scrapes, and burn injuries heal faster when zinc is present. Fast recovery can be useful when healing from surgeries. Healthy blood requires one part zinc to every seven parts copper.

Healthy skin will be rich in zinc. In animal studies, parakeratotic lesions appear when zinc levels in the skin become severely low. These symptoms are characterized by a thickening, or hyperkeratinization, of the epithelial cells of the skin, including impaired regeneration of new cells. In prolonged deficiencies, scaling and cracking of animal paws, including deep fissures, eventually result, along with hair loss and dermatitis. In 1975 a study of the six enzymes that involve glycolysis in the skin of rats showed a 30-50% decline in enzymatic activity when zinc levels were low.

It is clear that zinc helps with skin nucleic acid and collagen synthesis. Zinc helps keep skin clear by stimulating antibody responses to help ward off infections that are trying to enter the body through skin pores and cells. Zinc ointments can be used in the treatment of some forms of acne.

According to Dr. Todd, zinc helps to further the healing process in skin, and some optical tissues are derived from the same tissues that produce skin. Researchers have observed how salmon and other animals that were fed a zinc-deficient diet developed cataracts. If zinc is deficient, vitamin A is unable to move into the optical tissues where it can be utilized.

Zinc and vitamin A work well together. Zinc is non-toxic, and if it is supplemented, then vitamin A should be supplemented as well. At the Memorial Sloan-Kettering Cancer Service Center in New York City, Dr. Michael Bunk observed how mice tended to suffer from vitamin A deficiency symptoms when zinc was deficient. He concluded that zinc increases the mobilization of vitamin A from the liver, and also concluded that zinc was necessary for the epithelial cells to absorb and utilize vitamin A. These cells are used to cover surfaces, such as the skin, and can be found in mammary glands.

Some studies using animals have shown a reduction in the use of vitamin A during periods of zinc deficiency. When zinc levels are optimal, the concentration of vitamin A in the blood is optimized. Other animal studies have experimented with zinc's relationship to vitamin A by showing how synthesis of the retinol-binding protein known as R13P, which transports vitamin A through the blood, is impaired when zinc is lacking. This can eventually lead to decreased vitamin A being secreted from the liver.

When an enzyme is impaired due to a lack of its major metallic element, various bodily functions become at risk. For example, the alcohol dehydrogenase enzyme is responsible for the conversion of vitamin A alcohol (retinol) to vitamin A aldehyde (retinal), which is a process necessary for healthy vision. In 1973, researcher Arora observed decreased activity of this enzyme in lambs that were zinc deficient, which helped to explain why the animals were experiencing night-blindness.

Industrial applications of zinc include dipping steel alloys into melted zinc to prevent corrosion. This is called galvanization. Rust occurs when oxygen reacts with a heavy metal, such as steel, but steel will not rust after it is coated with zinc. Arteries are also susceptible to regular oxidative stress from oxidizing agents such as drugs and free radicals. Blood contains natural antioxidants, such as uric acid, ascorbic acid, and defensive proteins to limit this damage, but they are not 100%.

Zinc's ability to protect cells against dangerous oxidative damage is so profound that its benefits can be two-fold. Researchers at the University of Lodz in Poland studied how zinc interacts with DNA in both healthy and cancerous cells. They concluded that zinc not only helps to protect against DNA damage in healthy cells, but they also found that zinc increases its protection in cancerous cells. This shows why zinc should be used to prevent dangerous oxidative damage in normal cells and why it should be used in cancer therapy.

In a similar conducted by Oregon State University, researchers concluded that DNA integrity in the prostate is compromised during periods of zinc deficiency due to impaired function of zinc-containing proteins. Thus, modern research suggests that zinc protects the cells and DNA from damage, directly and indirectly, by activating enzymes that neutralize dangerous forms of oxygen and by working with proteins that protect the cells, all of which could help slow down the aging process.

Some studies show zinc's ability to protect cell walls, including keeping the tissues soft, thus preventing hardening of the arteries. Researchers from the University of Kentucky experimented with zinc's role in arterial cells. They discovered that when zinc levels were normal in these cells, the arteries were able to resist damaging cholesterol invasion. When zinc levels are low, the arterial cells became prone to damage from fat peroxidation.

Loss of appetite is one symptom of zinc deficiency. Sensory benefits from proper zinc levels include heightened senses of smell and taste. One study examined how zinc deficient rats consumed only one-third as much food compared to controlled rats. It was thought that the reduction in food consumption could be a result of diminished sense of taste, which can also result in eating disorders such as anorexia.

Skeletal growth is somewhat dependent on zinc. Some abnormalities observed in poultry experiments showed bones becoming shortened and thickened, along with a decreased width of epiphyseal cartilage when zinc was deficient. Similar studies in cows also revealed bowed hind legs and stiff joints. Overall, a zinc deficiency impairs bone collagen synthesis and hinders the zinc-dependent enzyme tibial collagenase.

Severe zinc deficiencies can affect the nervous system. In 1978, studies using laboratory rats showed how zinc deficiencies resulted in learning disabilities and emotional responsiveness. The zinc deficiencies were induced during gestation, lactation, or after weaning. Newborn monkeys experiencing zinc deficiency played less well with others and experienced impaired curiosities. This mineral has even been shown to enhance brain functioning. Women who supplemented with zinc have shown increases of 20% in mental capacity over a six-week period.

In general, zinc is required for the proper utilization of vitamins, physical and sexual growth and development, body tissues and fluids, immune strength, neutralization of free radicals, synthesis of DNA, cellular processes, and healing. It also helps with food absorption through the intestinal walls, stabilizes blood, assists with muscle contractions, and helps other minerals with the acid/alkaline balance. It is deficient in today's diets due to extreme food processing as well being missing from soils. Some observations show an 80% loss of zinc in white bread. Zinc is commonly lost through the kidneys, urine and skin. Zinc's high concentration in bodily fluids such as sweat makes it prone to loss during periods of exercise.

Other symptoms of zinc deficiency include lethargy, mental disturbances such as low academic performance, irregular menstrual cycles, nausea, bloating, diarrhea, abdominal cramps, fever, lowered libido, hypertension, paranoia, PMS, cavities, infertility, angina, bulimia, hair loss, miscarriages, stillbirths, thyroid disorders, depression, and anemia. Some have suggested larger conditions such as Alzheimer's disease, Crohn's disease, diabetes, eye diseases, and prostate cancer could be alleviated with proper zinc supplementation.

Common food sources of zinc include fruits and vegetables grown in mineral rich soils. Almonds, cashews, peanuts, sunflower seeds, and pumpkin seeds are all good sources. Mushrooms and many herbs also tend to have high levels of zinc.

Chapter 13

The Beneficial and Other Minerals in People

Boron

Boron has a long history that goes back many centuries. The famous Arab researcher Geber, who died in 776 A.D., first mentioned "boric acid," which was referred to in Middle Age writings as "Borach," "Bauracon," or "Baurach." Boric acid and borates were also known as precious commodities called Tinkal or Tinkar that were imported from Tibet. This element was originally used medicinally as a disinfectant and to treat burns.

Boron was first discovered and isolated by two French chemists, Louis-Jaques Thenard and Joseph-Louis Gay-Lussac, and then eventually by the English chemist Sir Humphrey Davy, in 1808. Since they were only able to isolate boron to only 50% purity, none of them recognized it as a new element. In 1824, it was the Swedish chemist Jöns Jakob Berzelius who became the first person to identify boron as an element. Decades later Moissan melted it down to its pure form.

Although it is not considered a metal, pure boron is hard and gray and melts at almost 4,000 degrees Fahrenheit. It is usually found in nature bound to other elements forming a compound, such as borax, boric acid (sassolite), ulexite, or boracite. Borax deposits were first found in Death Valley in 1881, where teams of 20 mules were used to haul out huge loads to a rail station 165 miles away.

Benefits of boron in animals were not discovered until 1981, wherein it was quickly identified as an essential nutrient. In 1990, boron was recognized as an essential nutrient in humans. Although it is mainly stored and utilized in bones, boron is found in trace amounts in most tissues. In human bone tissue, studies performed on cremated ash have shown boron concentrations to be between 16 and 138 ppm.

Boron works alongside calcium, magnesium, phosphorus, and vitamin D in building and maintaining strong bones and in the calcification of teeth. Over and over, research consistently shows how boron enhances the absorption and utilization of calcium and these other nutrients, so that loss of bone strength can easily be attributed to a boron deficiency.

Some studies show that calcium levels in tissues become low when boron is deficient. Forrest H. Nielsen of the Department of Agriculture's Grand Forks Human Nutrition Research Center examined calcium's need for boron. For 63 days he studied the effects of a low-boron diet on five men and five women on bone-preserving estrogen therapy, and four postmenopausal women who were not given estrogen. After the results were recorded, the subjects took 3 mg boron for the next 49 days. Although the first part of the study resulted in low levels of calcium in their blood when boron was deficient, the second part of the study resulted in both calcium and copper levels in the blood improving to healthy levels after the boron was added.

Boron is required to form estrogen and vitamin D, and it improves the utilization of copper. However, to make matters even more interesting, when magnesium is deficient boron utilization suffers. Although this mineral is still being investigated, boron contributes to bone formation in both men and women and seems to protect against magnesium and calcium losses by increasing their absorption.

An investigation into the relationship between boron and magnesium was conducted using 12 postmenopausal women between the ages of 48 and 82. When boron was supplemented, urinary loss of both calcium and magnesium declined. When magnesium was low, phosphorus loss accelerated, except when boron was supplemented. It was concluded that boron is paramount in preventing bone loss by being able to help the body avoid losing other elements. Researchers also noted an interesting observation during this experiment: the subjects were less mentally alert during periods of boron deficiency.

Another study investigated the effects of boron on hormones such as estrogen. After only eight days of boron supplementation, women's loss of calcium was reduced by 40%, magnesium loss by 33%, and the women experienced less phosphorus excretion through their urine. There is some evidence that women suffering from osteoporosis who take supplemental boron experience an increase in their serum hormone levels. The women who supplemented with boron doubled their amount of estradiol 17B versus women on estrogen replacement therapy. Boron is believed to enhance estrogen's role in bone strength by utilizing vitamin D into an active form necessary for calcium.

Other areas of the body also seem to benefit from boron, including teeth enamel. Also, the amount of boron found in hair resembles the amount found in tissues. During birth, concentrations of boron in blood plasma are unusually high, and will resume normal rates in less than a week following the birth. Mother's milk contains an average of 10% the amount of boron as that found in blood.

Considering boron's usefulness in bone metabolism, hormone therapy, and enzymatic activities, it should come as no surprise that deficiencies of boron have been linked to osteoporosis and tooth decay. Boron also aids cartilage formation and repair. In fact, some have observed that boron deficiencies aggravate arthritis and other joint conditions. Without boron, calcium, magnesium, and phosphorus levels begin to subside. Some observe decreased memory and mental functions during periods of boron deficiency. Without sufficient boron, some research has observed weaker cell walls and membranes. Brittle bones, carpal tunnel syndrome, loss of libido, hormonal imbalance, muscle pain, memory loss, receding gums, and fragile cartilage are all signs of possible boron deficiencies.

Water soluble boron is commonly found in pears, apples and grapes, and can usually be found in nuts, legumes, and green, leafy vegetables.

Germanium

Named for the country of Germany, germanium is a relatively new trace element whose existence was first predicted by Dmitri Mendeleyev years before the German scientist Clemens Winkler actually discovered it in 1886, who gave it the name "germanium." It is largely used in the semiconductor industry. During the mid-1900s this element was used extensively in radios due to its chemical tendency to act as a semiconductor by capturing radio waves. An atom of germanium is organized in a way that allows it to regularly transfer electrons, making it a great conductor of electricity and radio. These characteristics make germanium chemically related to silicon and carbon.

In living tissues, germanium is still under investigation. Thus, germanium remains a trace element until it is determined to provide health benefits that make it essential. Some of the scant research available on germanium indicates that when it is in ionic form its metallic electrochemical properties help to raise the activity level of various organs and tissues by expediting oxygen uptake. People who require higher oxygen levels should take supplemental germanium. Germanium even shows characteristics of helping the body excrete toxic materials, including infectious agents.

Germanium is found in soils (especially alkaline) and other materials, such as igneous rock, sandstone, ocean water, and limestone. In 1950, a Japanese chemist named Dr. Kazuhiko Asai discovered germanium in ancient plant fossils. His later studies linked the healing properties of ancient herbs to their high amounts of germanium. In fact, many herbs are accumulators of germanium. Herbs that are credited with high amounts of germanium that range from 100 to 2,000 ppm include: garlic, aloe, comfrey, chlorella, ginseng, watercress, Shiitake mushrooms, pearly barley, sanzukon, sushi, waternut, boxthorn seed, and wisteria knob. Years ago, Russian researchers credited germanium with having anti-cancer properties.

Germanium affects the immune system, osteoporosis, arthritis, and asthma. This element provides defense against infectious agents such as viruses, bacteria, and fungi by activating the manufacture of natural killer cells and T-suppressor cells. Some symptoms of germanium deficiency include cardiovascular problems including hypertension, leukemia, neuralgia, and even softening of brain tissues. Someday, germanium could very well be taken from the list of beneficial minerals and added to the list of essential minerals.

When germanium is in the form of a chelated supplement, only about 30% of it can be absorbed in the human body, while the rest is excreted within seven days. Good plant sources of water soluble germanium include tomatoes, garlic, and most fruits and vegetables that are grown in mineral rich soil.

Gold

Gold has been used as a commodity in trading for over 5,500 years and has been sought after for its luster. It is a soft metal that can be shaped into various tools, utensils, pottery, jewelry, and many other uses. Royal people have adorned themselves with gold for many centuries. In nature, gold is usually bound with other elements to form compounds, but it can be found as free ions if has been absorbed into plants that grow in areas that contain veins of gold.

There is approximately one milligram of gold dissolved in every ton of ocean water. It conducts electricity and heat and does not corrode. Gold is a good reflector of infrared radiation and is used to dissipate heat. It can be spread extremely thin—the facemasks of astronauts who walk in outer space are covered with a layer of gold so thin that it is transparent, to protect against sunlight that is not being filtered by Earth's atmosphere.

Gold has a long history of medicinal use in both Eastern and Western traditions. Gold was prescribed for longevity, rejuvenation, and relaxation in India and China for hundreds of years.

Gold has also been used to support the nervous, reproductive, and glandular systems. In the 16th century Paracelsus used gold to treat epilepsy and by the 17th century it was used regularly to treat the nervous system. Gold was also listed in the new pharmacopoeias as a treatment for depression, feelings of melancholy, fevers, fainting, and epilepsy—what we would call neurological or psychiatric disorders today.

By the 19th century, doctors had some success with using gold to cure syphilis. This was highlighted in a research report by J. A. Chrestien, a notable physician of the time, who published "Researches and observations on the effects of preparations of gold in the treatment of many diseases and notably in syphilitic maladies" (1821). Chrestien first began using gold instead of mercury for the treatment of syphilis and noticed that treatment with gold also came with feelings of vitality, enhanced intellectuality, stimulation of various glands as well as increased sexual performance.

In 1879 James Compton Burnett published a long historical account of the use of gold, going back to 2,500 BC. He noted neurological and glandular applications for gold, such as sterility, diseases in female reproductive organs, and epilepsy. In his book, he noted that Samuel Hanemann, who founded homeopathy, "…mentions nearly thirty authors (1698-1730) who praise gold as a valuable remedy in various diseases such as melancholia…"

Burnett continues, "Gold is an excitant…The patients feel an indescribable sense of well-being, they feel themselves lighten (as they express it), so that we may say that gold possesses hilariant properties. The intellectual faculties are more active…Some are of the opinion that gold belongs to that class of noble metals, such as silver and copper, which exert a powerful influence on the nervous system." Finally, by the end of the 19th century, gold was being used as a treatment for the nervous system.

In 1894, S. Potter published an article based on the 1890 U.S. Pharmacopoeia, stating that gold helps to promote healthy appetite and digestion, stimulates the nervous system, and produces a noticeable increase in mental exhilaration and a sense of well-being. Long-term benefits of gold may induce aphrodisiac effects in both men and women, and impotence may be cured by it. In fact, the 1899 Merck Manual lists gold as an aphrodisiac on page 187.

Leslie E. Keeley (1832-1900) is credited with using gold, sodium, and chloride to cure addictions to morphine, opium, cocaine, and alcohol. In 1897, he published a report titled "Opium: Its Use, Abuse, and Cure." During his practice of treating drug addictions, he said: "In opium patients whose bodies are covered with nodulations, sores, pimples, blotches, tumors, and ulcers…remarkable effects have been produced by the use of gold. The sores rapidly heal up and pass away…"

An 1894 editorial in the Chicago Tribune noted Dr. Keeley's incredible record of accomplishment by highlighting his 90% success rate and over 1,000 cases of people being cured from their drug addictions. Unfortunately, Keeley's successful formula was a closely guarded secret. After his death, many of the people he treated formed various clubs in an effort to provide support and continue spreading the word about the use of gold. However, after Keeley's death in 1900, the use of gold to treat alcoholism declined.

By the beginning of the 20th century gold was once again being touted as a powerful sexual and nervous system stimulant, and Keeley's cure for alcohol and opium addictions started to become accepted. In the 1942 edition of the Stedman's Practical Medical Dictionary, S.T. Garber includes gold as a treatment for epilepsy, headaches, and as a nerve sedative.

It is clear that gold was used for centuries in the nervous, reproductive, and glandular systems in observations, testimonials, and in individual cases. With the advent of modern medicine, gold began to disappear from the pharmacopoeias, except for the treatment of rheumatoid arthritis.

In recent years, some interesting experiments observed once again the roles of gold in sexual organs. In 1977, the journal Pediatric Research published an article titled, "Trace elements (zinc, cobalt, selenium, rubidium, bromine, and gold) in human placenta and newborn liver at birth." They measured gold and other trace elements and found gold to be three times more concentrated in human placenta than in liver tissue. However, other trace elements, such as selenium, zinc, and cobalt, were found in higher amounts in the liver tissue, so they concluded that gold is not an essential trace element.

In 1984, other researchers found high concentrations of gold in male semen. They stated: "...this is the richest source of gold reported in biological materials." In that same year, other researchers found high concentrations of gold along with zinc and copper in the hair of newborn infants. They suggested that levels of gold, copper, and zinc will temporarily increase during certain periods of development in-utero, but after time these levels will eventually decrease.

Examinations of blood and various human tissues reveal small amounts of gold, usually in the order of just a few ions. Heart tissues were observed to contain 0.0338 ngs of gold, while researcher Vanoeteren found a range of 0.72 to 1.6 ngs of gold in lung tissues from six different participants. Kjellin investigated gold's presence in the brain and found gold concentrated in the gray matter (0.024), white matter (0.040), cerebrospinal fluid (0.0062), whole blood (0.055), and serum (0.080) ng/g. Hair samples have shown gold in trace amounts—0.036 to 0.055 mcg/g.

Gold compounds such as gold sodium thiomalate and gold thioglucose should not be taken. Compounds such as these become problematic when they pass through the kidneys and liver, and people with blood diseases are also cautioned to avoid gold compounds. Some toxic reactions to gold compounds have included urine albumin, bloody urine, aplastic anemia, susceptibility to hepatitis infection, and pneumonitisin. Water-soluble gold taken as a supplement or from eating various plants is the best form of this element that will optimize its absorption and utilization in the cells. The body will excrete excess water-soluble gold along with other elements that may go unused, most commonly through the urine and feces.

Traces of gold ions can be found throughout most soils, having been broken down by weathering agents, water, and microbial processes, and absorbed into plant tissues. In an article published in Social Science Medicine (1989), Dr. Harry Warren of the Department of Geological Sciences at the University of British Columbia explained that gold was first discovered in honeybee pollen in 1981, with a surprisingly high amount of 0.9 ppm. Later, investigations found two plants that are consistently high in gold, namely Phacelia sericea and Dryas drummondi. These plants can contain concentrations of gold that are 25-50 times higher than surrounding plants, while the Indian mustard plant (Brassica juncea) can store up to 100 times more gold than most plants. However, further research on these and surrounding plants are limited since they grow at over 6,000 feet in elevation throughout British Columbia, usually too high for honeybees. A taste of honeybee pollen will dissolve quickly on the tongue, allowing for any mineral elements to become quickly absorbed into the tongue's tissues.

Observations into gold having human benefits include many different mental benefits, including a general "euphoric" feeling experienced by supplement users. Some people have reported that after prolonged periods of water-soluble gold supplementation, gold appeared to raise their energy levels. Gold can also help brain function, night sweats, and feelings of depression, despair, fear, and frustration. It has also been used to counteract feelings of sorrow, anguish, hot flashes, and seasonal attitude disorders. This element has even been linked to providing deep REM sleep and extended, peaceful dreaming.

One of the most profound functions of gold on the human body is its ability to repair damaged DNA. Our DNA can become damaged from free radicals or toxins, and since our cells are completely reproduced every seven years, if our DNA is damaged then we reproduce a damaged person over and over, getting worse and worse with every passing 7-year cycle, a phenomenon known as aging. Gold acts as a pure amalgam, which allows it to bind with other elements very easily, and some have observed its ability to repair damaged DNA, which prevents us from reproducing an inferior product every seven years.

Gold has a reputation for helping with arthritis and active joint inflammation, especially when taken with aspirin. It is not necessarily an analgesic, but does have some anti-inflammatory effects. Gold is known to help with glandular functions, chills, circulatory and digestive processes, and helps neutralize sodium fluoride poisoning. Other uses for gold include asthma, skin disorders, cancer, and lupus.

Lithium

Lithium was first discovered in 1817 by Johann August Arfvedson, and was later isolated by William Thomas Brande and Sir Humphrey Davy. It makes up only 0.0007% of Earth's crust and is usually found bound to other elements. In industrial applications, lithium is mixed into ceramics and glasses, including mirrors in telescopes, and is used in creating lightweight metal parts for aircraft.

Lithium is the lightest alkali metal and its ions are freely mobile in the soil. Soil samples have measured as high as 30 ppm but widely vary. In oceanic plant life, lithium has been measured at 5 ppm and land plants at 0.1 ppm, depending on which plant is being sampled and what soil it was grown in. Ocean animals have measured 1 ppm, while land animals have measured 0.02 ppm. Fresh water has been found to have 0.0011 ppm and ocean water, 0.18 ppm. Human tissues have shown between 2 and 200 ng/g net weight.

Lithium is widespread around the world. High concentrations of lithium were found in hair samples of university students in Tijuana, Mexico, while hair samples from residents of Munich, Germany, contained the lowest concentrations. Interestingly, hair samples of average adults have been observed to be almost 400 times higher than in violent inmates who were incarcerated in Texas, Oregon, Florida, and California.

Researchers Schrauzer and Schrestha conducted a 10-year study on lithium supplementation in drinking water of 27 Texas counties. Counties that supplemented their drinking water with lithium, even as little as 70-170 mcg per liter, experienced significantly fewer suicides, burglaries, rapes, homicide, and crimes involving drug abuse, as well as arrests for possession of opium, cocaine, and other illegal mind-altering drugs. The researchers concluded their investigation by stating, "These results suggest that lithium at low dosage levels has a generally beneficial effect on human behavior… increasing the human lithium intakes by supplementation, or the lithiation (adding lithium) of drinking water is suggested as a possible means of crime, suicide, and drug-dependency reduction at the individual and community level." It should also be noted that the amount of lithium found in vegetables is strikingly close to the lithium levels found in those Texas counties who experienced lower criminal activity following an increase in lithium concentrations.

There is still a big hurdle in understanding the benefits of lithium due to people's fears about it. There are a lot of misperceptions about lithium, and many people might find the idea that vegetables contain lithium or even that they would benefit from ingesting a lithium supplement, to be unpleasant. Many research studies document surprising benefits of lithium. Clinical use of lithium has usually involved treatment for various mental illnesses.

Epidemiological studies have shown a negative correlation between lithium in drinking water and admittance to psychiatric institutions. Since its introduction by researcher John Cade, lithium salts have been used the world over to treat manic-depressant patients for over 40 years. According to Dr. Myrna M. Weissman, a psychiatrist at Columbia University, "Depression is a worldwide phenomenon happening at younger and younger ages." Clinical depression has almost doubled with each new generation since 1915. In 1935, the average age range of those clinically diagnosed with depression was their late 20's. However, in 1955 the age range had already dropped to 15-20. On average, approximately 25% of women and 10% of men will develop some form of depression.

Dr. Melvyn Werbach found considerable evidence that lithium can reduce unusual aggressive behaviors in children, such as self-mutilation. Children who experience either Conduct Disorder or Aggressive Type Disorder, as well as brain-injured and mentally retarded patients with aggressive, self-combative or self-destructive disorders, have been treated successfully with lithium.

It is thought that lithium affects many metabolic pathways and organ functions, including the regulation of hormonal activity. For example, Graves's disease, also known as hyperthyroidism, is a condition that is characterized by an enlarged thyroid that secretes too much hormone. Researchers at the Mayo Clinic examined the effects of lithium in Grave's patients as far back as 1972. Their published results documented high doses of lithium in 10 patients, showing that hormonal secretion declined 20-30% to more normal levels within only five days.

With regards to treating depression, some experiments have used lithium to treat people who are trying to recover from alcohol and illegal drug addictions. The alcoholics that have been treated and their family members report improved moods, reduced temper in men, less depression and irritability in women, and an overall lessened desire for alcohol within 6-8 weeks of supplementation. An article in the British Journal of Addiction that studied high doses of lithium reported that "both controlled and uncontrolled experiments show that symptoms of both alcoholism and affective disturbance are reduced in patients treated with lithium."

These same researchers also reviewed 10 successful trials of lithium supplementation over the next 26 years in Grave's patients. They stated their conclusions: "A small number of studies have documented its (lithium's) use in the treatment of patients with Grave's disease…its efficacy and utility as an alternative anti-thyroid (treatment) are not widely recognized. Lithium normalizes (thyroid hormone) levels in one to two weeks…" However, the researchers also warned, "toxicity precludes its use as a first-line or long-term therapeutic agent."

Some users of lithium supplements report relief from cluster headaches. These types of headaches can show up at very inconvenient times, and sufferers experience merciless pain followed by a short hiatus. An investigation into lithium's effects on cluster headaches was performed using 19 men. Within just two weeks, eight of the men felt an 85% decline in the number of headaches. Four of the subjects had both cluster headaches and psychiatric symptoms and all four had nearly complete relief from all of their conditions. The other seven subjects experienced only a small amount of relief.

An unusual benefit of lithium involves a heightened sense of direction, commonly known as "spatial memory." Short-term memory functions such as where you last put your keys could be improved when lithium is present. Observations have centered on laboratory rats in mazes in an effort to study the effects of short-term memory showing how subjects repetitively maneuver through a maze. Studies have compared rats supplemented with and without lithium and found that lithium improved the spatial memory functions within only 24 hours of supplementation.

Research indicates that lithium can protect and even renew damaged brain cells, as well as preserve the gray matter that is normally expected to decline with age. For many years it has been standard medical belief that once the brain reaches a state of maturation, it begins to decline and shrink in size for the remainder of the person's life. In 2000, an article in the Lancet ran the headline "Lithium-induced increase in human brain gray matter." Although it didn't make an immediate groundbreaking impact, the significance of this article and studies that followed is profound. According to this report, researchers at Wayne State University in Michigan observed lithium's ability to preserve and initiate new brain cells. In a study involving 10 participants supplemented with high doses of lithium, eight participants experienced an average of 3% growth in brain gray matter within just one month.

According to Dr. Jonathan V. Wright, MD, brain cells are always at risk of damage from various toxins, sometimes referred to as excitotoxins. These toxins can be a result of ordinary brain functioning and are produced every day, eventually wearing down the brain cells. Another form of brain cell damage results from various cell receptors that have become over-activated. Lithium helps to normalize this activity and can even help produce bcl-2, which is a protective brain protein, found in most animals and all human brain cells.

However, lithium can also help prevent strokes and protect against damage incurred from prescription drugs. If minerals in the blood are lacking and a blood clot occurs that serves the brain, the blood flow to that area is decreased. If the arterial clog is large enough, the lack of blood to that area of the brain could result in a stroke with extreme damage to the brain cells. Studies examining animals show less brain cell damage when lithium was present. The overall area of damage was smaller due to the protective abilities of lithium.

One of the most remarkable studies on lithium and damaged brain cells occurred in laboratory rats. In this study, researchers induced strokes in two groups of rats. One group had already supplemented with lithium for 16 days while the other group did not supplement at all. After inducing strokes, autopsies revealed that the rats that supplemented with lithium experienced 56% less brain cell damage when compared to the control group.

In the nervous system, lithium has been found to generate DNA replication in nerve cells, which precedes cellular formation. Even more importantly, the new brain cells are able to communicate, known as "signaling," with the older cells without any difficulty. Scientists measure the health of brain cells by its level of N-acetylaspartate (NAA), an amino acid found in high concentrations in neurons. When NAA is lacking, it is thought that nerve functioning has diminished. A study was performed using 19 participants that were all given supplemental lithium. Fourteen experienced measurable increases in NAA, four subjects had little change, and one subject had no measurable change. It is thought that lithium influences two signal-carrying pathways, and some researchers have observed it reconstructing signaling pathways in need of repair.

Lithium is known to have to some protective effects on brain cells. A major development in the treatment of Alzheimer's disease involves keeping brain cells protected from toxins. Some have investigated lithium's ability to minimize the damage and secretion of the destructive beta-amyloid protein plaques that coat the brains of Alzheimer's patients. Evidence also shows its ability to limit the formation of other destructive proteins that are over-produced, including tau protein and neurofibrillary tangles, which are the hallmark of Alzheimer's disease. Even aluminum particles found in this disease can bind with lithium ions, making them easier to remove from the body.

One study observed lithium inhibiting the reproduction of viruses, including the herpes virus, Epstein-Barr virus, measles virus, the cytomegalovirus, and the adenovirus. A double-blind study showed that lithium consistently reduces the number of herpes episodes per month, the average duration of each episode, the total number of days infected per month, and the severity of the symptoms. The placebo responded by increasing three of the four severity measures.

Lithium has also shown an ability to boost the immune system by increasing the number of white blood cells, especially in people who have undergone chemotherapy radiation. White blood cells are used to ward off infections such as bacteria and viruses. When the number of white blood cells decreases, the body becomes more prone to sicknesses.

Lithium stimulates stem cells found in bone marrow, resulting in the formation of platelets and eventually the production of white blood cells, even in those who continue chemotherapy treatments.

A group of researchers tested lithium and its effects on early growth and development in goats and rats. During the postnatal period of 0-6 months, extreme lithium deficiencies resulted in low birth weight and impaired weight gain. Females experienced higher rates of both miscarriage and postpartum mortality. The rats did not suffer permanent growth conditions for the first three generations. However, they did experience reproductive abnormalities and low survival rates. Autopsies revealed that most of these tissues lacked lithium; however, lithium remained in constant normal supply in the brain, even long after the element was no longer being supplemented.

Other studies show that lithium relieves symptoms associated with fibromyalgia, a condition characterized by pain and stiffness. A small study using three women who wouldn't respond to conventional treatments showed measurable improvement after lithium supplementation. Others have used lithium to treat anorexic women. Even though zinc is more widely accepted in treating anorexia, treatment with lithium has also shown good results. A small study involving two women suffering from anorexia supplemented lithium and resulted in weight gains of 20 and 26 pounds in only six weeks.

Most of the results in these studies used unusually high amounts of lithium—much higher than what would normally be considered for a daily supplement. Lithium can be found in extremely trace amounts in naturally grown foods, but food may not be a reliable source. Rather, a lithium supplement in its ionic, water-soluble state should be taken occasionally. It is generally accepted that a lithium supplement should not be taken on a daily basis, unless undergoing a short-term protocol under the supervision of a professional therapist.

Just like any other mineral element, lithium should be taken in its water-soluble ionic form and not as part of a compound. According to Dr. Werbach, results of an uncontrolled study show that "Low doses of lithium derived from vegetable concentrates may have a powerful effect on mental state and behavior. Thirteen depressed patients with bipolar disorder were treated with natural lithium derived from vegetable concentrates. All improved in about 10 days and there were no adverse effects. After six weeks, they were taken off of lithium and all regressed to their former depressed state within three days. Two days after lithium was resupplied, their depressions lifted again."

According to the widely used college textbook Chemistry, The Central Science (8th Edition), lithium was first discovered in 1817 and lithium salts were widely believed to have "mystical healing powers." At that time, some claimed to include lithium in products that were touted as being a fountain of youth. Eventually in 1927, Mr. C. L. Briggs started to sell a soft drink that contained lithium, known as "Bib-Label Lithianated Lemon-Lime Soda." He later changed the name of the soda to Seven-Up©. Seven-Up© used to contain a form of lithium called lithium citrate and was sold as a beverage that claimed to provide "an abundance of energy, enthusiasm, a clear complexion, lustrous hair, and shining eyes." During the 1950s, concerns from the Food and Drug Administration resulted in its removal as an ingredient. However, around the same time neurological experiments were starting to show lithium's benefits on psychotic treatments, including therapeutic effects on mental disorders such as bipolar affective disorder and manic depression. Research has shown that lithium helps smooth out such mood swings.

Chemistry, The Central Science further states that the therapeutic effects of lithium were accidentally discovered by an Australian psychologist named John Cade in the 1940s. Using uric acid, he showed how manically depressed laboratory animals were able to reverse their psychotic mood swings when treated with lithium salt. It was later realized that the uric acid was not to be credited, but rather the lithium ions contained in the salt were responsible for such reversal. It wasn't until the 1970s that lithium was used regularly in psychological treatments. Studies show that as high as 70% of those who take supplemental lithium experience positive results. Lithium ions have proven to be the most effective treatment of certain mental disorders, even though it is still not entirely understood how this element is able to perform such remedial effects.

Nickel

"Nickel" is the German word that means "Old Nick," which is another name for the devil. The Swedish chemist Axel Fredrik Cronstedt first discovered nickel in 1751. The world's largest deposit of nickel is located in the Sudbury region of Ontario, Canada. This massive deposit is thought to be the remnants of an ancient meteorite impact.

Nickel is a hard and corrosive metal. Along with gold, it can be electroplated onto the surfaces of other elements to form a protective coating. When added to glass, nickel provides a green color. It is used to produce some batteries and coins. If nickel is added to other alloys, it improves its strength and helps resist corrosion. This dense metal is used to manufacture vaults, armor plates, and heavy machine parts.

Along with other heavy metals such as iron, aluminum, copper, gold, silver, and molybdenum, nickel can be found in plants such as legumes and cereal grains. Plants such as these need nickel ions in order for their seeds to germinate. It wasn't until 1987 that researchers finally acknowledged nickel's health benefits in plants and recognized it as an essential micromineral.

Research illustrates the benefits of nickel in both plants and animals. Nickel assists plants in the uptake and absorption of nitrogen and iron from the soil and is the metallic element needed to activate some plant enzymes. In animals, nickel is recognized as a beneficial micromineral, even while its exact functions are still being identified. Studies involving nickel deficiencies in animals have shown very surprising symptoms.

Farm animals such as cows, chickens, sheep, and goats that are fed nickel-free diets appear to suffer from abnormal rates of growth, development, and decreased red blood cell production. Other studies using laboratory rats have resulted in abnormal growth, lower iron content in blood, poor zinc absorption, birth defects resulting in high mortality rates, delayed puberty, and skin conditions. Goats and rats showed signs of improper utilization of other elements such as calcium, iron, zinc, and vitamin B12, while guinea pigs, goats, and rats consistently showed reproductive malfunction and slowed growth rates.

Though nickel provides enough health benefits to be considered an essential trace element for humans, a prominent specific role has yet to be identified. What is known so far seems to point towards increased utilization of other elements such as gastrointestinal absorption of iron and zinc, and participation in enzymatic and metabolic activities. Nickel assists in the metabolism of lipids and hormones, and plays a strong role in cellular activities such as cell membrane integrity and membrane metabolism. Nickel deficiencies have resulted in abnormal growth rates and impaired reproductive, skin, and liver functions.

Metalloenzymes need nickel as a cofactor, such as one enzyme responsible for the metabolism of branched-chain amino acids and odd-chain fatty acids, while other enzyme systems need nickel to be activated. Some research has shown this element's ability to decrease the need for vitamin B12. In fact, during tissue samples showing vitamin B12 deficiency, the body responds with a higher demand for nickel to compensate, which could imply that nickel and the element cobalt have similar working properties.

As with any other element, when nickel is ingested as a compound, risks of hazardous toxicity can result. Less than 10% of metallic nickel is useful to the body if swallowed. Metallic nickel is an industrial waste and is known as an environmental pollutant. Nickel carbonyl is one example of a nickel compound that is a toxic industrial chemical. In order for nickel to have positive health benefits, only nickel ions should be considered from foods such as plants. Examples of foods that commonly contain nickel are nuts, grains, oats, peas, beans, and even chocolate. Nickel should also be found in fruits and vegetables grown in mineral rich soil.

Rubidium

Two German scientists, Robert Bunsen and Gustav Kirchoff, first discovered rubidium in 1861 and named it after the Latin word for deep red, rubidus. They discovered rubidium while analyzing a compound that emitted deep red lines never before seen through their spectroscope. Later, Bunsen was able to isolate rubidium, and today it is obtained as a byproduct from refining lithium. Compounds of this element have very little industrial applications, although recent discoveries of large rubidium deposits could pave the way for more uses, but only after our understanding of this element's usefulness is recognized.

Rubidium is an "ultratrace" element that is very widespread, including seawater (120 parts per billion) and Earth's crust (100 parts per million). This element is in the potassium family group and its ions do not accumulate toxically in any particular organ or tissues. Normal adults carry 300 ppm in any of their body's tissues, which is the highest among all ultratrace elements, totaling around 360 milligrams for a healthy man.

Since rubidium is not considered an essential or beneficial nutrient, and due to its extreme trace amounts, it is considered an ultratrace element. However, it might be the most useful ultratrace element of all. Some reports have shown blood tests with higher-than-expected levels of rubidium in children, which suggests that it could have an essential role, especially since its presence in living tissues is higher than in the environment.

Although rubidium may not yet be considered "essential" in living tissues, it does have some characteristics of usefulness. Rubidium and cesium both share close physicochemical characteristics with potassium. These three elements appear to have some exchangeable characteristics. Some research shows that either rubidium or cesium can replace potassium as a nutritional substitute, with little evidence of toxicity. Specifically, this is true in the growth and development of yeast and of sea urchin eggs. During the 1800s, Ringer showed how rubidium could replace potassium in its influence on heart contractions in frogs. Interchangeable characteristics have even been observed in bacteria, algae, fungi, and some invertebrates, although it remains unclear if higher animals such as humans can benefit in this manner.

Shared characteristics between rubidium and potassium in rats include prevention of lesions in kidneys and muscles, and allowing for normal rates of growth. Rats fed up to 200 micrograms of rubidium did not show signs of toxicity. However, when the rats were fed over 1,000 micrograms, reproduction, growth and survival were abnormal. Most studies show that rubidium is not an essential element in rats, although some results continue to show its usefulness in partially replacing potassium.

Rubidium ions are usually concentrated in areas outside the cell where they contribute to nerve and muscle activities. Once rubidium was identified as having close characteristics with potassium, studies began to indicate that it had some function in neurophysiological activities. Samples of heart tissue show higher amounts of rubidium in muscle tissues that surround that heart than in conductive tissues.

In the brain, rubidium's presence is scattered, depending on functional regions, and can decrease with age. This element apparently can quicken the turnover of brain norepinephrine. One researcher suggested that since rubidium causes electroencephalogram activation in animals such as monkeys, a deficiency of rubidium could result in low wave power values in dialysis patients, since this element quickly diffuses through artificial kidney tissues. It appears that rubidium can have an influence on electrocardiograms.

Rubidium ions even resemble potassium in their patterns of absorption, utilization, and excretion. Inside the cells, rubidium and potassium apparently share a transport system; they both permeate across cellular membranes at almost identical rates. These two elements are so close in chemical composition that they may even share ion channels. This is unusual since most elements have their own ion channels and rates of transport across membranes, making them easy to identify and monitor during observations.

Foreign studies of rubidium show that most Finnish foods contained 0.5-5 mcg of rubidium and the average daily intake was over 4 milligrams. The same studies were conducted in England, which showed average daily intakes of 4 milligrams per day, while the United States varied between 1-5 mg per day. Italians averaged 2.5 mg per day. Rubidium should always be taken in the same form that is found in plants. Brazil nuts, for example, are usually high in rubidium.

Silver

Silver has been used to make tools, china, and other metal products for over 5,000 years. It is obtained through its own deposits and can be found in and around deposits of gold, copper, and lead. Silver is the world's best metal conductor of electricity and it is used in the production of circuit boards and electrical contacts. It has been used to create coins, jewelry, china, and silverware, as well as other decorative products. Silver is great at reflecting light, so it is used to capture reflected images on photographic film. Silver is bound with iodine to create silver iodide, a compound that is used to seed clouds to produce rain.

Silver is found scattered in very low concentrations throughout nature, including rocks, soils, ocean water, marine and land plants, tissues of aquatic and land organisms, and has even been found in tortoise shells. Research studies on food samples from fruits and vegetables have yielded very little silver. In fact, in many studies the amount of silver either goes undetectable or contains well less than one part per million, an amount so small its benefit is usually insignificant.

Various types of Chinese health care have used silver for over 8,000 years. Probably the most well-known characteristic of silver is its use as an antibiotic. For years, silver has been known to have anti-fungal, anti-bacterial, and anti-viral properties.

Although silver may not show up on the list of essential nutrients, it does possess characteristics worth mentioning that make it invaluable for medicinal uses. In an article called "Silver: Our Mightiest Germ Fighter," Science Digest reported that silver is an effective antibiotic that destroys over 650 infectious organisms and prevents resistant strains from developing. The article also reported that silver is totally non-toxic to humans at normal rates of ingestion.

Silver specifically destroys microscopic organisms that are nitrogen-breathing, or "anaerobic," organisms. Fortunately, the friendly bacteria found in human intestines are oxygen-breathing, or "aerobic," and are not susceptible to being destroyed by silver. Silver has been reported to disable some enzymes that infectious microorganisms need for respiration. It is thought that silver's unique valence charge is responsible for the effectiveness of destroying such organisms.

Ancient folk remedies included placing silver utensils or silver coins in water or milk during long periods of travel to prevent bacterial infection or spoilage at room temperature. Wealthy people used to eat on "silverware" in an attempt to have some silver in their diets and were commonly known as the "blue bloods." Silver can be placed in water dispensers to keep the water sterile and the spout clean, which also helps prevent slime from building up around the spout. Silver has also been used as a food preservative in canning.

Silver has many other applications that are worthy of mention. In the British Medical Journal, J. Mark Hovell found silver to be beneficial in "restoring the patency of the Eustachian tubes and for reducing nasopharyngeal catarrh." He also found it successful when treating oral and ear infections.

Silver is used in 70% of the burn centers in the United States. Dr. Charles Fox of Columbia University created a silver product called silver sulfadiazine (marketed as Silvadene®). This product has been used successfully in treating infections such as malaria and cholera, and even stops the herpes virus from replicating cold sores and fever blisters. Silver was used intravenously to treat kidney infections without any irritation or skin discoloration. At one point, silver was applied to the eyes of newborn infants to ensure the baby's eyesight if it was suspected the mother had gonorrhea.

A solution of water-soluble silver is clear, non-toxic, has very little taste, will not build up in human tissues, and may even reach the lymph system. When taken internally, water-soluble silver ions absorb quickly into the body's cells and are not susceptible to the acids and alkalis of the stomach, which allows them to pass unchanged into the intestines.

Many people use silver on a regular basis to boost their immune system. It is not present in all body fluids such as sweat, but silver and zinc's presence in the blood can prevent infections from occurring. Although it is believed that the body's immune system does not include spinal fluid, some have reported relief from back pain as a result of using silver supplementation to rid infections.

The use of non-toxic water soluble silver as an antibiotic in home applications includes use as an oral rinse, topical, nasal, rectal and vaginal applications, and it can even be applied directly into eyes and ears. It destroys disease-causing organisms after only a few minutes. This form of silver does not hurt, sting, or burn in any way. It has also been used topically on warts, open sores, and applied directly or mixed with other medicinal agents to combat acne, eczema, or other skin conditions. Some people even report adding silver to their shampoos as an antiseptic and to assist with dandruff.

In 1917 Sir Malcolm Morris of the British Medical Journal reported that water-soluble silver does not pose a risk or have drawbacks when compared to silver compounds, such as skin discoloration or irritation. He stated that silver works against inflammation and helps with healing and he used it with great success against enlarged prostate, hemorrhoids, and bladder irritations.

Common symptoms of silver deficiency include weak immune system and infections from bacteria, fungi, and viruses.

Tin

Tin has been used for 5,500 years. It comprises a mere 0.001% of Earth's crust and is found in large deposits in mining operations throughout Malaysia. Tin avoids corrosion and is even used as a protective coating for other heavy metals. Tin compounds are used to produce solder and pewter, as well as super-conductive wires. Tin salts are dissolved and sprayed onto glass to provide an electrically conductive coating during the manufacture of frost-free windshields. Tin is also a component of stannous fluoride, a compound in toothpastes.

Tin is considered a heavy metal and is a member of the fourth main chemical group of elements on the Periodic Table of Elements. Its chemical properties resemble other elements such as lead, germanium, silica, and carbon. Researcher Schroeder explained that out of the 30 most common trace elements in existence, tin is 21st in the universe,

17th on Earth's crust, 12th in the oceans, and 8th in human tissue. Some have gone on to say that tin is 10th in the plant kingdom, 5th in the lymphatic system, and is preceded by only zinc and iron in the thymus. At the cellular level, each cell contains around 106 to 108 ions of tin—a number comparable to iodine, cobalt, selenium, and chromium.

Tin is still being investigated today to determine its benefit, if any, on human nutrition. As early as 1964, researchers argued about whether or not it provided any benefits at all. Many of the early studies were based on the fact that tin was not found in infants shortly after childbirth and showed no evidence that tin played any important roles. So far, the few studies that have been performed continue to show that tin is commonly found in most tissues.

Autopsies have been performed in an effort to find what elements were located in what tissues of the body. In 1964, researchers Tipton and Shafer sampled lung tissues of cadavers who died of accidental deaths. Although trace amounts of tin were found in the brain, blood vessels, heart, liver, kidneys, ovaries, muscles, stomach, testes, spleen, adrenal glands, and uterus, it was discovered that 137 out of 140 showed less than 5 to 920 mcg of tin per gram in lung tissues. Interestingly, the prostate showed traces of tin but no other trace elements were found there, and none was found in the thyroid. The researchers also concluded that concentrations of tin do not tend to vary with regard to age, sex, or geographical location, and tend not to decline with age.

Another study using autopsies performed by researcher Cook investigated tin levels of 150 cadavers who died of accidental deaths. Using 29 different tissues, it was reported that this sample had very high tin levels, as high as 5 to 72 ppm, and averaged 23 ppm throughout. Overall, tin was discovered in 75% of all sampled tissues, except muscle and brain tissues. Later studies have shown extremely trace amounts in the heart and spleen of fetuses, while other studies have shown no tin existing in stillborns. Even today, there is still no definitive evidence of the role of tin in newborns. What is known is that minerals analyses that are capable of detecting mineral levels below 10 ppm with accuracy continue to show the presence of tin in human tissues. However, its exact role is still being investigated.

Research conducted so far has centered on the effects of tin in laboratory rats. Researcher Schwarz observed stimulation of growth rates, eventually meeting the criteria necessary to be considered an essential nutrient. He also suggested that tin could have a significant role in the heme oxygenase enzyme, which breaks down heme in kidneys, as well as functioning in the tertiary structure of proteins or other substances.

A study conducted by Yokoi provided strong evidence that tin plays some roles in growth. One group of rats were fed diets with only 2 mg/g of tin, and another group was fed a much smaller 17 ng/g of tin. The rats fed the lesser amount of tin experienced stunted growth, impaired food utilization, hearing loss, male pattern baldness, and fluctuations in levels of minerals in its organs. Other rats fed as little as 1-2 ppm have experienced as much as 60% increase in growth rate.

Symptoms of tin deficiency can include hearing loss, male pattern baldness, reduced hemoglobin synthesis, and hair loss. When tin is taken as a water soluble mineral supplement, some have reported stimulation in hair growth and reflexes. Schwarz hypothesized that tin could be an oxidation-reducing catalyst and serve to activate some enzymes. Deficiencies in this trace element have resulted in depressed growth rates and a diminished reproductive system. Tin is also thought to have an affect on the pigmentation of teeth.

What conclusions can be drawn so far is that supplementation of tin in rats that were already lacking in riboflavin improved their growth rates, although they were not quite optimal growth rates. It has not yet been concluded, however, if tin deficiency results in sub-optimal growth rates in animals. Although tin may provide some small benefit, without reasonable data, tin should not necessarily be considered an essential trace mineral at this time.

Vanadium

Named after the Scandinavian goddess Vanadia, vanadium was first discovered in 1801 by a Mexican chemist named Andres Manuel del Rio. He sent samples of vanadium ore along with a letter detailing his explanation to the Institute de France in Paris for analysis. However, his letter was lost in a shipwreck and the Institute was only able to receive his sample. A brief note was also included that described how Rio thought this new element resembled chromium. However, Rio took back his claim after he received a letter from the Institute that disputed it.

In 1830, the Swedish chemist Nils Gabriel Sefstrom accidentally rediscovered vanadium while he was examining iron. But it wasn't until 1867 that the English chemist Sir Henry Enfield Roscoe first isolated it. Today, vanadium compounds are commonly used in nuclear power and to manufacture tubes and pipes for the chemical industry. Since vanadium is a heavy metal, most of its use can be found in the manufacture of steel.

Vanadium is the 21st most abundant element found throughout Earth's surface, comprising around 150 mg/kg, or 0.02%, of metals in the crust. Soils usually average around 100 ppm of vanadium, while samples of ocean water have shown 0.002 ppm and samples of fresh water have revealed 0.001 ppm. Marine plants and land plants are also very similar in their vanadium concentrations, 2.0 to 1.6 ppm, respectively.

In 1971, vanadium became one of the most recent elements to be added to the list of essential trace minerals. Extensive research on vanadium is lacking, but it does seem to act similarly to chromium by regulating insulin and glucose levels. Vanadium functions like insulin because it alters cellular membrane functions for ion transport processes, which increases the cell receptor's sensitivity to insulin. Early research shows that vanadium enhances the performance of insulin by stimulating glucose transport and oxidation, glycogen deposit in the liver, and enhancing the performance of insulin in DNA synthesis. Interestingly, both chromium and vanadium activate enzymes associated with glucose tolerance factor.

Supplementing diabetics with vanadium has shown some promise. A compound form of vanadium was invented over 100 years ago that resulted in reduced glucose levels in 2 out of every 3 diabetic patients. However, a group of Type I patients who supplemented with this compound did not see consistent effects on glucose levels, but they did see a reduction in daily insulin requirements by 14%. Type II patients, however, who supplemented with vanadium experienced higher insulin sensitivity, which resulted in improved glycogen levels and liver deposit. When the study was completed, improvements in insulin and glucose levels remained for almost two weeks.

Because insulin is not orally active, this hormone must be injected directly into the bloodstream. Researchers have tried to find an alternative that would mimic insulin by making it easier for patients to receive treatment. In 1992, researchers from the University of British Columbia, John H McNeill, Chris Orvig, V.G. Yuen, and H. R. Hoveyda, discovered a form of vanadium that seemed to show a faster rate of absorption, and significantly less toxicity from previous vanadium derivatives that were not as absorbable. Tests using laboratory rats resulted in decreased glucose levels to near normal. They also experienced weight loss and proper fluid consumption.

Dr. R.J. Schamherger reported in the Journal of Advancements in Medicine that small doses of a vanadium compound given to diabetic rats improved their glucose levels without interrupting their food consumption or causing weight gain. It was especially noted that glucose levels were not improved by caloric restrictions; thus, the benefits of vanadium supplementation did not influence body weight. He concluded that these benefits are probably attributed to vanadium's role in the liver and tissues. If mineral supplementation is to be considered in the future, for best results vanadium should be combined with chromium.

Besides its ability to alter glucose levels and insulin sensitivity, vanadium has also been observed to function in blood transport. It helps prevent excess cholesterol deposits in blood vessels and in the nervous system. It also works to normalize blood pressure, all of which reduces the likelihood of a heart attack. Studies have shown lowered blood cholesterol in plasma samples following vanadium supplementation. Vanadium has even been credited with increasing the contractile force of the heart muscle, commonly known as the "Inotropic effect." One form of vanadium called vanadyl sulfate appears to accelerate increases in muscle size and density.

Vanadium assists the formation of cartilage and muscle and it helps with cellular division. This element has the reputation of having anti-carcinogenic properties. Tumor growth in mice ceased after supplementing with 25 mcg of vanadium. In fact, there was a decrease in tumor incidence, average tumor count per rodent, and sustained tumor-free time long after completion of the study. Some symptoms of vanadium deficiency in animals show infertility, thyroid malfunction, low fluid retention, decreased growth and fat metabolism, and abnormal growth of teeth, hair, and bones.

Common food sources of vanadium include parsley, radishes, dill seeds, black pepper, whole grains, and most other fruits and vegetables grown in mineral rich soil.

Silicon

In 1824, the Swedish chemist Jons Jacob Berzelius first discovered silicon when he heated chips of potassium in a silica container, then washed away the remaining byproducts. This element is the 7th most abundant element in the universe, and is the 2nd most plentiful element in Earth's crust. Silicon dioxide is the most abundant compound in Earth's crust, and is usually found as sand but can also be found as rock crystal, amethyst, opal, flint, quartz, and jasper. This compound is used largely to manufacture glass. Silicon can be produced by heating sand with carbon.

Other types of silicon compounds are used as abrasives, in soap manufacturing, adhesives, and even as an egg preservative. It can also be found in polishing agents, glass, bricks, lubricants, medical implants, and electrical insulators.

Silicon is known as the "beauty mineral" due to its beautifying effect on skin, hair, and nails. A deficiency of silicon is usually exhibited in dry, brittle hair, easily broken nails, reduced strength in blood vessel tissues, and loss of skin elasticity. Some cardiovascular conditions can be attributed to low silicon levels. Along with calcium and other elements, silicon helps with the hardening and developing of the bones. Abnormalities of the bones and skull can result from a prolonged deficiency of silicon, which can be passed onto the next generation.

Platinum

Platinum was used for centuries by the ancient inhabitants of South America but it wasn't noticed by modern scientists until 1735. It is commonly found around gold deposits, especially in and around the Ural Mountains, Columbia, and the western United States. It can also be obtained from nickel mining operations around the Sudbury region of Ontario, Canada. Antonio de Ulloa is credited with the modern rediscovery of platinum.

This heavy metal resists corrosion and is used in jewelry and electrical contacts. Its ability to resist high temperatures explains why it is used today in jet engines. It can even be found in catalytic converters and exhaust systems of automobiles.

During the 1970s, platinum was an ingredient in the dyes that were used during breast cancer x-ray examinations. Repeated use of this dye resulted in the lumps shrinking and eventually disappearing. People credited the platinum in the dye. This element may have properties that are anti-viral, anti-bacterial, and anti-fungal.

Platinum and gold are two elements that are commonly found in bee pollen. Platinum concentrations in pollen range anywhere from six parts per billion to four parts per million. Platinum and gold can be found in plants growing throughout British Columbia over 6,000 feet in elevation, although these plants are at higher altitudes that would prevent honeybees from existing in that area.

Platinum can be found in trace amounts in various soils (and therefore in plants) around the world. It is not found on any list of essential nutrients, but many people have reported positive health benefits when taking platinum supplements.

People who have regularly supplemented with water soluble platinum report relief from pain such as headaches, PMS, and back pain. It can help various states of mental aptitude, such as mental alertness, concentration, high energy, conditions of over-sensitivity, and even insomnia. Interestingly, users of water-soluble platinum have even reported having dreams in vivid color. Circulatory problems, including cold feet, have been reported as platinum deficiencies. Other examples of platinum deficiencies include nerve damage, chronic fatigue syndrome, cancer, glandular dysfunction, and neuralgia.

Indium

Indium is named after the bright blue line in its spectrum and was first discovered and identified in 1863 by two German chemists, Ferdinand Reich and Hieronlymus Theodor Richter, who stumbled upon indium inadvertently while looking for thallium. A brilliant blue line was emitted through their spectrum, revealing the presence of something new and undiscovered. Industrial uses include using it to coat the bearings of high-speed motors since it aids lubricants. It can even be used in conjunction with germanium to produce transistors.

Although some people estimate that indium is about as plentiful as silver, most believe that it is a very rare element that is found in extremely small quantities in soils around the world, making it very possible that it will be found in some agricultural crops.

Scant research provides some clues into the role of indium in health. Yukawa constantly detected the presence of indium in human tissue samples, ranging anywhere from 0.01 to 0.07 mcg/g. In hair samples, researcher Tornza observed indium present at an average of 0.0045 mcg/g.

Laboratory mice have responded to indium. When drinking water was supplemented with indium, the mice experienced lower occurrences of cancerous tumors than mice that supplemented with scandium, rhodium, chromium, yttrium, or gallium. The mice also exhibited healthier levels of copper and chromium in various organs, such as the heart and kidneys, when indium was present.

This element seems to support the body's hormone systems, including the body's two master hormone producers, the pituitary and hypothalamus glands. These master hormone glands have both responded to the presence of indium. Their roles in the body are to provide the appropriate amount of hormones for various bodily processes and mental states. When these two glands are working optimally, the body's other hormone-producing glands also work properly, making the entire hormone system function properly.

Water soluble indium is considered non-toxic when taken orally. People who have supplemented with water soluble indium report immediate benefits, such as increased energy levels, less need for sleep, and an elevated sense of confidence and well-being. They also report benefits from long-term supplementation, including normalized blood pressure, less feeling of stress, a return to normal body weight, and improvement in Attention Deficit Disorder. Indium also appears to have an effect on the absorption of other minerals and fluids, which could strengthen the immune system. Most of these benefits are attributed to the increase and optimal functioning of the hormone system. Some symptoms of indium deficiency could include mental behavior such as depression and lack of energy, as well as obesity and some glandular disorders.

Arsenic

Many believe that arsenic was first discovered in 1250 by Albertus Magnus, a German alchemist. Arsenic occurs freely in nature, although it is usually found in various compounds. Early Chinese, Egyptian, and Greek civilizations mined various arsenic compounds.

Today, arsenic is mixed with germanium to produce transistors. When this element is found in compounds or in states other than ionic, it can be poisonous. Arsenic compounds are major ingredients in rat poisons and pesticides.

The ionic form of arsenic that is found in soils is known as "arsenate." Therefore, some plants may contain small amounts of water-soluble arsenate, a cation that can sometimes compete with phosphate for cellular absorption in some plants and possibly humans.

A deficiency of arsenic can depress growth and impair the reproduction process. Arsenic may also provide some benefit in the breakdown of methionine to labile methyl, tarine, and the polyamines. It should be realized that many of the elements considered essential today were once considered "toxic" and dangerous. Eventually, after considerable research discovered their functions in plants and human cells, many of them are now listed as "essential" or at least "beneficial." If water soluble arsenate instead of arsenic compounds is ever studied extensively in human tissues, perhaps eventually it, too, could one day be acknowledged as a beneficial nutrient and will no longer be considered a toxic element.

Gallium

In 1871, Dmitri Mendeleyev found a gap in his Periodic Table of Elements, and first proposed the idea of gallium's existence. Only four years later, the French chemist Paul-Emile Lecoq de Boisbaudran actually discovered the element. Gallium can be found in various geologic compounds and is used as a byproduct of burning coal. Today gallium is used alongside mercury inside thermometers, due to its high temperature range of liquidity. The semiconductor industry uses gallium to produce transistors. Another gallium compound is used to produce laser light from electricity. This element is even used by scientists to build huge observatories that study neutrinos (particles created on the sun during the nuclear fusion process).

Gallium is not a well-known element. However, some observers have found gallium to modulate brain chemistry and provide some anti-cancerous properties.

Praeseodymium

The German chemist Carl F. Auer von Welsbach first discovered praseodymium in 1885 while tinkering with didymium. Compounds of this element can include magnesium, which are used to make parts for aircraft engines. Praseodymium is used to make flint for lighters, studio lights for the film-making industry, and can give glass a yellowish color. When used alongside didymium, this element makes glass for welders and glass blower's goggles.

Thulium

Thulium comes from the word Thule, which was the original name for Scandanavia. It was first discovered by Per Theodore Cleve in 1879. It is one of the rarest of all naturally-occurring trace elements. As of yet, there are no known commercial or industrial uses for this element.

Neodymium

Carl F. Auer von Welsbach, a German chemist, discovered neodymium in 1885. It is used to make flint for lighters, and is also used to make didymium glass, which glass welders wear, and to make the goggles used by glass blowers. When added to glass, neodymium removes iron contaminants, and can also provide violet, red, or gray colors. Scientists use this element to make the glass in spectrometers or artificial rubies in lasers.

Lanthanum

Lanthanum was first discovered in 1839 by the Swedish chemist Carl Gustaf Mosander while he was searching for impurities in his cerium samples. Only 0.0018% of Earth's crust is comprised of this element. The film-making industry uses lanthanum compounds inside their studio lights. It can even be found in flints for lighters, and is an important ingredient in the glass inside camera lenses.

Samarium

Although Jean Charles Galissard de Marignac, the Swiss chemist, first observed samarium in 1853, it was actually Paul-Emile Lecoq de Boisbaudran, a French chemist, who first isolated samarium in1879. Samarium was named after the Russian mine official, Colonel Samarski.

Compounds of this element are used in the film-making industry inside studio lights. Samarium is used to produce flints for lighters and is added to glass to absorb infrared radiation. Samarium compounds are also used in various ethanol processes.

Europium

In 1896, the French chemist Eugene-Antole Demarcay discovered europium while studying samarium. In 1901, he isolated this element for the first time. There are many rare Earth elements, but europium is the most reactive, making it relatively unusable in manufacturing processes, although it can be used occasionally as an additive in plastics to make lasers. This element is currently being investigated for possible uses in nuclear reactors.

Ytterbium

Ytterbium was originally found by Carl Gustaf Mosander in 1843 in Ytterby, Sweden, an area known for extremely rare elements. In 1877, however, Jean Charles Falissard de Marignac isolated it and is credited with its discovery. Ytterbium is sometimes mixed into steel, or it can also be used in radiation X-ray machines.

Cadmium

Friedrich Strohmeyer, a German chemist, is credited with the discovery of cadmium in 1817. Cadmium can be electroplated onto other metals like zinc to prevent corrosion. Its compounds are used in the production of rechargeable nickel-cadmium batteries and the nuclear power industry uses cadmium to make control rods. Other industries use this element to make pipes, electrical parts, and low friction bearings that require high resistance to fatigue. When mixed with sulfur, cadmium sulfide becomes a yellow powder that is used in pigments. When bound with phosphorus, blue, green, and black phosphors are created, which are used to manufacture television sets.

Deficiencies in this trace element have resulted in depressed growth rates and a diminished reproductive system.

■ ■ ■

Some of these elements are extremely rare and not always found in soil samples or have not yet been found in plant tissues. The body may not need much at all and could probably function just fine without them. However, rather than conclude that they do not serve any purpose, it would be wise to heed the counsel of Emanuel Epstein who explained that researchers using rare trace elements in plants use the terms "apparently nonessential" or "now known to be essential." Although it is easy to conclude that the human body does not need much of these elements, it remains unclear if all of these elements have been investigated independently. However, what little data is available seems to conclude that when ions of these extremely rare elements are found together, they help to enhance cell growth, which can extend life.

Chapter 14

Minerals and Our Health

Scientists estimate that there are over 60 trillion cells in an adult body, each type of cell having its own unique set of functions. As much as five percent of the cell is comprised of various minerals that provide both functional and structural support. Each cell determines the optimal quantities of every mineral that it will contain; any less than this optimum and the cell's overall integrity is compromised, weakened, and becomes prone to disease.

According to Forrest H. Nielsen, PhD, of the United States Department of Agriculture, in just the past 30 years there has been an increase in the amount of research that recognizes the health benefits of microminerals, suggesting that many of them are more important to human health than was previously realized. According to Dr. Earl Mindell, most of our present understanding of minerals results from research conducted throughout the 19th and 20th centuries. For example, in 1928 only three elements were considered essential microminerals, namely iron, iodine, and copper. During the 1950s, selenium was considered "toxic" and was supposed to be avoided. Upon further analysis, its benefits eventually became recognized and it later made the list of essential microminerals. Boron and vanadium didn't even make the list until the 1980s.

The body has far more use for minerals than for any other nutrient, including vitamins, calories, carbohydrates, or protein. A United States Senate document No. 264, published in 1936, explains: "Our physical well-being is more directly dependent upon minerals we take into our systems than upon calories or vitamins, whereupon the precise proportion of starch, protein, or carbohydrates we consume." The document continues to stress the overall importance of minerals by saying: "It is bad news to learn from our leading authorities that 99 percent of the American people are deficient in these minerals, and a marked deficiency in any one of the more important minerals actually results in disease. Any upset of the balance, any considerable lack of one or another element, however microscopic the body requirement may be, and we sicken, suffer, and shorten our lives."

Minerals are not produced by plants or animals, therefore they are always considered inorganic. Their responsibilities are innumerable and an understanding of their full benefits to the human body is beyond the scope of this book. It is understood, however, that minerals are needed in order for vitamins to function. They also play key roles, both directly and indirectly, in the creation and regulation of hormones and amino acids, as well as activating enzymes. Minerals can also regulate fluid balance, digestion, proper brain and heart functions, blood sugar balance, and the immune system. They also influence nerve transmission, muscle contraction, blood formation, tissue rigidity, cell structure and integrity, and energy and protein metabolism. The body can create some vitamins, but minerals must be supplied through the diet, and the body can go for longer periods of time without vitamins than it can without minerals.

■ ■ ■

Various health practitioners have used both vitamins and minerals successfully in their practice. Dr. Todd attributes loss of color vision as an early sign of vitamin A deficiency. Also, patients with glaucoma have responded well to vitamin A supplementation. His findings have concluded that zinc must be present in order for the eye to utilize vitamin A, while vitamin E can help prevent toxic by-products that may result from vitamin A metabolism. In 1983, the National Institutes of Health determined that vitamin E was essential in the regular functioning of the retina, which could help to explain his successful treatment using this vitamin. Dr. Todd has also credited successful glaucoma treatments to manganese supplementation.

Other optical tissues and membranes respond to nutritional supplementation. Some research suggests that cataracts are a direct result of both mineral and vitamin deficiencies, which explains why calcium has been used in the treatment of cataracts since the 1950s. Dr. Todd has also observed that vitamin E and selenium have dramatic effects on cataracts, since selenium and vitamin E work well together, and selenium is an important mineral to one of the enzyme systems in the eye.

The body has many different chemical functions inside cells, and in order for these functions to operate, a protein macromolecule known as an enzyme is used to act as a catalyst. According to Molecular Cell Biology, almost every chemical reaction in a cell is carried out by a class of proteins called enzymes. Enzymes are responsible for increasing the rates of reactions by helping to lower the activation energy required for these chemical reactions, thus giving them the name "catalysts." These enzymes usually require mineral ions in order to be activated; some enzymes require several different ions in order to both be activated and function properly. It is thought that between 25-35% of all enzymes involve an ion from one of the metals. Enzymes require mild conditions in cells in order to function optimally: 98.6 °F (37 °C) and a pH of 6.5-7.5.

Although some enzymes are found in blood, in the digestive tract, and spread throughout the space between cells, most enzymes are located inside cells, all depending on which function they carry out. Some cells even have their own unique enzyme system, while some types of enzymes are found throughout all cells. Depending on which tissue is being analyzed, there may be anywhere from 1,000-4,000 different enzymes present inside cells carrying out various chemical reactions. Again, their activation and ability to carry out their critical functions is often based on the presence of certain mineral ions (some minerals activate more enzymes than others).

Some examples of chemical reactions that are carried out in the body include digestion and healing. It is possible for these and other processes to occur without enzymes, but they would occur much more slowly. Enzymes exist to speed up these processes in a timely manner, or else these processes would be too slow to sustain life. Enzymes also help these processes occur using less energy than if they were left on their own.

Minerals also play a strong role in cardiovascular health by regulating the volume of blood that pumps through the vessels to maintain adequate blood pressure. Dr. Alexis Carrel demonstrated this phenomenon by keeping a heart beating outside the body in a solution of mineral ions. It is believed that by supplying any cell with the appropriate concentration of minerals, the cell will be able to carry out its processes and establish its electrical balance.

During 2002, a research charity known as Natural Justice, an organization that was established in 1991 to study social and physical causes of crime, coordinated a study with the University of Oxford to determine the effects of nutrition on social behavior. Together, they studied the effects of nutrition on 230 maximum-security juvenile offenders. In this study, one group was given supplemental vitamins, minerals, and essential fatty oils, and the other group was given a placebo. They monitored the number and type of offenses committed by each group and compared them to the previous nine months of behavior. Interestingly, those who took the nutritional supplements experienced a 25% reduction in offenses, while those who took the placebo experienced no change at all. Serious offenses, such as violence, were reduced by 40%. Bernard Gesch at the University of Oxford stated, "The supplements just provided vitamins, minerals and fatty acids found in a good diet which the inmates should get anyway. Yet the improvement was huge." The results were published in the British Journal of Psychiatry.

■ ■ ■

There has been a lot of discussion in recent years surrounding free radicals. A free radical is a dangerous and highly reactive molecule or atom that has an unpaired electron in its outer electron shell, and is attributed to many different degenerative diseases. Free radicals are constantly being formed in our bodies as byproducts during normal metabolism, even in healthy bodies. Free radicals are also formed from toxic carcinogenic substances, such as tobacco, or they can be formed from radiation. In fact, radiation damage is due to the tremendous increase of free radicals, and causes the same damage that occurs from toxic substances or from a degenerate diet.

According to Dr. Todd, free radicals can be characterized as an accident looking for a place to happen if they are not contained. If left uncontrolled, free radicals can wreak havoc inside the body, causing serious degenerative diseases, such as cancer, arthritis, hardening of the arteries, heart disease, and premature aging.

Dr. George Redmon, PhD, ND, explains that lysosomes are small particles inside cells that contain enzymes. However, if these lysosomal membranes are ruptured by free radicals that have gained entry into the cell, the enzymes it holds will be released. This causes severe damage to the surrounding tissues, which can result in inflammatory conditions such as Rheumatoid arthritis flares.

When a free radical attacks a cell, the cell membrane is affected first, causing it to lose its function and to leak mineral ions out of the cell, while allowing mineral ions that are supposed to remain outside the cell, as well as other fluids and products, to enter in. It is thought that loss of chromium in this manner contributes to adult onset diabetes. Also, the gradual loss of potassium and magnesium ions exiting the cell, and the influx of sodium and calcium ions which are supposed to remain outside the cell, is thought to disrupt the overall fluid balance and contribute to hypertension. Free radicals have also been attributed to collagen damage, involving the cross-linkage of collagen molecules and the gradual loss of elasticity. Collagen damage can also be seen as wrinkled skin, hypertension, and stiff joints.

Dr. Robert D. Willix, Jr., MD, an open heart surgeon, revealed that scientists during the 1980s observed a colony of bacteria that could survive the toxic environment of radioactive waste water. In general, radioactivity creates a cascade of free radicals. But these bacteria produced a high amount of antioxidants, as much as 50 times more than normal, and were able to survive the brief period of radioactivity.

Fortunately, our bodies also have ways to counteract free radicals. Dr. Todd recounts an experience he had with another researcher, who used phase light photography to film a type of white blood cell known as a lymphocyte that was produced by the immune system. His observations showed how it moves in and out of cells at will as it goes about its daily routine through the opening and closing of the cell membranes. However, upon entry, if it was discovered that the cell had been infected with destructive free radicals, the lymphocyte would form a torpedo-like shape and plunge deep into the cell's nucleus and immediately explode. The lymphocyte and the cancerous cell were immediately destroyed before the cancer had a chance to mutate and multiply. It is thought that we produce these types of cancerous cells every day through the normal routine of cellular processes, but the lymphocytes in our immune system destroy them before they are able to reproduce and grow. The body has systems in place that are meant to protect against infectious agents such as viruses and bacteria, and it makes sense that the body has a natural defense against free radicals, too.

According to Dr. Redmon, certain enzymes and other nutrients are also able to keep them under control, provided that the body has enough to work with. Two powerful enzyme systems, SOD and glutathione peroxidase, are both well-known for being powerful antioxidants. In fact, without these two enzyme systems, disease and death quickly result. All air-breathing organisms must be prepared to deal with free radicals and must have evolved enzymes to combat them.

Free radicals are used to produce energy by small organelles inside cells known as mitochondria. Eventually, free radicals inside the mitochondria are neutralized by the SOD enzyme, which contains manganese as its metal ion. The SOD enzyme will also subdue free radicals found outside the mitochondria, but for antioxidant activities outside the mitochondria it needs zinc and copper. Glutathione peroxidase is another enzyme that destroys free radicals, and it requires four ions of selenium in order to be activated. Silicon is another element that acts as an antioxidant because it protects collagen against cross-linkage damage from free radicals.

The effectiveness and activity level of these enzyme systems is largely dependent upon the presence of mineral ions. However, other nutrients have their own ways of providing antioxidant protection. Beta-carotene and vitamins C and E provide antioxidant protection by donating one of their electrons to free radicals in an effort to quickly stabilize them. Singlet oxygen is considered the most destructive free radical. It is widely understood that its most effective scavenger is water soluble beta-carotene. Yellow and dark green vegetables, along with a wide variety of fruits, are rich in minerals and beta carotene.

■ ■ ■

Perhaps the most important concept regarding the usability of minerals is not only what form they are in, but what allows them to remain soluble in the body. During the processes of physical and chemical weathering and the activity of microorganisms' to break down rocks into smaller and smaller particles, the minerals will eventually dissolve into their smallest possible size, the atom, after which they will either gain or lose one of their electrons, thus becoming electrically charged particles known as ions. This occurs in the soil as weathering forces and microorganisms in the soil break down the rocks to liberate the minerals independently.

After the minerals finally dissolve into ions, and as long as they remain water soluble by not binding with anything, they remain available for absorption into plant or animal cells. Solubility is a measure of how much an element has dissolved, releasing its ions into a solution. This is what determines their "availability." After all, a mineral can be present, but not necessarily available.

Some of the biggest advantages of soluble minerals is that they remain non-toxic, are easily absorbed in the body, or they are excreted out of the body if they are not needed. Regardless of which element is being considered, if the element is in the same form as that found in plants, there should be no risk of toxicity. If the body determines it does not need the particular element, it will promptly excrete it out of the body with no toxic accumulation whatsoever. This is what makes water solubility so critical.

The availability of minerals to continue being soluble and therefore available is largely determined by the pH level. As previously stated in Chapter 2, the availability of minerals for plant uptake is heavily dependent upon the pH of the soil, because in a dissolved state, all minerals have certain limitations on how long they will remain soluble, thus available for absorption. Once the pH range moves out of an element's solubility range, it will begin to bind with other elements, forming a compound, and become unavailable for absorption.

The most common classes of soil pH are the following:

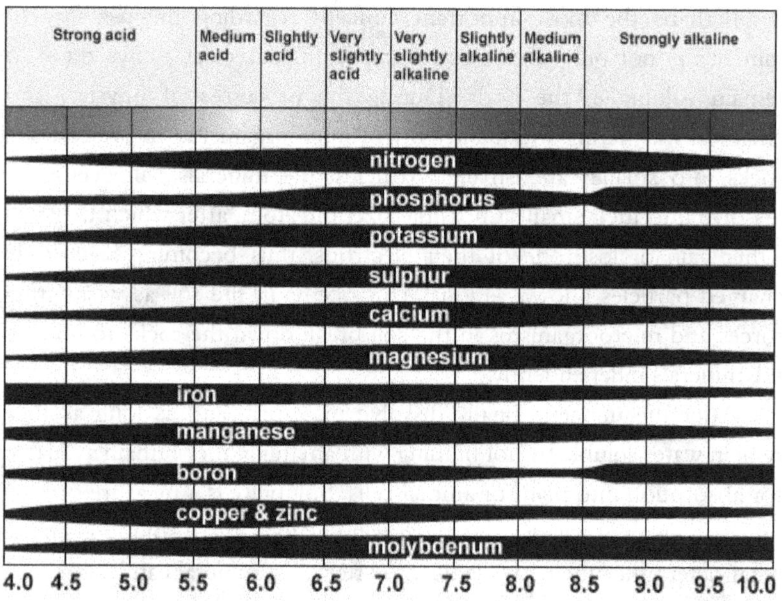

Generally, a pH level between 6.0 and 7.0 is an optimal range that maximizes the availability of as many minerals as are present. The solubility of minerals is important in that it allows the element to remain in a form that the body can either use or excrete if it does not need it. The pH level of blood is between 7.35 and 7.45, which is a neutral range that protects elements from becoming insoluble as they are transported throughout the body. However, if the pH range becomes too acidic or too alkaline, certain minerals will be affected, causing them to become bound to other elements, a chemical reaction known as "precipitation." When precipitation occurs, ions bind with other elements and create compounds and are then they are no longer soluble.

A strongly acidic environment with less than 5.5 pH causes calcium, magnesium, nitrogen, potassium, sulfur, and phosphorus to become insoluble. However, an acidic environment in this range allows cationic (positively charged) ions such as zinc, copper, manganese, cobalt, boron, aluminum, and iron to be highly soluble. It is widely accepted that the human body should have a neutral pH range, rather than leaning toward acidic or alkaline, in order to maximize the solubility potential of the minerals it may have in its tissues.

When the pH range is moderately alkaline above 7.8, calcium, molybdenum, and magnesium are soluble and readily available. However, if the pH level becomes more acidic, their ions will start to bind with other elements forming compounds, and they will become no longer water soluble. Iron, copper, zinc, manganese, boron, aluminum, manganese, and phosphorus are all soluble in acidic soils and will lose their solubility if the pH range becomes too alkaline. Generally, metallic elements such as iron, copper, zinc, aluminum, silver, gold, and manganese all remain soluble in acidic environments since they become highly corrosive, while non-metallic elements such as calcium, sodium, and phosphorus become more soluble in more alkaline environments.

Phosphorus is more soluble between 6.5 and 7.0 pH range, and outside of this pH range it can begin to precipitate and form solids with other elements. For example, raising the pH from 6.0 to 6.4 increases the availability of phosphorus by 48% and nitrogen by 11%. Once the environment becomes greater than 7.0 pH, boron availability begins to decline. If the pH range increases above 7.0, solubility of manganese is limited. Manganese is more soluble and ready for absorption into living cells in pH range below 6.5.

To summarize, precipitation is a term that describes when minerals start to lose their solubility as the pH range fluctuates. When an element precipitates, the extreme pH range is causing the ions to bind with other elements to form compounds and become insoluble. Precipitation can occur in any environment, whether in soil or inside plant or animal cells, and every mineral is prone to becoming insoluble. Since pH ranges can quickly change, these processes occur constantly.

When soils are acidic, farmers try to increase the pH range of soils through a process called "liming." Liming involves adding ground up limestone (calcium carbonate) to the soils since lime is naturally alkaline. This process adds calcium and magnesium to the soils, which will eventually be broken down from their compounds into ions. However, excess calcium carbonate can cause the environment to become too alkaline, referred to as calcareous. In calcareous soils, the excess calcium carbonate needs to be removed from the soil or acids must be added to dissolve the carbonates in an effort to decrease the pH back to a neutral range.

The pH level also influences the activity of microorganisms. According to Donald Cickelhaupt of the SUNY College of Environmental Science and Forestry, bacteria that break down organic matter in soils are hindered in strongly acidic soils, thus preventing organic matter from decomposing, effectively preventing the minerals from re-entering the soils.

According to Drs. Rachel Casiday and Regina Frey of the Department of Chemistry at Washington State University in St. Louis, Missouri (2005), nutrients must be soluble. The solubility of nutrients is critical to keeping them dissolved and in their ionic state. This provides for absorption through intestinal walls, distribution through blood, and movement into various cells in the body. If the ions are not needed upon consumption, their ionic status allows them to be either synthesized into an organic molecule depending on the needs of the body, stored for later use in fat cells, or excreted through the urine. None of these fates are possible unless the consumed mineral is an ion. Any other form of a mineral, or a pH range that causes the mineral to precipitate, will yield a useless form of the element, which can result in toxicity.

After considering all the things that make minerals important to our health, the best way to receive minerals in the right form is to consume a plant-based diet, including plenty of fruits, vegetables, nuts, and seeds in their natural, raw state. This allows the mineral ions in the plants to be absorbed quickly and efficiently in the body. When it comes to passage across a cellular membrane and absorption into a cell, particle size and its electrical charge are the key factors. It is the opinion of the author that the best mineral supplement would consist of individual mineral ions in the same form and bearing the same electrical charge as they are found in plants.

Therefore, the ideal mineral supplement should be prepared through an ionization process that would liberate ions into a solution of clean water and be allowed to diffuse throughout the entire solution. A solution of water would allow the ions to remain electrically charged, water-soluble, and held in suspension indefinitely. Whenever an element is ionized, it has its own naturally-occurring positive or negative charge that will result. For example, ionized potassium, calcium, zinc, and magnesium naturally become positively charged, while elements such as iodine, molybdenum, fluorine, and selenium naturally become negatively charged. Whichever element is being prepared should be allowed to fall into its natural ionic state. Also, since each element has its own chemical behavior and can react or bind with other elements, then ideally each element should be prepared in its own solution and not mixed with ions of other elements.

Both supplementation and research using ionic minerals prepared in a solution of water will yield dramatic results when compared to compound minerals commonly found in pills or powders. When taken orally, they will be 100% absorbable and results should be felt within minutes. For a list of elements and their most common ionic charge, see Appendix A.

When soluble nutrients are absorbed, they pass through the intestinal lining and enter the bloodstream, which carries these nutrients to various parts of the body. Solubility determines their ultimate fate inside the body. A mineral's solubility allows it to be transported throughout the watery blood plasma, stored in fat cells, or promptly discharged out of the body if it does not need it.

■ ■ ■

A critical understanding of the role of ions involves a closer look at cells. Cells are the smallest living organisms and are found in both plant and animal tissues. Although both plant and animal cells have their differences in their various biological functions, as well as differences in the content and structure of the cells, they both require the presence of mineral ions in order to carry out their processes. As a layer of protection, and as a way to regulate the amount of nutrients that will enter or exit the cell, most plant and animal cells have cell walls that contain tiny pores that allow ions to pass through. These transport mechanisms are known as ion channels and protein transport carriers. Ion channels exist in both plant and animal cell walls, and are responsible for allowing both positively and negatively charged ions to be transported in and out of the cell by opening or closing. Four of the macrominerals, calcium, sodium, potassium, and chloride, make up the most commonly found ion channels.

Once inside the cells, ions carry out various cellular processes, including the activation of enzymes, production of carbohydrates, proteins, and other organic substances needed by the living organism. Essentially, it becomes the prerogative of the living organism to do what it may with the ion. In some circumstances, the ion can be joined with other manufactured products to create various forms of organic substances that will be used in various biological processes, while other circumstances may require the ion to be put into storage in fat cells in animal tissues, or stored in vacuoles in plants. Other biological processes may require the ion to be bound with other ions to create a compound or a larger particle, such as a colloid. But how the ions will be used inside a cell should always be left up to the needs of the cell.

Furthermore, only ions and water are allowed into the cell. This is the critical responsibility of both the ion channels and the protein transport mechanisms. A healthy cell wall prevents particles such as toxins, viruses, and particles of matter larger than an ion, such as colloids or chelated particles, from entering. However, the presence of some viruses, synthetic products such as drugs or supplements, or even malnutrition, can make these ion channels either work inoperably or even become larger—thus allowing particles usually restricted—to enter.

Ions are usually found in a solution of water inside plants, whether it is the leaves, seeds, nuts, fruits, or vegetables. Since ions are water soluble, water becomes the easiest and most effective agent for their transport and storage. It only makes sense that supplemental minerals must first be ions, and then must be provided in a solution of water. When ions are not found in water, it is likely that the ions will have precipitated and bound together into a compound, thus losing their water solubility and possibly their charge.

■ ■ ■

Each one of the naturally-occurring elements on the Periodic Table came from humble beginnings. In order to understand how each element was originally created, one needs to understand the evolution of stars. The first stars that form a universe are giant balls of hydrogen, comprising 70% hydrogen and 28% helium. All the atoms in the universe that are heavier than hydrogen and helium are produced inside stars. The elements were forged from hydrogen and helium inside these dense and extremely hot masses of gaseous energy. The pressure and temperature in the core of a star is so hot, sometimes exceeding billions of degrees, that hydrogen atoms fuse together to create helium. This hydrogen fusion energy gives off the light and glow of a star we see at night.

After billions of years, the star eventually runs out of hydrogen to burn, and it begins to burn its supply of helium, a process that will create heavier elements. Once the helium supply runs out, the star begins to burn everything else that it possesses. Eventually the burning of helium becomes so intense that it forces electrons to create other elements. In fact, this extremely hot burning process is what creates all the different elements that we are familiar with today. It takes three helium atoms to form carbon, and if one more atom of helium is added oxygen will form. The next three elements created in stars happen to be the group of elements necessary to form life—carbon, nitrogen, and oxygen.

Ultimately, all the remaining elements on the Periodic Table of Elements will soon be forged. The next to form are sulfur, argon, chlorine, potassium, calcium, and scandium. At one billion degrees, carbon is forged. The burning pace becomes faster and faster. At three and a half billion degrees, silicon burns. As the heat becomes more and more intense, heavier elements begin to form, such as titanium, vanadium, chromium, followed by manganese, cobalt, nickel, and finally iron. Once the heavy element iron is forged, no other elements can be forged inside the star from iron. Therefore, any star that relies on fusion reaches the end of its cycle after the creation of iron. The fusion process cannot continue. There is nothing more to burn. Radiation continues to leave the exterior of the star, but the inside has no more fuel to burn.

Suddenly, disaster is waiting to happen as the life of the star quickly nears an end. All of the energy it has created makes it a disaster waiting to happen. Iron cannot fuel the inner furnace, and the star begins to collapse on itself and die. It is estimated that our sun's hydrogen supply will be depleted approximately five billion years from now.

A star's death is dramatic! The inner core begins to collapse and the intense energy that has been created moves outward faster and faster, sending waves back through the star. Eventually, the star blows up in a huge cosmic explosion that is estimated to be as bright as 4 billion suns. This is known as a "supernova." As the supernova explodes, the remaining other elements on the Periodic Table are forged from the shockwaves. Some of the elements that have been forged so far are radioactive. However, during the explosion, stable elements heavier than iron are forged. Neutrons bombard iron at such force that copper, zinc, gallium, silver, gold, platinum, cobalt, germanium, uranium, arsenic, zirconium, and the rest, were all created from the shockwaves during this huge explosive supernova. For example, neutrons bombard iron, forming gold. Some of the gold will be formed into lead, while some of the neutrons will then bombard lead to make all the elements up to uranium. For each one hundred billion atoms of hydrogen in the universe, there is one uranium atom. Ultimately, all of the elements are created.

These particles of matter were scattered throughout the universe where some eventually collected together to form planets. Smaller particles continued to travel aimlessly, unless they eventually crashed as meteorites upon other planets around the galaxy. When astronomers study comets, they are studying matter left over from a supernova, or the "Big Bang."

But just one star cannot produce enough of these heavy elements by itself to form all the necessary ingredients to produce life. Rather, the universe had to concentrate enough of these newly forged elements from areas scattered throughout the universe to organize and settle on this planet. Whether our planet formed from a collection of elements as a result of natural scientific events over billions of years, or the divine hand of Providence gathered material from around the universe to form our planet, the end result is the same. Neil de Grasse Tyson, an astrophysicist and director of the Hayden Planetarium in New York City, and host of the PBS documentary Origins, has stated: "We are not simply in the universe; we are born from it. We are literally children of the stars."

We are all stardust. This is one of the most profound realizations that came out of the 20th Century. Every atom that exists in our bodies and anywhere else on this planet was formed in a dying star. The carbon and nitrogen in our bodies, calcium and magnesium in our bones, iron and copper in our blood, potassium and zinc in our cellular fluids, and even the chloride and sodium in our brain cells, were all created individually billions of years ago through hot, explosive cosmic activity that eventually settled on a newly organized planet that became Earth.

Ultimately, after minerals were carried throughout the universe, having created various planetary formations, participated in dynamic geological changes over billions of years, heaved up onto the planet's outer crust, been broken down by weathering forces to their ionic state, were absorbed into plants, carried out photosynthesis and other forms of plant metabolism, contributed to the plant's fruit and vegetable formation, and entered the cells of a human, they are eventually excreted by the body and enter the cycle once again. There is no end to this cycle.

From the Big Bang to your cells, minerals are responsible for not only the creation of our planet, but also the formation of life, as well as the maintenance and continued existence of all living organisms since the first arrangement of complex chains of amino acids, to the rise of bacteria, lower and higher plants, sea creatures, and all animals and humans. Although the minerals that have been delivered to Earth are likely to remain here, they will enter, exit, and re-enter the mineral cycle over and over, repeating the process of benefiting both plants and animals again and again.

Appendix A

Ionic forms (most common) of selected naturally-occurring elements that may be found in soils and therefore in plant tissues:

ELEMENT:	(Valence) **CATIONS (+)** **ANIONS (-)**	**SIZE** **(Å)****
1. Oxygen	O2, H2O	0.73
2. Nitrogen	NH+, NO3-	0.13
3. Carbon	CO2	0.91
4. Calcium	Ca++	0.99
5. Magnesium	Mg++	0.66
6. Potassium	K+	1.33
7. Phosphorus	HPO4=H2PO4-	0.38
8. Sulfur	SO42-	0.37
9. Copper	Cu+, Cu++	0.73
10. Iron	Fe++, Fe+++	0.64
11. Manganese	Mn++	0.46
12. Zinc	Zn++	0.74
13. Boron	H3BO3¬	0.23
14. Molybdenum	MoO4- -	0.65
15. Chlorine	Cl-	1.67
16. Sodium	Na+	0.97
17. Cesium	Cs+	1.67
18. Arsenic	AsO++++	0.58
19. Chromium	Cr+++,CrO4--	0.52
20. Iodine	I-	1.33
21. Indium	In+++	0.81
22. Germanium	Ge++, Ge++++	0.53
23. Lithium	Li+	0.68
24. Vanadium	V+++++	0.59
25. Gallium	Ga+++	0.62
26. Beryllium	Be++	0.31
27. Titanium	Ti++++	0.60
28. Tin	Sn++	0.69
29. Selenium	Se--	1.16
30. Rubidium	Rb+	1.47
31. Gold	Au+	0.85

32. Silver	Ag+	1.26
33. Palladium	Pd++	0.86
34. Mercury	Hg2++	1.02
35. Bromine	Br-	1.14
36. Bismuth	Bi+++, Bi+++++	1.03
37. Lead	Pb++, Pb+++	1.19
38. Antimony	Sb+++, Sb+++++	0.76
39. Aluminum	Al+++	0.51
40. Cadmium	Cd++	0.97
41. Platinum	Pt++, Pt++++	0.62
42. Strontium	Sr++	1.13
43. Barium	Ba++	1.35
44. Nickel	Ni++	0.69
45. Cobalt	Co++	0.74
46. Fluorine	F-	0.71
47. Silicon	Si++++	0.42

*Also occurs in small amounts as anions.

**The size of an ion will depend, based on its nuclear charge, number of orbitals, and the number of electrons. Measurement is the diameter represented in Angstroms (Å).

Appendix B

Many Compound Minerals are Industrial Chemicals

The following list will describe what many mineral salts/chelates used in supplements actually are and what they are used for when not in supplements:

1. **Boric acid** is the rock known as sassolite. Used in weatherproofing wood, fireproofing fabrics, and as an insecticide.
2. **Calcium ascorbate** is calcium carbonate processed with ascorbic acid and acetone. It is a manufactured product used as a 'non-food' supplement.
3. **Calcium carbonate** is the rock known as limestone or chalk. Used in the manufacture of paint, rubber, plastics, ceramics, putty, polishes, insecticides, & inks. Used as a filler for adhesives, matches, pencils, crayons, linoleum, insulating compounds, & welding rods.
4. **Calcium chloride** is calcium carbonate and chlorine and is the byproduct of the Solvay ammonia-soda process. It is used for antifreeze, refrigeration, & fire extinguisher fluids. Also used to preserve wood & stone. Other uses include cement, coagulant in rubber manufacturing, dust control of unpaved roads, freezeproofing coal, & increasing traction in tires. Also spread on icy roads to melt ice.
5. **Calcium citrate** is calcium carbonate processed with lactic and citric acids. It is used to alter the baking properties of flour.
6. **Calcium gluconate** is calcium carbonate processed with gluconic acid (which is used in cleaning compounds). It is used in sewage purification and to prevent coffee powders from caking.
7. **Calcium glycerophosphate** is calcium carbonate processed with dl-alpha-glycerophosphates. It is used in dentrifices, baking powder, & as a food stabilizer.
8. **Calcium hydroxyapatite** is crushed bone and bone marrow. It is used as a fertilizer.
9. **Calcium iodide** is calcium carbonate processed with iodine. It is an expectorant.
10. **Calcium lactate** is calcium carbonate processed with lactic acid. It is used as a dentrifice and as a preservative.
11. **Calcium oxide** is basically burnt calcium carbonate. It is used in bricks, plaster, mortar, stucco, and other building materials. It is also used in insecticides & fungicides.

12. **Calcium phosphate tribasic** is the rock known as oxydapatit or bone ash. It is used in the manufacture of fertilizers, milk-glass, polishing powders, porcelain, pottery, and enamels.
13. **Chromium chloride** is a preparation of hexahydrates. It is used as a corrosion inhibitor and waterproofing agent.
14. **Chromium picolinate** is chromium III processed with picolinic acid. Picolinic acid is used in herbicides.
15. **Copper aspartate** is made from the reaction between cupric carbonate and aspartic acid (from chemical synthesis is a manufactured product used as a 'non-food' supplement.
16. **Copper (cupric) carbonate** is the rock known as malachite. It is used as a paint and varnish pigment, plus as a seed fungicide.
17. **Copper gluconate** is copper carbonate processed with gluconic acid. It is used as a deodorant.
18. **Copper sulfate** is copper combined with sulfuric acid. It is used as a drain cleaner and to induce vomiting; it is considered as hazardous heavy metal by the City of Lubbock that can contaminate the water supply.
19. **Dicalcium phosphate** is the rock known as monetite, but can be made from calcium chloride and sodium phosphate. It is used as a 'non-food' supplement.
20. **Ferric pyrophosphate** is an iron rock processed with pyrophosphoric acid. It is used in fireproofing and in pigments.
21. **Ferrous lactate** is a preparation from isotonic solutions. It is used as a 'non-food' supplement.
22. **Ferrous sulfate** is the rock known as melanterite. It is used as a fertilizer, wood preservative, weed-killer, and pesticide.
23. **Magnesium carbonate** is the rock known as magnesite. It is used as an antacid, laxative, and cathartic.
24. **Magnesium chloride** is magnesium ammonium chloride processed with hydrochloric acid. It fireproofs wood, carbonizes wool, and as a glue additive and cement ingredient.
25. **Magnesium citrate** is magnesium carbonate processed with acids. It is used as a cathartic.
26. **Magnesium oxide** is normally burnt magnesium carbonate. It is used as an antacid and laxative.
27. **Manganese carbonate** is the rock known as rhodochrosite. It is used as a whitener and to dry varnish.

28. Manganese gluconate is manganese carbonate or dioxide processed with gluconic acid. It is a manufactured item used as a 'non-food' supplement.

29. Manganese sulfate is made from the reaction between manganese oxide and sulfuric acid. Used in dyeing and varnish production.

30. Molybdenum ascorbate is molybdenite processed with ascorbic acid and acetone. It is a manufactured item used as a 'non-food' supplement.

31. Molybdenum disulfide is the rock known as molybdenite. It is used as a lubricant additive and hydrogenation catalyst.

32. Potassium chloride is a crystalline substance consisting of potassium and chlorine. It is used in photography.

33. Potassium iodide is made from HI and KHCO3 by melting in dry hydrogen and undergoing electrolysis. It is used to make photographic emulsions and as an expectorant.

34. Potassium sulfate appears to be prepared from the elements in liquid ammonia. It is used as a fertilizer and to make glass.

35. Selenium oxide is made by burning selenium in oxygen or by oxidizing selenium with nitric acid. It is used as a reagent for alkaloids or as an oxidizing agent.

36. Selenomethionine is a selenium analog of methionine. It is used as a radioactive imaging agent.

37. Silicon dioxide is the rock known as agate. It is used to manufacture glass, abrasives, ceramics, enamels, and as a defoaming agent.

38. Vanadyl sulfate is a blue crystal powder known as vanadium oxysulfate. It is used as a dihydrate in dyeing and printing textiles, to make glass, and to add blue and green glazes to pottery.

39. Zinc acetate is made from zinc nitrate and acetic anhydride. It is used to induce vomiting.

40. Zinc carbonate is the rock known as smithsonite or zincspar. It is used to manufacture rubber.

41. Zinc chloride is a combination of zinc and chlorine. It is used as an embalming material.

42. Zinc citrate is smithsonite processed with citric acid. It is used in the manufacture of some toothpaste.

43. Zinc gluconate is a zinc rock processed with gluconic acid. Gluconic acid is used in many cleaning compounds.

44. Zinc lactate is smithsonite processed with lactic acid. Lactic acid lactate is used as a solvent.

45. Zinc orotate is a zinc rock processed with orotic acid. Orotic acid is a uricosuric (promotes uric acid excretion).

46. Zinc oxide is the rock known as zincite. It is used as a pigment for white paint and as part of quick-drying cement.

47. Zinc phosphate is the rock known as hopeite. It is used in dental cements.

48. Zinc picolinate is a zinc rock processed with picolinic acid. Picolinic acid is used in herbicides.

49. Zinc sulfate can be a rock processed with sulfuric acid. It is used as a corrosive in calico-printing and to preserve wood.

Appendix C

The following is a comparison of "Essential" and "Beneficial" minerals between plants and humans. The list of elements considered essential for plants is not the same as those considered essential for humans.

PLANTS	PEOPLE
Essential Elements:	
Macronutrients	
Calcium	Calcium
Magnesium	Chloride
Nitrogen	Magnesium
Phosphorus	Phosphorus
Potassium	Potassium
Sulfur	Sodium
	Sulfur
Micronutrients	
Boron	Chromium
Copper	Cobalt
Chloride	Copper
Iron	Fluorine
Manganese	Iodine
Molybdenum	Iron
Nickel	Manganese
Zinc	Molybdenum
	Selenium
	Zinc
Beneficial Elements:	
Aluminum	Boron
Cobalt	Germanium
Sodium	Gold
Silicon	Lithium
	Nickel
	Platinum
	Silicon
	Silver
	Tin
	Vanadium

Honorable Mention Elements:

Cadmium	Arsenic
Cerium	Bromine
Chromium	Cadmium
Iodine	Lead
Lanthanum	Mercury
Lead	
Mercury	
Titanium	
Vanadium	

Bibliography

Chapter 1 References

1. Hankin, Rosie. Rocks, Crystals, Minerals, Barnes & Noble Books, New York, 2004.
2. The History Channel. "Meteors: Fire in the Sky," 2005.
3. Hazen, Robert M. "Life's Rocky Start," Scientific American Magazine, April, 2001.
4. Grady, Monica. Catalogue of Meteorites, 5th Edition, Natural History Museum, Cambridge University Press, London, 2000.
5. Britt, Robert Roy. "Ancient Impact Turned Part of Earth Inside-Out." June 4th, 2004. Article also appeared in the June 3rd issue of Nature.
6. Benner, Steven. "UF Study Suggests Life on Earth Sprang from Borax Minerals," University of Florida News, January 8th, 2004.
7. Rocksforkids.com. "How Rocks & Minerals Are Formed," 2003.
8. Idaho Public Television. "Investigating Rocks and Minerals in Your World," http://idptv.state.id.us, 2004.
9. Idaho Public Television. "Rocks and Minerals: Facts," http://idptv.state.id.us, 2004.
10. Vernon, Ron. Beneath Our Feet: The Rocks of Planet Earth, Cambridge University Press. 2000.
11. Brown, Theodore L, LeMay, Jr., H. Eugene, Bursten, Bruce E. Chemistry: The Central Science, 8th Edition, Prentice Hall Publishing, 2000.
12. Singer, Michael J. and Munns, Donald N. Soils: An Introduction, 3rd Edition, Prentice Hall Publishing, 1996.
13. Fairbanks Museum and Planetarium. "Down and Dirty," 2004.
14. Hynes, Erin. Rodale's Improving the Soil, Rodale Press, 1994, by Weldon Russell Pty Ltd.
15. Brown, Paul. "Britain Being Battered by Waves Hurling Giant Rocks," The Guardian, 2004.
16. "Soil," Microsoft□ Encarta□ Online Encyclopedia 2004 http://ca.encarta.msn.com □ 1997-2004 Microsoft Corporation. All Rights Reserved.
17. Hinkson, David. "New Ideas for Nutritional Healing" audiotape, WaterOz Corporation, 2001.

18. Whiting, Dr. Stephen E. "How Your Body Uses Minerals," Institute of Nutritional Science.
19. Spector, Christy. "The Story of Rocks and Soil," Soil Science Education, Goddard Space Flight Center, 2004.
20. Ohio Department of Natural Resources. "Ohio Outdoor Notebook," 2004.
21. Cooper, John. "Soil and How to Treat It," Texas A&M University.

Chapter 2 References

1. Roper, Dr. Terry R., and Combs, Sherry. "Mineral Nutrition of Fruit Crops," Department of Horticulture, University of Wisconsin-Madison, 2004.
2. Hynes, Erin. Rodale's Improving the Soil, Rodale Press, 1994 by Weldon Russell Pty Ltd.
3. Cooper, John. "Soil and How to Treat It," Texas A&M University.
4. Singer, Michael J., and Munns, Donald N. Soils: An Introduction, 3rd Edition, Prentice Hall Publishing, 1996.
5. Alexander, Martin. "Biodegredation of Chemicals of Environmental Concern," 1981, from Soil Productivity Variables.
6. Brown, Theodore L, LeMay, H. Eugene, Jr., and Bursten, Bruce E. Chemistry: The Central Science, 8th Edition, Prentice Hall Publishing, 2000.
7. Hopkins, William G. Introduction to Plant Physiology, John Wiley & Sons, Inc. 1995.
8. Mader, Sylvia S. Biology, 6th Edition, McGraw Hill Publishing, 2004.
9. Rosenberg, Chris. "Uptake and Transport of Nutrients," Biology.
10. University of Arkansas-Little Rock. "Water and Mineral Transport," Biology Department, 2004.
11. Stiles, Warren C., PhD. "Nitrogen Management in the Orchard," and "Phosphorus, Potassium, Magnesium, and Sulfur Soil Management," Tree Fruit Nutrition, Good Fruit Grower Publishing, 1994.
12. Shaw, Marty. "Tree Nutrition," Adams Business Media.

Chapter 3 References

1. Hopkins, William G. Introduction to Plant Physiology, John Wiley & Sons, Inc., 1995.
2. Singer, Michael J. and Munns, Donald N. Soils: An Introduction, 3rd Edition, Prentice Hall Publishing, 1996.

3. Cooper, John. "Soil and How to Treat It," Texas A&M University.
4. Epstein, Emanuel. Mineral Nutrition of Plants: Principles and Perspectives, Academic Press, 1972.
5. The Department of Environmental Transport Regions. "The Draft Soil Strategy for England – A Consultation Paper," March, 2001.
6. University of Arkansas-Little Rock. "Water and Mineral Transport," Biology Department, 2004.
7. Rosenberg, Chris. "Uptake and Transport of Nutrients," Biology.
8. Marschner, Horst. Mineral Nutrition of Higher Plants, 2nd Edition, Academic Press, 2002.
9. Mader, Sylvia S. Biology, 6th Edition, McGraw Hill Publishing, 2004.
10. University of Arkansas-Little Rock, "Water and Mineral Transport." Biology Department, 2004.
11. "Plasma Membrane," Microsoft□ Encarta□ Online Encyclopedia 2004 http://ca.encarta.msn.com □ 1997-2004 Microsoft Corporation. All Rights Reserved.
12. Nelson Thornes Limited, "Biology Teacher's Reference," 2004.
13. Rom, Curt, PhD. "Fruit Tree Growth and Development," Tree Fruit Nutrition, Good Fruit Grower Publishing, 1994.
14. Fallahi, Esmaeil, PhD. "Root Physiology, Development and Mineral Uptake," Tree Fruit Nutrition, Good Fruit Grower Publishing, 1994.
15. "Soil," Microsoft□ Encarta□ Online Encyclopedia 2004 http://ca.encarta.msn.com □ 1997-2004 Microsoft Corporation. All Rights Reserved.
16. Gray, Barry, "Plant Nutrition," June 2002.
17. Penalosa, Dr. Javier. "Absorption and Transport Systems," Buffalo State College, 2004.
18. Nelson Thornes Limited, "Molecules & Cells." Information Question Sheet: Transport across Membranes, 2004.
19. Epstein, Emanuel. Mineral Nutrition of Plants: Principles and Perspectives, Academic Press, 1972.
20. University of the Western Cape, Department of Biodiversity & Conservation Biology, 2005.
21. Alberts, Bruce, Johnson, Alexander, Lewis, Julian, Raff, Martin, Roberts, Keith, and Walter, Peter. Molecular Biology of the Cell, Fourth Edition, Garland Publishing, 2002.
22. Salisbury, Frank B., and Ross, Cleon W. Plant Physiology, 4th Edition, Wadsworth Publishing Company, 1992.
23. Stern, Kingsley R. Introductory Plant Biology, 8th Edition, McGraw-Hill Publishing, 2000.

Chapter 4 References

1. Marschner, Horst. Mineral Nutrition of Higher Plants, 2nd Edition, Academic Press, 2002.
2. Hopkins, William G. Introduction to Plant Physiology, John Wiley & Sons, Inc, 1995.
3. Mader, Sylvia S. Biology, 6th Edition, McGraw Hill Publishing, 2004.
4. University of Arkansas-Little Rock. "Water and Mineral Transport," Biology Department, 2004.
5. Epstein, Emanuel. Mineral Nutrition of Plants: Principles and Perspectives, Academic Press, 1972.
6. Thomas, Dr. James, and Lung, Dr. Oliver. "Photosynthesis," Department of Biological Sciences, University of Lethbridge, 2001.
7. "Photosynthesis," Microsoft□ Encarta□ Online Encyclopedia 2004 http://ca.encarta.msn.com □ 1994-2004 Microsoft Corporation. All Rights Reserved.
8. Rom, Curt, PhD. "Fruit Tree Growth and Development," Tree Fruit Nutrition, Good Fruit Grower Publishing, 1994.
9. "Phloem," Microsoft□ Encarta□ Online Encyclopedia 2004 http://ca.encarta.msn.com □ 1994-2004 Microsoft Corporation. All Rights Reserved.
10. Cooper, John. "Soil and How to Treat It," Texas A&M University.

Chapter 5 References

1. Rom, Curt, PhD. "Fruit Tree Growth and Development," Tree Fruit Nutrition, Good Fruit Grower Publishing, 1994.
2. Morgan, Dorothy. "The Orchid House," University of Waterloos.
3. Street, Jimmy J., and Kidder, Gerald. "Soils and Plant Nutrition," University of Florida Cooperative Extension Services, 1997.
4. Stern, Kingsley R. Introductory Plant Biology, 8th Edition, McGraw-Hill Publishing, 2000.
5. Salisbury, Frank B., and Ross, Cleon W. Plant Physiology, 4th Edition, Wadsworth Publishing Company, 1992.
6. Marschner, Horst. Mineral Nutrition of Higher Plants, 2nd Edition, Academic Press, 2002.
7. Cooper, John. "Soil and How to Treat It," Texas A&M University.
8. Epstein, Emanuel. Mineral Nutrition of Plants: Principles and Perspectives, Academic Press, 1972.
9. Wild Oats Market. "A New Day for Organics," 2002.

10. Kirby, Alex. "Organic Farming a 'Realistic Choice,'" BBC News, May 30, 2002.
11. Thomas, David M. "Mineral Depletion in Foods over the Period 1940 to 1991," The Nutritional Practitioner, 2001, 2.1:27-29.
12. The Department of Environmental Transport Regions. "The Draft Soil Strategy for England – A Consultation Paper," March, 2001.
13. Whiting, Dr. Stephen E. "How Your Body Uses Minerals," Institute of Nutritional Science.
14. Hynes, Erin. Rodale's Improving the Soil, Rodale Press, 1994, by Weldon Russell Pty Ltd.
15. Stiles, Warren C., PhD. "Nitrogen Management In the Orchard," Tree Fruit Nutrition, Good Fruit Grower Publishing, 1994.
16. Hopkins, William G. Introduction to Plant Physiology, John Wiley & Sons, Inc., 1995.
17. Canberra Organic Growers Society. "Nutrient Deficiencies in your Plants: How to Identify and Correct Them—Organically," 2003.
18. Ludwick, A. E., PhD. "Phosphorus and Potassium Fertilizer Sources," Mexico Potash and Phosphate Institute, Tree Fruit Nutrition, Good Fruit Grower Publishing, 1994.
19. Roper, Dr. Terry R., and Combs, Sherry. "Mineral Nutrition of Fruit Crops," University of Wisconsin-Madison, 2004.
20. Dixon, Bob. "Managing Disease with Nutrients," California-Arizona Farm Press, 1996.

Chapter 6 References

1. Hynes, Erin. Rodale's Improving the Soil, Rodale Press, 1994 by Weldon Russell Pty Ltd.
2. Hopkins, William G. Introduction to Plant Physiology, John Wiley & Sons, Inc., 1995.
3. J&L Garden Center. "Plant Nutrient Information," Bountiful, Utah, 2004.
4. Epstein, Emanuel. Mineral Nutrition of Plants: Principles and Perspectives, Academic Press, 1972.
5. Marschner, Horst. Mineral Nutrition of Higher Plants, 2nd Edition, Academic Press, 2002.
6. Morgan, Dorothy. "The Orchid House," University of Waterloos.
7. Peryea, Frank J., PhD. "Boron Nutrition in Deciduous Tree Fruit," Tree Fruit Nutrition, Good Fruit Grower Publishing, 1994.

8. Roper, Dr. Terry R., and Sherry Combs. "Mineral Nutrition of Fruit Crops," Department of Horticulture, University of Wisconsin-Madison, 2004.
9. Stiles, Warren C., PhD. "Phosphorus, Potassium, Magnesium, and Sulfur Soil Management," Tree Fruit Nutrition, Good Fruit Grower Publishing, 1994.
10. Barrow, Jim. "Understanding Soils and Nutrients, Part 3," Newsletter of the Wildflower Society of Western Australia, 1999.
11. Street, Jimmy J., and Gerald Kidder. "Soils and Plant Nutrition," University of Florida Cooperative Extension Services, 1997.
12. Salisbury, Frank B., and Cleon W. Ross. Plant Physiology, 4th Edition, Wadsworth Publishing Company, 1992.
13. Neilsen, D., PhD, and Neilsen, G.H., PhD. "Tree Fruit Zinc Nutrition," Agriculture Canada Research Station, Tree Fruit Nutrition, Good Fruit Grower Publishing, 1994.

Chapter 7 References

1. Cooper, John. "Soil and How to Treat It," Texas A&M University.
2. Epstein, Emanuel. "Mineral Nutrition of Plants: Principles and Perspectives," Academic Press, 1972.
3. Marschner, Horst. Mineral Nutrition of Higher Plants, 2nd Edition, Academic Press, 2002.
4. Time Life Books. Pests & Diseases, Time Life, Incorporated, 1995.
5. Agrios, George N. Plant Pathology, Academic Press, New York and London, 1969.
6. Ultra Gro Plant Food Newsletter. Ultra Gro Plant Food Company, Volume 2-10, June 2000.
7. Stebbins, Robert L., PhD. "Diagnosing Sick Orchards," Tree Fruit Nutrition, Good Fruit Grower Publishing, 1994.
8. Dixon, Bob. "Managing Disease with Nutrients," California-Arizona Farm Press, 1996.
9. Stern, Kingsley R. Introductory Plant Biology, 8th Edition, McGraw-Hill Publishing, 2000.
10. Singer, Michael J., and Munns, Donald N. Soils: An Introduction, 3rd Edition, Prentice Hall Publishing, 1996.
11. Agro-K Corporation, "Nutrients and Their Role in Plant Disease," 2005.

Chapter 8 References

1. The Duval Collection of Gems and Minerals. The University of Houston, 2004.
2. Hall, Dr. Jeff. Department of Veterinary Medicine, Utah State University, 2004.

Chapter 9 References

1. Redmon, George, PhD, ND. "Minerals: What Your Body Needs & Why," Avery Publishing Group, 1999.
2. Mindell, Earl, R.Ph, PhD. What You Should Know About Trace Minerals, Keats Publishing, Inc. 1997.
3. Nielsen, Forrest H. "Ultratrace Elements of Possible Importance for Human Health: An Update," United States Department of Agriculture, Agricultural Research Service, Grand Forks Human Nutrition Research Center, Grand Forks, North Dakota.
4. Farish, Donald J. Human Biology, 1st Edition, Jones and Bartlett Publishers, 1993.
5. Jefferson Lab. "It's Elemental," 2005.
6. Greene, Winston W., BA, BS, DC. "General Discussion of Minerals," 2005.
7. Higdon, Jane, PhD. The Linus Pauling Institute, Oregon State University, 2001.
8. Pikilidou MI, Lasaridis AN, Sarafidis PA, Befani CD, Koliakos GG, Tziolas IM, Kazakos KA, Yovos JG, Nilsson PM. "Insulin sensitivity increase after calcium supplementation and change in intraplatelet calcium and sodium-hydrogen exchange in hypertensive patients with Type 2 diabetes." Diabet Med. 2009 Mar;26(3):211-9.
9. Rodale, J.I., with Taub, Harald J. Magnesium: The Nutrient that Could Change Your Life, Pyramid Books, New York, 6th Printing, 1971.
10. Hinkson, David. "New Ideas for Nutritional Healing" audiotape, WaterOz Corporation, 2001.
11. Levitan, Irwin B., and Kaczmarek, Leonard K. The Neuron, Second Edition, Oxford University Press, 1997.
12. WaterOz Corporation. Various newsletters and general catalog from 2001-2004.
13. Lodish, Harvey, Baltimore, David, Berk, Arnold, Zipursky, S. Lawrence, Matsudaira, Paul, and Darnell, James. Molecular Cell Biology, Third Edition, Scientific American Books, 1995.

14. Meletis, Chris, ND. "Chloride: The Forgotten Essential Mineral," 2004.
15. Whiting, Dr. Stephen E. "How Your Body Uses Minerals," Institute of Nutritional Science, 2004.
16. Todd, Gary Price, MD. Nutrition,Health & Disease, Whitford Press, 1985.
17. Kaleita TA. "Neurologic/behavioral syndrome associated with ingestion of chloride-deficient infant formula," Pediatrics, 1986, October, 78(4):714-5.
18. Dreosti, Ivor E., PhD, D. Sc. Nutrition Reviews, Vol. 53, No 9.
19. Werbach, Dr. Melvyn R., MD. "Nutritional Influences on Aggressive Behavior," Journal of Orthomolecular Medicine, Volume 7, Number 1, 1995.
20. Rylander R, Bonevik H, Rubenowitz E. "Magnesium and calcium in drinking water and cardiovascular mortality." Scand J Work Environ Health. 1991 Apr;17(2):91-4.
21. HealthDay News. "Magnesium Maintains Memory," December 1, 2004. Courtesy of Yahoo! News.
22. Journal of the American Medical Association. June 13, 1990.
23. International Medical Veritas Association. Medical News. "Magnesium in Modern Medicine." February 20, 2006.

Chapter 10 References

1. Jefferson Lab. "It's Elemental," 2005.
2. Pasek, Matthew A. University of Arizona Planetary Sciences Department and Lunar and Planetary Laboratory. See Lori Stiles, "Meteorites could have supplied the Earth with Phosphorus."
3. Lauretta, Dante. University of Arizona professor of planetary sciences. Also see Lori Stiles, "Meteorites could have supplied the Earth with Phosphorus."
4. Higdon, Jane, PhD. The Linus Pauling Institute, Oregon State University, 2001.
5. Redmon, George, PhD, ND. Minerals: What Your Body Needs & Why, Avery Publishing Group, 1999.
6. United States Department of Agriculture. "Soil Quality Indicators: pH," Prepared by the National Soil Survey Center in cooperation with the Soil Quality Institute, NRCS, USDA, and the National Soil Tilth Laboratory, Agricultural Service, USDA, January, 1998.
7. Whiting, Dr. Steven A, "How Your Body Uses Minerals," 2004.

8. Greene, Winston W., BA, BS, DC. "General Discussion of Minerals," 2005.
9. WaterOz Corporation, Various newsletters and general catalog from 2001-2004.
10. Todd, Gary Price, MD. Nutrition, Health & Disease. Whitford Press, 1985.
11. Jefferson, James W, "Potassium Supplementation in Lithium Patients: A Timely Intervention or Premature Speculation?" Journal of Clinical Psychiatry, 53:10 October, 1992.
12. Hinkson, David, "New Ideas for Nutritional Healing" audiotape, WaterOz Corporation, 2001.

Chapter 11 References

1. Jefferson Lab. "It's Elemental," 2005.
2. Greene, Winston W., BA, BS, DC. "General Discussion of Minerals," 2005.
3. Mindell, Earl, R.Ph, PhD. What You Should Know About Trace Minerals, Keats Publishing, Inc., 1997.
4. Redmon, George, PhD, ND. Minerals: What Your Body Needs & Why, Avery Publishing Group, 1999.
5. WaterOz Corporation. Various newsletters and general catalog from 2001-2004.
6. Todd, Gary Price, MD. Nutrition, Health & Disease, Whitford Press, 1985.
7. Farish, Donald J. Human Biology, 1st Edition, Jones and Bartlett Publishers, 1993.
8. Higdon, Jane, PhD. The Linus Pauling Institute, Oregon State University, 2001.
9. Hinkson, David. New Ideas for Nutritional Healing audiotape, WaterOz Corporation, 2001.
10. Rogers, Sherry A., MD. "Copper: The Missing Link in your Diet," 2004.
11. Prohaska, J.R., and Failla, M.L. "Copper and Immunity," in Nutrition and Immunology Vol. 8, Human Nutrition: A Comprehensive Treatise, (D.M. Klurfeld, ed.), (1993) Plenum Press, New York, NY.
12. Whiting, Dr. Steven A. "How Your Body Uses Minerals," 2004.
13. McDowell, Lee Russell. Minerals in Animal and Human Nutrition, Academic Press, 2003.

14. Fluoride Action Network. Various articles and reports, part of the American Environmental Health Studies Project (AEHSP), 2005.
15. International Program on Chemical Safety (IPCS INCHEM). "Fluorides," 1996.
16. Yiamouyiannis, Dr. John. Fluoride: The Aging Factor (2nd Edition), Health Action Press, 1986.
17. Zhao LB, Liang GH, Zhang DN, and Wu XR Lu-Liang. "Effect of a High Fluoride Water Supply on Children's Intelligence," Fluoride 1996; 29(4):190-192.
18. Klein, Wolfgang. "DNA Repair and Environmental Substances," Zeitschrift fur AngewanilteRader und Klimaheilkunde, Volume 24, No. 3, pp. 218-223 (1977).
19. Mohamed, Aly and M.E. Chandler. "Cytological Effects of Sodium Fluoride on Mice," Fluoride, Vol. 15 No. 3, pp. 110-118 (1982).
20. Chhabra S, and Hora A. "Reproductive insufficiency in women with iodine deficiency," The Journal of the Institute of Obstetrics and Gynaecology Trust, 1996; 16:242-243.
21. Hetzel, Basil S. "The Control of Iodine Deficiency," American Journal of Public Health, 1993, 83:4.

Chapter 12 References

1. Jefferson Lab. "It's Elemental," 2005.
2. Redmon, George, PhD, ND. Minerals: What Your Body Needs & Why, Avery Publishing Group, 1999.
3. Greene, Winston W., BA, BS, DC. "General Discussion of Minerals," 2005.
4. WaterOz Corporation. Various newsletters and general catalog from 2001-2004.
5. Mindell, Earl, R.Ph, PhD. What You Should Know About Trace Minerals, Keats Publishing, Inc. 1997.
6. Higdon, Jane, PhD. The Linus Pauling Institute, Oregon State University, 2001.
7. Pollitt, E. "Iron Deficiency and Cognitive Function," Annual Review of Nutrition, 13 (1993), pp. 521-37.
8. Reuters Health News. "Low Iron Levels May Contribute to ADHD," December 15, 2004. Archives of Pediatric and Adolescent Medicine; 158:1113-1115. Courtesy of Yahoo! News.

9. Werbach, Dr. Melvyn R., MD. "Nutritional Influences on Aggressive Behavior," Journal of Orthomolecular Medicine, Volume 7, Number 1, 1995.
10. Kerr, Martha. "Restless Leg Syndrome Tied to Mental Woes," Reuters News, October 31, 2005. Courtesy of Yahoo! News.
11. Freeland-Graves, Jeanne. "Manganese: an Essential Nutrient for Humans,"' Nutrition Today, November-December, 1988, pp. 13-19.
12. Gottschalk, L.A. "Content Analysis of Verbal Behavior, significance in clinical medicine," Springer-Verlag Publishing, 1986.
13. Todd, Gary Price, MD. Nutrition, Health & Disease. Whitford Press, 1985.
14. Enemark, John H., PhD. "Molybdenum-Containing Enzymes," Research Summary, University of Arizona Department of Chemistry, 2004.
15. Schrauzer, Gerhard N., PhD., White, D.A. "Selenium in human nutrition: dietary intakes and effects of supplementation," Bioinorganic Chemistry, April, 8(4):303-318, 1978.
16. Taylor, Ethan Will, PhD. "Selenium and Viral Diseases: Facts and Hypothesis," Journal of Orthomolecular Medicine, December, 1997.
17. Mertz, W. "Review of the Scientific Basis for establishing the essentiality of trace elements," Biological Trace Element Research, Volume 66, pages 185-191, 1998.
18. National Cancer Institute. "Antioxidants and Cancer Prevention: Questions and Answers," July 28, 2004.
19. National Institute for Health. "Dietary Supplement Fact Sheet: Selenium," 2005.
20. Combs, Gerald, Turnbull, Bruce, and Clark, Larry. "Effects of Selenium Supplementation for Cancer Prevention in Patients with Carcinoma of the Skin," Journal of the American Medical Association, December 25, 1996.
21. Whitaker, Julian. MD's Health & Healing newsletter; Vol. 7, No.2, Feb 1997.
22. Lang, Susan. "Selenium Supplements Can Reduce Cancer Rates, New Study Shows," Cornell University, January 7th, 1997.
23. American Journal of Gynecology. "Low Selenium Linked to Pregnancy Complication," November, 2003. Courtesy Reuters Health News.
24. University of Miami. "Study Finds Selenium Affects Survival in HIV/AIDS," University Press Release, September, 1997. Printed in the Journal of AIDS.

25. Konz, K.H., Haap, M., Xia, Y., Mill, K.E., Walsh, R.A., and Burk, R.F. Department of Medicine, Vanderbilt University.
26. van der Torre, H.W., J. Veenstra, H. van de Pol, H. van Steenbrugge, S. Pelupessy and G. Schaafsma. The Ockhuizen Department of Nutrition,TNO-CIVO Toxicology and Nutrition Institute, The Netherlands.
27. Journal of Agricultural and Food Chemistry. "Selenium-Enriched Broccoli and Cancer Prevention," 2001; 49:2679-2683.
28. Rutz, Dan. "Selenium: New Entry In fight Against Prostate Cancer," CNN Senior Medical Correspondent, June 17, 1999.
29. Connell P., et al. "Zinc attenuates tumor necrosis factor-mediated activation of transcription factors in endothelial cells," J Am College Nutrition 1997; 16: 411-417.
30. McDowell, Lee Russell. "Minerals in Animal and Human Nutrition," Academic Press, 1992.
31. Mares-Perlman, J.A., et al. "Zinc Intake and Sources in the U.S. Adult Population 1976-1980," Journal of the American College of Nutrition, 14:4, 1995.
32. Associated Press. "Zinc Improves Memory of 7th-Graders," April 26, 2005.
33. Rauscher, Megan. "Zinc Helps Teens Think," April 6, 2005, Reuters Health.
34. A.D.A.M., Incorporated. "Zinc," 2002.
35. Neurology. January 1, 2008.
36. British Medical Journal, "Folic acid fortification and congenital heart disease," BMJ 2009338:b1144, 12 May 2009.
37. Sliwinski T, Czechowska A, Kolodziejczak M, Jajte J, Wisniewska-Jarosinska M, Blasiak J. "Zinc salts differentially modulate DNA damage in normal and cancer cells." Cell Biol Int. 2009 Apr;33(4):542-7. Epub 2009 Feb 28. Department of Molecular Genetics, University of Lodz, Poland.
38. Yan M, Song Y, Wong CP, Hardin K, Ho E. "Zinc deficiency alters DNA damage response genes in normal human prostate epithelial cells." J Nutr. 2008 Apr;138(4):667-73. Department of Nutrition and Exercise Sciences, Oregon State University.

Chapter 13 References

1. Blaurock-Busch, E., PhD. "The Clinical Effects of Boron (B)," Townsend Letter for Doctors and Patients, #172, pages 56-57.

2. Jefferson Lab. "It's Elemental," 2005.
3. Greene, Winston W., BA, BS, DC. "General Discussion of Minerals."
4. Newnham, R.E. "'Essentiality of Boron for Healthy Bones and joints,'" Environmental Health Perspectives, 102: supplement November 1994.
5. WaterOz Corporation. Various newsletters and general catalog from 2001-2004.
6. Nielsen, Forrest H. "Facts and Fallacies about Boron," Nutrition Today, May-June, 1992.
7. Richards, Douglas G., McMillin, David L., Mein, Eric A., and Nelson, Carl D. "Gold And Its Relationship to Neurological/Glandular Conditions," Meridian Institute, International Journal of Neuroscience, 2002, Volume 112, pages 31-53.
8. Mahdihassan, S. "Cinna-bar gold as the best alchemical drug of longetivity, called Makaradhwaja in India," American Journal of Chinese Medicine, Volume 13.
9. Temkin, O. "The falling sickness. A history of epilepsy from the Greek's to the beginnings of modern neurology," 1971, Baltimore, Johns Hopkins Press.
10. Niel, J. G., and J. A. Chrestien. "Recherches et observations sur less effets des peparations d'or dud r. Chretien dans le traitement de plusieurs maladies, et notamment dans celui des maladies syphilitiques," 1821, Paris, Gabon: J. A. Chresien.
11. Burnett, J. C. "Gold as a remedy in disease, notably in some forms of organic heart disease, angina pectoris, melancholy, tedium vitae, scrofula, syphilis, skin disease, and as an antidote to the ill effects of mercury," 1879, London: Gould.
12. Richards, Douglas G., David L. McMillin, Eric A. Mein, Carl D. Nelson. "Gold And Its Relationship to Neurological/Glandular Conditions," Meridian Institute, International Journal of Neuroscience, 2002, Volume 112, pages 31-53.
13. Potter, S. O. L. "A compend of material medica, therapeutics, and prescription writing, with especial reference to the physiological actions of drugs," 1894, Sixth Edition, 1902. Philadelphia: P. Blakiston's Sons & Co.
14. Keeley, L. E. "Opium: Its use, abuse and cure," 1897, Chicago: The Banner of Gold, Co. Reprint New York: Arno Press; 1981.
15. Higby, G. J. "Gold in medicine: A review of its use in the West before 1900," Gold Bulletin, Volume 15, 1982.

16. Garber, S. T. Stedman's Practical Medical Dictionary, Baltimore: Williams &Wilkins, 1942.
17. Alexiou, G., Gramanis, A. P., Grimani, M., Papaevengelou, G., Koumantakis, E., and Papadatos, C. "Trace elements (zinc, cobalt, selenium, rubidium, bromine, gold) in human placenta and newborn liver at birth," Pediatric Research, Volume 11, pages 646-648.
18. Skandan, K. P., and Abraham, K. C. "Presence of several elements in normal and pathological human semen samples and its origin," Andrologia, Volume 16, pages 587-588, 1984.
19. Kauf, E., Wiesner, W., Niese, S., and PlenertW. "Zinc, copper, manganese and gold content of the hair of infants," Acta Paediatrica Hung, Volume 25, pages 299-307, 1984.
20. Warren, Harry V. "Gold and Arthritis," Soc. Sci. Med., Vol. 29, N0. 8, 1989.
21. Hinkson, David. New Ideas For Nutritional Healing audiotape, WaterOz corporation, 2001.
22. Schrauzer, G.N., et al. "Lithium in Scalp Hair of Adults, Students, and Violent Criminals," Biol.Trace Ele. Research., 34:161.1992.
23. Schrauzer GN, Shrestha KP, "Lithium in drinking water and the incidences of crimes, suicides, and arrests related to drug addictions." Biol Trace Elem Res. 1990 May;25(2):105-13.
24. Werbach, Dr. Melvyn R., MD. "Nutritional Influences on Aggressive Behavior," Journal of Orthomolecular Medicine, Volume 7, Number 1, 1995.
25. Wright, Jonathan V. M.D. "Lithium fights crime and some of your most nagging health concerns," and various newsletters, Tahoma Clinic, Nutrition and Healing.
26. Brown, Theodore L, LeMay, H. Eugene, Jr., Bursten, Bruce E. Chemistry: The Central Science, 8th Edition, Prentice Hall Publishing, 2000.
27. Moore, G.J., Bebchuk, J.M., Wilds, I.B., Chen, G. & Manji, H.K. "Lithium-induced increase in human brain gray matter," Lancet 356, 124 1−1242, 2000.
28. Thomson Reuters. "If it doesn't kill you: Arsenic helps in cancer." June 2, 2007.

Chapter 14 References

1. Redmon, George, PhD, ND. Minerals: What Your Body Needs & Why, Avery Publishing Group, 1999.

2. Nielsen, Forrest H. "Ultratrace Elements of Possible Importance for Human Health: An Update," United States Department of Agriculture, Agricultural Research Service, Grand Forks Human Nutrition Research Center, Grand Forks, North Dakota.
3. Mindell, Earl, R.Ph, PhD. What You Should Know About Trace Minerals, Keats Publishing, Inc. 1997.
4. Todd, Gary Price, MD. Nutrition, Health & Disease. Whitford Press, 1985.
5. Lodish, Harvey, Baltimore, David, Berk, Arnold, Zipursky, S. Lawrence, Matsudaira, Paul, and Darnell, James. Molecular Cell Biology, Third Edition, Scientific American Books, 1995.
6. Farish, Donald J. Human Biology, 1st Edition, Jones and Bartlett Publishers, 1993.
7. United States Department of Agriculture. "Soil Quality Indicators: pH," prepared by the National Soil Survey Center in cooperation with the Soil Quality Institute, NRCS, USDA, and the National Soil Tilth Laboratory, Agricultural Service, USDA. January, 1998.
8. Singer, Michael J. and Munns, Donald N. Soils: An Introduction, 3rd Edition, Prentice Hall Publishing, 1996.
9. N-Rich Plant Food, Incorporated. "Major and Minor Plant Food Elements," 2004.
10. Bickelhaupt, Donald. "Soil pH: What It Means," State University of New York, College of Environmental Science and Forestry, 2004.
11. Casiday, Rachel, and Frey, Regina. "Nutrients and Solubility," Department of Chemistry, Washington University—St. Louis, 1999.
12. BBC News. "Healthy Eating 'Can Cut Crime,'" June 25th, 2002.
13. Public Broadcasting Service. Origins: Fourteen Billion Years of Cosmic Evolution, hosted by Neil deGrasse Tyson, 2004, WGBH, Boston.
14. Alles, David L. "The Origin of the Elements," Western Washington University, 2005.

Appendix A References

1. Barbalace, Kenneth, Roberta Barbalace, and Julia Barbalace, Service provided by www.environmentalchemistry.com.
2. Brown, Theodore L, H. Eugene LeMay, Jr., Bruce E. Bursten. Chemistry: The Central Science, 8th Edition. Prentice Hall Publishing, 2000.

3. Danish Environmental Protection Agency, The Elements in the Second Rank, Environmental Project Number 770, 2003.
4. Epstein, Emanuel. Mineral Nutrition of Plants: Principles and Perspectives. Academic Press, 1972.
5. Stevens, Robert G., PhD. Washington State University. Soils: A Part of the Production System, Tree Fruit Nutrition. Published by Good Fruit Grower, Yakima, Washington, 1994.

Appendix B References

1. Budvari S, et al eds. The Merck Index, "An Enclyopedia of Chemicals, Drugs, and Biologicals, 12th ed." Merck Research Laboratories, Whitehouse Station (NJ), 1996.
2. Anagisawa KY, Rendon-Angeles JC, Shizawa NI, Ishi SO. Topotaxial replacement of chlorapatite by hydroxy during hydrothermal ion exchange. Am Mineralogist 1999;84:1861-1869.
3. Vitamin-Mineral Manufacturing Guide Nutrient Empowerment, Volume 1. Nutrition Resource, Lakeport (CA), 1986.
4. Hojo Y, Hashimoto I, Miyamoto Y, Kawazoe S, Mizutani T. In vivo toxicity and glutathione, ascorbic acid, and copper level changes induced in mouse liver and kidney by copper (II) gluconate, a nutrient supplement. Yakugaku Zasshi 2000;120(3):311-314.
5. City of Lubbock, July 18th, 2002.
6. Patrick J. "What most people don't know about vitamin C." The Alacer Health Report, Foothill Ranch (CA), 1994.

INDEX

C

ABOUT THE AUTHOR

Ryan Kane has degrees in Business and Economics and has a professional background working as a fraud investigator. He loves the outdoors and in his spare time he enjoys researching unique subjects and finding creative ways to present them to anyone who is interested.

www.ingramcontent.com/pod-product-compliance
Lightning Source LLC
Chambersburg PA
CBHW062153270326
41930CB00009B/1520

* 9 7 8 0 5 7 8 1 6 6 1 1 7 *